SECRET MEDICINES
from Your
GARDEN

"Rare are those herbalists who understand the perfection of balance when knowledge is based both upon the wisdom that has survived the passing of millennia and knowledge that is affirmed with the modern tools of research and analysis. I encourage you to take the intimate journey Ellen Evert Hopman offers you in *Secret Medicines from Your Garden*. Her opening sentence resounds as a truth in my own life as well. And from that sentence onward, as she shares her own journey into the study of herbal medicine, she will engage you as a trusted friend and as someone who goes out of her way to always speak with clarity. The recipes and preparations are delicious, the medicinal information trustworthy, and the historical references reflect academic accuracy. This book should go home with you. And then? Let Ellen take you on a wonderful journey into our herbal world."

PAUL BEYERL, MASTER HERBALIST, AUTHOR OF *THE MASTER BOOK OF HERBALISM,* AND FOUNDER OF THE HERMIT'S GROVE

"This is the most tantalizing type of herb book—the kind I love most—filled with lore and history, myth and magic, and the author's own rich experiences weaving the tales together. We are led on a most unique multidimensional journey to the heart of herbalism. Along the way we are taught how to use plants for medicine, daily well-being, ritual, and ceremony."

ROSEMARY GLADSTAR, HERBALIST, FOUNDER OF UNITED PLANT SAVERS, AND AUTHOR OF *PLANTING THE FUTURE: SAVING OUR MEDICINAL HERBS*

"Just like in nature where you encounter the same herb many times but in different ways, Ellen Evert Hopman's new book takes you on a spiraling exploration into the world of healing plants. Your first encounter is a taste, the next a healing brew, and then a story as if around a campfire. She also shares, for the first time in print, the brilliant herbal formulation technique of the late (great) herbalist William LeSassier. What a delight to journey with Ellen as she shares her extensive experience and knowledge of the rich diversity found in each plant!"

PAM MONTGOMERY, HERBALIST, EDUCATOR, AND AUTHOR OF *PLANT SPIRIT HEALING* AND *PARTNER EARTH*

"Ellen Evert Hopman is a master herbalist who understands both the physical and spiritual nature of plants. In *Secret Medicines from Your Garden* she draws on her extensive experience and brings us a wonderful book that is so much more than the average herbal. Packed full of practical guidance, accessible information, and useful recipes, this original and beautifully illustrated book takes us deep into nature and teaches how plants can nourish both body and soul. Ellen is making a significant contribution to contemporary plant wisdom. Highly recommended for anyone interested in plant spirits, herbal lore, and plant magic."

CAROLE GUYETT, MEDICAL HERBALIST,
CELTIC PRIESTESS, AND AUTHOR OF *SACRED PLANT INITIATIONS*

"Like a box of bonbons, this collection of arcane and useful herbal lore will delight and entertain you, no matter your mood. *Secret Medicines from Your Garden* courses through bee-humming meadows and skirts hedgerows guarded by rowan woods, while eating flower sandwiches and pouring libations for the fairies. You will love this new and wonderful treasure from the enchanted pen of Ms. Hopman."

SUSUN S. WEED, AUTHOR OF THE WISE WOMAN HERBAL SERIES

"Her eyes opened to the power and beauty of nature first by the Franciscan community near Assissi in northern Italy and subsequently by the New Age community of Findhorn in Scotland, Ellen Evert Hopman felt called to work with plants in all their forms and guises. After an herbal apprenticeship with William LeSassier, the visionary herbalist and creator of the Triune formulation system, she spent five years studying the herbal ways of Native American elders. Declaring herbalism a lifelong learning path, this book is a distillation of all the knowledge she has acquired from the natural world and its benefits for our physical, mental, and spiritual health. It is a fascinating, educational, and highly enjoyable read brimming with practical ideas, recipes, and rich in history as well an important reference work from an accomplished herbalist, author, and all around plant woman."

ALEX DOVER, MEDICAL HERBALIST

"This book is multifaceted, a gem that is full of information about our personal green paths that encompass medicine, food, religion, and ritual."

MARY PAT PALMER, REGISTERED HERBALIST AND DIRECTOR OF THE
PHILO SCHOOL OF HERBAL ENERGETICS, PHILO, CALIFORNIA

"A delightful collection of nature's wisdom translated into an easy-to-follow instructional book of herbal medicine. Ellen provides a great medicinal resource while inviting you to cultivate your intuition and connect with the spiritual components of plant medicine."

AVIVA D. WERTKIN, N.D., FOUNDER OF NATURAE MEDICAL

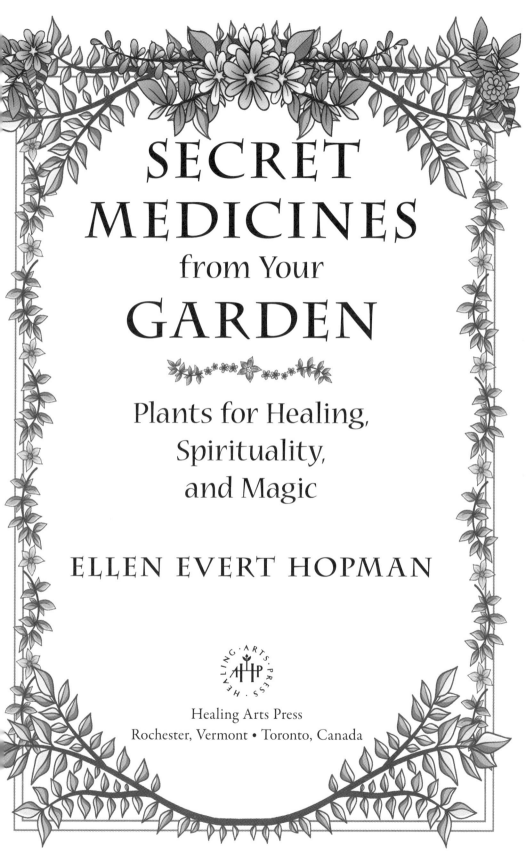

SECRET
MEDICINES
from Your
GARDEN

Plants for Healing,
Spirituality,
and Magic

ELLEN EVERT HOPMAN

Healing Arts Press
Rochester, Vermont • Toronto, Canada

Healing Arts Press
One Park Street
Rochester, Vermont 05767
www.HealingArtsPress.com

Healing Arts Press is a division of Inner Traditions International

Note to the reader: *This book is intended as an informational guide. The remedies,
approaches, and techniques described herein are meant to supplement, and not to be a
substitute for, professional medical care or treatment. They should not be used to treat
a serious ailment without prior consultation with a qualified health care professional.*

Library of Congress Cataloging-in-Publication Data
Hopman, Ellen Evert.
  Secret medicines from your garden : plants for healing, spirituality, and magic /
Ellen Evert Hopman.
     pages cm
  Includes bibliographical references and index.
  ISBN 978-1-62055-557-6 (paperback)—ISBN 978-1-62055-558-3 (e-book)
  1. Herbs—Therapeutic use. 2. Medicinal plants. 3. Mind and body. I. Title.
  RM666.H33H668 2016
  615.3'21—dc23
                                                                    2015027301
Printed and bound in the United States by Versa Press, Inc.

10 9 8 7 6 5

Text design and layout by Virginia Scott Bowman
This book was typeset in Garamond Premier Pro, Frutiger, and Gill Sans with
Charlemagne, Nuevo, and Myriad Pro used as display typefaces

To send correspondence to the author of this book, mail a first-class letter to the
author c/o Inner Traditions • Bear & Company, One Park Street, Rochester, VT
05767, and we will forward the communication, or contact the author directly at
www.elleneverthopman.com.

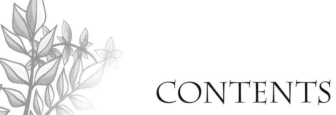

CONTENTS

Author's Note on How to Use This Book   vii

Foreword by Matthew Wood   ix

Acknowledgments   xiii

INTRODUCTION
Walking the Green Path—An Herbalist
Discovers Her Calling   1

PART ONE

A WILDCRAFTING PRIMER

1 The Signatures of Plants—Learning Nature's Alphabet   6

2 Herbs of Spring   20

3 Herbs of Summer   31

4 Herbs of Fall   41

5 Winter Cold and Flu Care, Naturally!   51

6 Bug Stuff—Plants to Repel Mosquitoes, Ticks, and Fleas   62

PART TWO

EXPLORING INVISIBLE DIMENSIONS
OF THE PLANT WORLD

7 Magic of the Dragon and the Hag—Dracaena and Mullein   68

8   Animal Spirit Medicines   76

9   Herbal Astrology   112

10 Working with Plant Spirits   119

PART THREE

ENJOYING NATURE'S BOUNTY

11 Bee Medicine—The Splendors of Honey   126

12 Some Kitchen Medicines   141

13 Hedgerows Are Food, Medicine, and Magic   154

14 Deciduous Trees for Healing   162

15 Conifers for Healing   181

PART FOUR

FORMULA MAKING

16 General Formulas—From Tinctures to Poultices   198

17 Constitutional Prescribing—Plants to Build, Cleanse,
    and Tone the Organs and Systems of the Body   211

Glossary of Herbal Contraindications   281

Sources and Resources   297

Index of Plants by Common Name   306

Index of Plants by Scientific Name   316

Index of Health Concerns   326

General Index   331

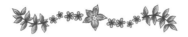

AUTHOR'S NOTE
ON HOW TO USE THIS BOOK

In the event of a medical situation please seek the assistance of a competent health professional. Persons on medications prescribed by a health professional should always seek advice before ingesting herbal preparations. Please consult a naturopathic physician or search online for "herb and drug interactions" or "drug and herb contraindications" before combining herbs and allopathic medicines.

Any dosages mentioned are for an adult weighing approximately one hundred and fifty pounds. Amounts should be halved for a child who weighs seventy-five pounds, and quartered for a child of thirty pounds. Infants can get the benefits of herbal remedies via their mother's breast milk.

Herbs and plants, particularly roots, should be soaked in cold water with sea salt or vinegar (about one tablespoon per quart of water) for about twenty minutes to remove parasites.

In horticultural usage, the abbreviations "subsp." (or "ssp."), "var.," and "f." are inserted before the subspecific epithet, variety, or form name. The abbreviations "sp." and "var.," when used without a following element, indicate that the species or variety is unknown or unspecified. The plural "spp." is used to refer to a group of species.

All of the artwork in this book—the color plates and the decorative line art—are illustrations from old botanicals and herbals published prior to 1923 and are therefore in public domain. These beautiful and timeless images illustrate many aspects of the plant, including root, flower, and seed, making them very useful to the aspiring herbalist.

FOREWORD
by Matthew Wood

Knowledge comes in threes according to the ancient Celts, and the herbal knowledge in this book comes in three dimensions. First, plants are healers, and *Secret Medicines from Your Garden* teaches us how to use them for healing in a great diversity of ways. Second, the lore of herbs is fascinating and, like the healing properties, almost without end. This book demonstrates that fact. It contains lore from all sorts of sources. Finally, herbs are fun. Although modern drug companies—with their disinformation campaigns on the Internet and control of the media—would like us to hesitate and bow down to the gods of seriousness, the truth is otherwise. Herbalism can be a fun, do-it-yourself project. Our little green friends are safe—if well selected or directed by a good book such as this one. Herbs are lore-filled-fascinating-fun-healing. And that is the main point of this book.

Looking at the book as a whole, however, we see that it is also an account of a journey, a master herbalist's notebook, and an autobiography written in green script. We find here not the facts of Ellen's life, but the things that thrilled her. And we feel the thread of the writer's experience and life running through the pages, unifying diverse lessons into a flowing and almost living narrative.

Ellen Hopman is an herbalist, Druidess, student, teacher, writer, and lore mistress, and all those facets contribute to this master herbalist's journey–notebook–green-script–autobiography. This book could only have been written by one who has been collecting information—and using it—for a very long time.

Ellen reveals that she was called. A real teacher does not brag; she just mentions what happened. Ellen simply describes how the green path called her and took her on a lifetime journey. And something of that calling enters into this book.

This is my favorite Ellen Evert Hopman book precisely because it is *not* one more herbal written in an organized manner—herb by herb or condition by condition—but flows from topic to topic, giving us a kaleidoscopic view of herbalism that reflects, in a real sense, what it feels like to be an herbalist. This book is closer to the green world in its unorganized, raw, primal origins, before human beings drew up boxes and organized it for their own consumption. I could relate to it so deeply; it could have been my story or that of any other herbalist revealing the things that thrilled us on the path. Here Ellen unwinds the organization enough to see the raw green woods that inspire each and every savant of this art.

But if the reader wants organizational themes, you can also find these—collected like little treasures—in chapters such as "The Signatures of Plants" and elsewhere. If the reader wants scientific evidence, look at the sources listed in the bibliography. And if the reader simply wants a fun read, just plunge into any chapter, anywhere.

Ellen is an experienced herbalist who has worked with thousands of people, but we can tell a true doctoress of the art because she can heal unintentionally, by mistake, and after the lights have been turned off. Ellen healed me in just such a manner.

I had enjoyed the winding California road that took me from Ukiah down into the Anderson Valley and on to the herb school and home of my friend, Mary Pat Palmer, just past the small village of Philo. My back was extra stiff from the drive over the moderately dangerous roads of the California coastal ranges, but I'd suffered from back pain for over forty years. One particular type of pain I considered incurable. The muscles attaching to the iliac crest had grown stiff a long time before, compensating for other stiff muscle groups. Then small cysts of cartilage, fats, and serous fluid had developed at the juncture of the bone and the muscle. I'd heard from chiropractors and massage therapists that these are "sometimes curable" with a lot of work.

Ellen had just taught a class at Mary Pat's the month before and I was shown a bottle of salve the class had made from the characteristic local trees of the area—Ellen is a tree herbalist, one more feather in her hat. The ingredients were Oak, Black Walnut, Bay Laurel, Eucalyptus, and Redwood. A note on the bottle opined that it might be helpful for the lungs and pain.

"Ridiculous," I thought. "What a waste of time to just throw together a bunch of local trees. What was Ellen thinking?" I am, however, a big believer in Bay Laurel, which gives me great dreams (it contains DMT) and is an excellent muscle relaxant. So I smeared a bunch of the green salve across the top of my iliac crest. Wow! The pains I had always felt across there melted in seconds. In a few weeks the cysts had disappeared. For the first time in decades I could reach my toes.

How was this possible? Ellen might rely on her special relationship with the spirits of the trees, but I needed an explanation. There must be a synergism of trees: Oak bark to remove scar tissue, Black Walnut to remove effusions of serum, Bay Laurel to relax the muscles and probably direct the formula, Eucalyptus to diffuse the remedies through the tissues, and Redwood for—I think—dissolving fats in the cyst. But it took a magician to put the group together and leave them on the table for me after she'd left the theater.

Thank you, Ellen.

MATTHEW WOOD has been a practicing herbalist for nearly thirty-five years and is an internationally known and traveled lecturer and author in the field of herbal medicine. He is the author of *The Book of Herbal Wisdom* and five other works. He has a master's degree in herbal medicine from the Scottish School of Herbal Medicine and is a registered herbalist (American Herbalists Guild). He is particularly experienced with Western herbal medicines, especially Native American and folk medical traditions.

ACKNOWLEDGMENTS

A big thank-you to my primary teacher, William LeSassier, for his excellent apprenticeship many years ago, to author and herbalist Matthew Wood, who introduced me to animal medicines, and to the Plant Foragers group (http://groups.yahoo.com/group/PlantForagers/) for their spirited discussions and love of all plants. Thanks to Lewis Blake for comments about Hickory nut milk, and thanks as always to Joyce Sweeney for her help. Thanks to Dr. Patrick MacManaway, Scottish geomancer and dowser, for ideas on how to work with Land Spirits. A big thank-you to Alex Dover, BSc (Hons) in herbal medicine from the University of Westminster, London, for helping me confirm the energetics of plants and to Mary Pat Palmer of the Philo School of Herbal Energetics, Philo, California, for comments on Cannabis, a most misunderstood herb.

Most of all, a big thank-you to the Green Nations, the plants and trees that have sustained our bodies and spirits for millions of years:

A Blessing on the plants,
algae of the oceans,
wet mosses,
and Forest ferns.
A Blessing on the shady trees,
protective Oaks,
holly and rowan that feed the birds,
cedar and juniper,
spicebush and maple.
A Blessing on the fruitwoods,

and the woods that build our homes,
our furniture,
our sailboats and spoons,
and give us leaves for books.
A Blessing on the herbs of the fields,
damp in summer mornings,
and on all the plants that fill the table,
giving their lives in silent sacrifice:
the carrots and tomatoes,
the rice and the plums,
blessings on them all.
Deep in the forest, in a circle of trees
Is where they bless me,
close by a running brook and
weathered stone.
Quiet and still their beauty,
roots running deep,
I bless them and thank them
every day.

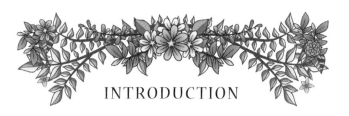

WALKING THE GREEN PATH

An Herbalist Discovers Her Calling

I never set out to be an herbalist. As a graduate student I was offered a scholarship to study art history in Rome. My plan was to explore Neoplatonism as it was expressed in Renaissance sculpture and to make a catalog of dolphins on baptismal fonts. Since early childhood I had been mystically inclined, and the iconography of the dolphins seemed fascinating. They were carved on the fonts because according to ancient tradition they ferried the souls of the dead across the water to the other world. Never mind that these were Christian baptismal fonts.

I dutifully began to photograph and read, spending days studying in the dim Hertziana and Vatican libraries and exploring ancient churches. But, being me, I soon felt a pull to go to the countryside. I took the train to Assisi, in Umbria, to look at the famous frescoes of Giotto in the local cathedral.

What I saw there were sumptuously laid-out depictions of the life of the saint known as Il Poverello, "the Poor One." I knew that Saint Francis had lived a life of dedicated simplicity and poverty, eating gruel with ashes mixed in and wearing simple brown robes. It seemed incongruous to me that there was gold leaf on the lavishly painted images. I ran into a monk in a brown wool cassock as I was leaving the church. "Where can I find out more about how Saint Francis actually lived?" I asked.

He looked at me for a moment before replying. "Go to San Masseo."

"What is San Masseo?" I asked.

"Don't ask any questions, just go," he said, pointing down the road.

I dutifully took off down the street. The road led out of town and eventually I saw a small wooden sign that pointed off to the right. There was a muddy little path through some bushes and then a small clearing where I saw groups of young men and women, mostly Germans, all roughly my age, lolling around on the grass.

"Have you come here to stay?" one of them asked in a friendly tone.

"I don't know," I replied.

I ended up staying for four days. Then I returned to Rome to pack up my belongings and took the train right back to Assisi.

Art history research was put on the back burner as I learned the ways of the Franciscan community I had stumbled upon. I soon began to take part in community activities such as baking bread in the stone oven and feeding the ducks and chickens that were given free rein to wander the kitchen and dining room.

I went to Mass twice a day (never telling anyone that I wasn't a Catholic) and on Wednesdays and Sundays I fasted. Those were the days when we were supposed to "wander in the wilderness," walking out of the community with no thoughts of a destination, because God would lead us to wherever or whomever we were supposed to meet.

I would clamber around the hillsides at those times, taking in the beauty of the flowers and trees and grasses, delighting in the bright green life that expressed itself in the ancient olives and tiny wildflowers. I never missed human companionship, feeling that the plants were my friends and companions.

One day I found myself on Mount Subasio, a place the saint himself used to frequent. (Keep in mind that this was a saint who once preached naked and who talked to wolves and birds. He also thought of the sun, moon, and fire as his brothers and sisters.)

I was wandering around up there, high above the tree line, when a sudden storm came up. Next thing I knew, there was thunder and lightning and snow coming down. I was terrified because I was all alone. What to do? So I did something that in hindsight was actually rather stupid—I found a tiny pine tree and wrapped myself around it for comfort. It was the only living thing on the mountainside other than the grass.

The storm passed quickly and I was soaked. I remember looking at my shoulders and seeing snow caked on them. The whole experience was so exhilarating that I sang out loud as I made my way back down the mountain.

Right across from the path to San Masseo was a little Romanesque church that Saint Francis had repaired with his own hands. Being pre-Gothic, it had no stained glass windows to let in the light. It was very dark in there as I slipped inside to rest and meditate.

I settled myself on a wooden bench in the darkness, and suddenly I heard a voice coming from inside and outside of my body all at once. "Everything you have been doing until now has been for status and intellect and to please your parents," the voice said. "You are supposed to be working with plants."

I instantly knew that this was true. I had felt a bond and a companionship with the herbs and grasses that went far beyond anything I had experienced in museums and dry libraries. I began to mentally throw out everything I was doing: the master's degree in art history, the thesis on dolphins on baptismal fonts, and my parents' ambition that I be a college professor.

As I mentally threw out each item I felt lighter and lighter. Soon my chest was glowing with a kind of inner fire. I walked back to the little community of San Masseo and told them what I had experienced. "You need to go to Findhorn, everybody there is just like you," a man said.

I knew that I was on a vision quest at that point and so I did not ask any questions. I went back to the States, sold all my possessions, and made my way to Findhorn, Scotland, one of the first New Age communities in the world. I spent five weeks learning about fairies and studying massage and flower essence counseling. Then I spent two weeks on Erraid and Iona in the Hebrides (islands that eventually inspired my second novel, *The Druid Isle*).

I came back to the States and immediately began an herbal apprenticeship with William LeSassier in New York City. After I finished my studies I set up a practice in Philadelphia and began writing herbal articles and doing radio shows.

My spiritual path was Earth based; I had found a group of like-minded people with whom I did rituals in nearby forests. I also began to study with Native American elders like Wallace Black Elk, Ron Evans, and others, deepening my relationship with the herbs and trees and grasses, and with the animals, rocks, water, and fire. After I had studied with the First Nations for five years, one of the elders said to me: "It's great that you are learning our ways and honoring our ancestors. But you need to honor your own." At the time I had no idea what he meant.

A client of mine happened to mention that she had met a Druid. She told me that she had been to several Pagan festivals but had not been terribly impressed. Then she met Isaac Bonewits and liked his clean robes and academic knowledge about the Celts.

The moment I heard the word *Druid* it was as if a harp string were being plucked in my heart. I had heard about the ancient Druids who once lived on Iona, but I had no idea that there were still Druids in this world. I knew deep inside that this was my path, and so I set out to find Druids.

I eventually located Isaac and ADF (A Druid Fellowship), the group he was forming. That was in 1983. By 1984 I was one of the first members. After two initiations, the second supervised by Isaac himself at Pagan Spirit Gathering in Wisconsin, I went on to cofound the Henge of Keltria in 1986 with four other people.

Lady Olivia Robertson of the Fellowship of Isis made me an Archdruidess of the Druid Clan of Dana after my first book, *Tree Medicine Tree Magic,* came out in 1991. In 1996 I started the Whiteoak mailing list and then became a cofounder and later co-chief of the Whiteoak Druid Order (Ord na Darach Gile) in 1997. Starting in the winter of 2013 I became Archdruidess of a new order called the Tribe of the Oak (www.tribeoftheoak.com).

And all along I taught and wrote about the plants. Herbalism is a lifelong learning path, one that is never finished. Certain plants are especially important to me and have nourished my soul and my body over the years. Over time others will make themselves known. Here in this book is a small selection of my favorite plant allies.

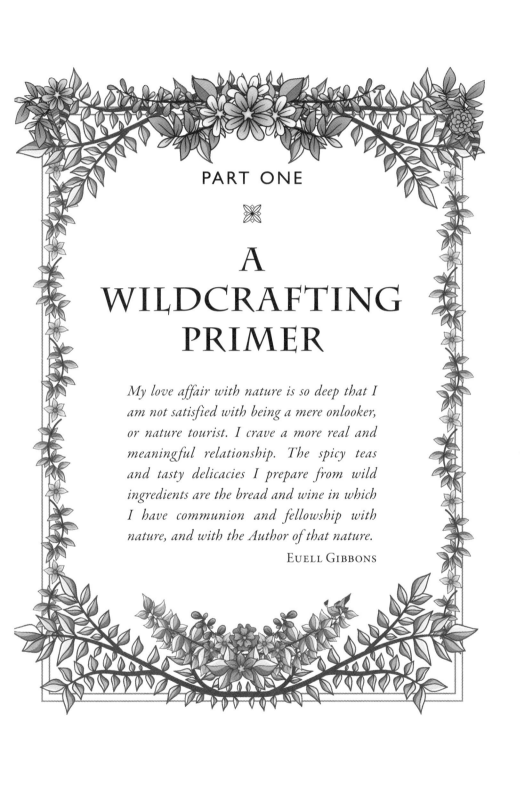

PART ONE

A WILDCRAFTING PRIMER

My love affair with nature is so deep that I am not satisfied with being a mere onlooker, or nature tourist. I crave a more real and meaningful relationship. The spicy teas and tasty delicacies I prepare from wild ingredients are the bread and wine in which I have communion and fellowship with nature, and with the Author of that nature.

EUELL GIBBONS

1

THE SIGNATURES
OF PLANTS

Learning Nature's Alphabet

There are those who say that they get messages from plants and that plants actually speak to them with a human voice, telling them the healing virtues of an herb. Others (like me) get pictures in their minds that seem to be another form of direct communication from the plant world. Over the millennia many other plant identification and communication systems that do not rely on the written word have been devised.

THE DOCTRINE OF SIGNATURES

Centuries ago in Europe, in a time before most people could read, a system called the "doctrine of signatures" was developed to catalog the language of plants. With this plant classification system in their head, illiterate people with no access to a printed herbal could encounter a plant they had never seen before and divine its medicinal properties.

I have successfully used this system to understand the medicinal properties of a plant, and it is great fun to look the plant up later to see if others have determined the same thing. The first thing is to get used to using all of your senses: touch, sight, smell, and taste. Next, be aware that this system works only with wild plants growing in their natural habitat, or with "invasives" that have chosen, without human intervention, to incorporate a certain set of light and soil conditions. Nonnative species that have been planted by humans do not give accurate readings!

Here is an overview of some elements of the doctrine of signatures. Once you have these in your mind, it's easy to ferret out the properties of an unfamiliar herb.

Habitat

Where is the plant growing, in sunlight or in shade? Plants that crave a lot of sun will generally bring dryness and heat into the body; examples include Elecampane (*Inula helenium*), Sunflower (*Helianthus annuus*). Plants that thrive in the shade tend to be cooling; examples include Elderberry (*Sambucus nigra, S. canadensis*), and Peppermint (*Mentha piperita, M. balsamea* Willd.).

Is the plant growing in a wet place or a dry place? Plants that thrive in damp areas will help with conditions such as rheumatism, fevers, colds, and coughs; examples include Willow (*Salix* spp.), Mint (*Mentha* spp.), Vervain (*Verbena hastata, V. officinalis*), Sweet Flag (*Acorus calamus*), Elderberry (*Sambucus nigra, S. canadensis*), Boneset (*Eupatorium perfoliatum*), Jack-in-the-Pulpit (*Arisaema triphyllum*), Skunk Cabbage (*Symplocarpus foetidus*), and Sundew (*Drosera rotundifolia, D. anglica, D. linearis*).

Plants that are used to dry up mucky soil will help dry mucous secretions; examples include Sunflower (*Helianthus annuus*), and Eucalyptus (*Eucalyptus globulus*).

Plants that grow in or around clear ponds and fast-moving brooks tend to be diuretic and will help clear the urinary tract of waste; examples include Horsetail (*Equisetum hyemale*), Bedstraw or Cleavers (*Galium aparine*), Mint (*Mentha* spp.), and Alder (*Alnus serrulata*).

Plants that thrive in gravel and rock formations will help clear stone-forming and catarrhal accumulations from the bronchial and alimentary systems; examples include Bearberry (*Arctostaphylos uva-ursi*), Horsetail (*Equisetum hyemale*), Peppergrass (*Lepidium virginicum*), Parsley (*Petroselinum crispum*), Shepherd's Purse (*Capsella bursa-pastoris*), Juniper (*Juniperus communis*), and Sassafras (*Sassafras albidum, S. variifolium*).

Does the plant grow in thin or disturbed soil? If thin soil, it is a plant that likes to struggle and will bring grit and strength to the body, such as Horsetail (*Equisetum hyemale*).

Alone or in a Group

Is the plant growing alone or in a group? Solitary plants are telling you they are powerful and need to be treated with cautious respect. For example, you will never see a field of Yarrow, but a field of Clover or Dandelion is often seen. Plants that grow in masses such as Red Clover (*Trifolium pratense*) are more gentle in action or esculent.

Does the plant grow near people or as far away as it can manage? Plants that grow on your doorstep, like Dandelion (*Taraxacum officinale*) and Plantain (*Plantago major*), can be used safely for a long time. Plants that grow in the deep woods, such as Goldenseal (*Hydrastis canadensis*) and Blue Cohosh (*Caulophyllum thalictroides*), have more specialized uses and should only be used for a short time period. Plants that grow in fields, the middle distance between house and forest, such as Yarrow (*Achillea millefolium*) and Saint-John's-Wort (*Hypericum perforatum*), can be used for a while but only during special seasons or for a certain period of time.

The Signatures of Stems and Roots

Does the plant have hollow stems? If so, it will help clean tubes in the human body such as the bronchi and alimentary tract; examples include Comfrey (*Symphytum officinale*), Onion (*Allium cepa*), Garlic (*Allium sativum, A. canadense*), Thyme (*Thymus serpyllum, T. vulgaris*), Irish Moss (*Chondrus crispus, Gigartina mamillosa*).

Check out the roots. Are they deep or shallow? Thick or thin? Plants with very thin, threadlike stems and roots, which imply the sewing up of lesions, are often skin healers; examples include Bedstraw or Cleavers (*Galium aparine*), Tormentil or Septfoil (*Potentilla tormentilla*), Cinquefoil (*Potentilla reptans*), Gold Thread (*Coptis greenlandica*).

Very fine and meshed roots are a signature for healers of the nervous system; examples include Valerian (*Valeriana officinalis*), Lady's Slipper (*Cypripedium calceolus, C. pubescens*).

Annuals have small thread-thin roots. These plants are mostly Fire and Air.* They do not live longer than one year and lack strong Earth energy; thus they are not grounding to the body and mind. However, they will help raise a person's spirits, lighten that person's outlook, and promote change. Their medicinal properties will be concentrated in the leaves and flowers.

Biennials are plants that grow over a two-year life cycle. They have large fleshy roots that store energy to get them through the dark, cold winter. In their first year they have no flowers or seeds and their healing virtue is concentrated in their roots. In their second year the energy moves to the flowers or berries and ultimately the seeds, which is where their medicinal properties will be found; examples include Carrots and Queen Anne's Lace or Wild Carrot (*Daucus carota*), Beets (*Beta vulgaris*), Burdock (*Arctium lappa*), Parsnip (*Pastinaca sativa*), Salsify (*Tragopogon* spp.), Raspberry (*Rubus idaeus*). These plants tend to have sweet roots that are nutritive due to their high carbohydrate content.

Perennials are plants that come back every year. Some, such as deciduous trees, Reeds (*Phragmites communis*), and Comfrey (*Symphytum officinale*), may appear to die back in the winter. Conifers, of course, stay green all year. These plants have very large and deep roots and more even energy distribution. Even in winter their twigs and roots will provide medicinal aid.

Leaf Shapes and Texture

Understanding the structure of leaves can point to the uses of a plant. For example, Liverwort (*Hepatica* spp.), used to heal liver conditions, has a leaf that is three-lobed, like the liver. Comfrey (*Symphytum officinale*) leaves have "cells" and tiny hairs that look like human skin as seen under a magnifying glass. It is one of the greatest skin healers and a healer of areas of the human body that have small hairs, such as the nose, throat, and intestines.

Plants with very soft leaves will often ease pain in a diseased

---

*For an explanation of the four elements—Earth, Water, Fire, Air—see the section "Classification according to the Four Humors," page 17).

or injured area; examples include Mallow (*Malva rotundifolia*), Horehound (*Marrubium vulgare*), Hollyhock (*Althaea rosea*), and Mullein (*Verbascum thapsus*), whose leaves were once used as a wound dressing.

Spotted leaves point to tumorous growths and pus sacks on infected lungs; examples include Saint-John's-Wort (*Hypericum perforatum*), Lungwort (*Pulmonaria officinalis*).

Overall Shape and Formations

Plants that help the eyes, such as Eyebright (*Euphrasia officinalis*), look like an eye, while the seeds of Skullcap (*Scutellaria* spp.) resemble a cap or helmet, pointing to its use to help sleeplessness, headaches, and nerve problems.

A skull-like shape reveals a brain healer, such as Walnut (*Juglans* spp.) and Skullcap (*Scutellaria lateriflora*).

Plants with a groin-like shape are used to overcome sterility and sexual lethargy; examples include Mandrake (*Mandragora officinarum*), Poke (*Phytolacca americana*), Ginseng (*Panax quinquefolius*), Bryony (*Bryonia dioica*).

Plants with long trailing root systems and vines that resemble veins and the nervous system of the body are often blood purifiers, nervines, and antispasmodics; examples include Sarsaparilla (*Smilax* spp.), Woodbine (*Lonicera periclymenum*), Licorice (*Glycyrrhiza glabra*), Bittersweet Nightshade (*Solanum dulcamara*), Grapes (*Vitis vinifera*), Hops (*Humulus lupulus*), Mints (*Mentha* spp.), Cinquefoil (*Potentilla reptans*), Dog Grass (*Agropyron repens*), Bearberry (*Arctostaphylos uva-ursi*).

Trees with bark that has openings and tears or "lenticels" are a signature for broken skin and thus skin healers; examples include Birch (*Betula* spp.), Elder (*Sambucus* spp.), Cherry (*Prunus* spp.), Sumac (*Rhus typhina*).

If a plant has thorns it is probably edible and evolved the thorns to protect itself; examples include Raspberry (*Rubus idaeus*), Blackberry (*Rubus villosus*), Rose (*Rosa* spp.). Thorns are also a signature for sharp pain. Thorny plants relieve pain, not by sedating it but by striking at the root cause of it. Hawthorn (*Crataegus* spp.), for example, is a tonic for angina and all manner of heart conditions. Other such plants are Prickly or Wild Lettuce (*Lactuca virosa, L. serriola*), Motherwort (*Leonurus cardiaca*), Blessed Thistle (*Cnicus benedictus*), and Raspberry (*Rubus idaeus*), which eases labor pains. Strawberry (*Fragraria* spp.) and Blackberry (*Rubus villosus*) contain malic and citric acids, which break up formations that lead to kidney and gall stones.

Hairy plants relieve "stitch in the side" types of pain; examples include Nettles (*Urtica dioica*), Sumac (*Rhus typhina*), Mullein (*Verbascum thapsus*), Currant (*Ribes* spp.), Hops (*Humulus lupulus*), Sundew (*Drosera rotundifolia, D. anglica, D. linearis*). Plants that sting stimulate internal circulation of fluids; examples include Ginger (*Zingiber officinale*), Nettles (*Urtica dioica*).

Plants with compact flower clusters can deal with an intense accumulation of pus in the throat and tonsils and are astringents for tonsillitis and sore throats; examples include Sumac (*Rhus typhina*), Self-heal (*Prunella vulgaris*), Hardhack (*Spiraea tomentosa*).

Wart-like growths and galls, such as growths on Sumac (*Rhus typhina*) and galls on Oak (*Quercus* spp.), contain tannins and gallic acid, which are astringent and pull together the edges of a wound.

Lichens and molds are useful for skin conditions such as psoriasis, which they resemble.

Moisture and Stickiness

Mucilaginous plants will soothe the throat; examples include Acacia (*Acacia* spp.), Tragacanth (*Astragalus adscendens, A. gummifer, A. brachycalyx, A. tragacanthus*), Irish Moss (*Chondrus crispus*), Hollyhock (*Alcea* spp.), Slippery Elm (*Ulmus fulva*), Mallow (*Malva rotundifolia*), Lungwort (*Pulmonaria officinalis*), Flaxseed (*Linum usitatissimum*).

Plants that contain a lot of resin are often healers of moist lesions, cuts, and ulcers; examples include Balsam of Peru or Tolu Balsam (*Myroxylon balsamum pereirae*), Benzoin (*Styrax* spp.), Mastic (*Pistacia lentiscus*), Pine (*Pinus* spp.), Myrrh (*Commiphora myrrha*), Turpentine (from *Pinus* spp.), Aloe (*Aloe* spp.). Plants with a sticky mucilaginous sap are also great itch healers; examples include Aloe

(*Aloe* spp.), Pine (*Pinus* spp.), Comfrey (*Symphytum officinale*). If they are very juicy and wet (*Aloe* spp.), they will help swell excretions and benefit the colon.

If a plant is very dry and lacking in juice, such as Sage (*Salvia officinalis*), it will be good for drying up secretions such as catarrh and breast milk.

A plant that sticks to itself will cling to and remove hardened mucus; examples include Sage (*Salvia officinalis*), Coltsfoot (*Tussilago farfara*), Horehound (*Marrubium vulgare*), Life Everlasting (*Gnaphalium obtusifolium, G. polycephalum*), Mallow (*Malva rotundifolia*).

Smell

Plants that are highly aromatic are also disinfectant and deodorizing; examples include Thyme (*Thymus serpyllum, T. vulgaris*), Rosemary (*Rosmarinus officinalis*), Lemon (*Citrus limon*), Juniper (*Juniperus* spp.). For bad breath and body odor, examples include Marjoram (*Origanum marjorana*), Mint (*Mentha* spp.), Rosemary (*Rosmarinus officinalis*), Anise (*Pimpinella anisum*).

Other aromatics are antiseptic, germicidal, and antibiotic; examples include Tansy (*Tanacetum vulgare*), Pennyroyal (*Mentha pulegium*), Sage (*Salvia officinalis*), Savory (*Satureja hortensis*), Fennel (*Foeniculum vulgare*), Basil (*Ocimum* spp.).

Plants that stink are used for indolent, foul ulcers; examples include Stinking Arrach (*Chenopodium olidum*).

Color

The color red points to the blood and the plant is likely a blood purifier or beneficial to the heart; examples include Red Clover (*Trifolium pratense*), Burdock (*Arctium lappa*), Rose (*Rosa* spp.), Raspberry (*Rubus idaeus*), Bee Balm (*Monarda fistulosa, M. punctata, M. fistulosa* var. *menthifolia, M. didyma*), Hawthorn (*Crataegus* spp.).

Yellow flowers are associated with the liver and gall, jaundice, and yellow bile; examples include Dandelion (*Taraxacum officinale*), Celandine (*Chelidonium majus*), Goldenseal (*Hydrastis canadensis*), Barberry (*Berberis vulgaris*), Lemon (*Citrus limon*).

White-blooming flowers point to bone healing; examples include Boneset (*Eupatorium perfoliatum*), Comfrey (*Symphytum officinale*).

Blue and purple flowers point to a plant that will improve the complexion and may also be a remedy for cyanosis (a blueness of the skin resulting from lack of oxygen in the blood and impaired arterial flow); examples include Joe Pye Weed (*Eupatorium purpureum*), Red Clover (*Trifolium pratense*), Vervain (*Verbena hastata, V. officinalis*), Burdock (*Arctium lappa*), Gentian (*Gentiana lutea*), Chicory (*Chichorium intybus*).

Nature in her kindness has given us a signature for poisonous herbs—the color maroon—which we can see, for example, in the berries and stems of Poke (*Phytolacca americana*), and the streaks of maroon found up and down the stems of Water Hemlock (*Cicuta* spp.), the herb that did in Socrates.

Taste

There is an old adage: "Bitter taste, sweet to the stomach, sweet taste, bitter to the stomach." Plants that are yellow and bitter, such as Dandelion (*Taraxacum officinale*), benefit the liver, while plants that are yellow and sweet, such as Astragalus root (*Astragalus membranaceus*) and Elecampane (*Inula helenium*), are building to the stomach, spleen, and pancreas.

Plants that are sour and taste like lemons are telling you they have a lot of vitamin C. Plants that taste like carrots have a lot of carotene or vitamin A. Lichens will taste of the minerals in the rock they are growing on. Spinach, high in iron, actually tastes like iron ore. Plants that taste like garlic contain sulfur and can help clear heavy metals out of the body.

Pain-killing plants will deaden the lower lip when tasted.

The Signatures of Foods

Slice a carrot and you will find radiating spokes that look like the human eye. Carrots contain vitamin A, which is very beneficial to eye health. Onion cells under the microscope look like human cells. They help clear waste from cells and cause tears, which clean the epithelial layers of the eyes. Tomatoes are red and have four chambers, just like a human heart. They, like all red fruits and vegetables, benefit the heart, blood, and circulation. Grapes hang in heart-shaped clusters. Grapes are great blood and lymph cleansers and contain resveratrol, which helps the heart.

Walnuts look like little brains, with left and right hemispheres and wrinkles that resemble the neocortex. Walnuts are known to improve brain function. Kidney beans actually do benefit the kidneys. Sweet potatoes resemble the pancreas and can help balance blood sugar levels. In Chinese medicine orange foods are said to benefit the Earth element and the pancreas.

Avocados are shaped like the female womb, and it takes nine months to grow an avocado from seed to fruit. In turn, avocados balance hormones, help women shed pregnancy weight, and prevent cervical cancers. Olives help the ovaries, which they resemble in structure. Pomegranates, which are larger but also resemble the ovary filled with blood and eggs, are cleansing to the female reproductive tract. Citrus fruits, such as grapefruits, oranges, and others, resemble mammary glands. They help move lymph in and out of the breasts.

Figs hang in clusters of two and are filled with seeds. They increase the number and motility of sperm.

The Contribution of Intuition

Once you have the basics down you can let your intuition lead you further. For example, when I sat before a Cardinal Flower (*Lobelia cardinalis*), I thought immediately of a fire engine, of burning, redness, fever, and sparks before the eyes. That seemed way too obvious and I didn't think it could be so easy. Then I went and looked it up in Clarke's materia medica, and here was what I found:

> There is a proving* of Lob. card. by S. D. R. Dubs, who took ten drops of the tincture in one dose. Dubs' symptoms have been confirmed by a second proving by Kopp (H. W., xxxi. 26). The acrid

---

*In homeopathy, a dilute amount of the herb, mineral, or other substance is taken until a "proving" or symptom picture results. The symptoms that appear in the provings are compared to those of a sick person; if properly matched, the person who takes the remedy will heal.

properties of the plant were immediately felt by Dubs, in burning in mouth and throat, which lasted a long time. Sticking and pricking sensation in various parts, especially left chest and left hypochondrium. Oppression of breathing. Headache at base of occiput burning in tongue and fauces. Many symptoms occurred at 8 a.m. Sleepy but difficulty in sleeping. A lady to whom Cooper gave one dose of Lob. cd. had "flashes of light before eyes every day for a week." It seems, he says, to have an action distinct from that of other Lobelias, since a dose of it brought back pains which had been relieved by Lob. dort.

THE ANCIENT CHINESE SYSTEM OF PLANT CLASSIFICATION

In addition to the system of classification by plant signatures, other systems also were used in ancient times. Thousands of years ago the Chinese developed a system of plant classification based on temperature, flavor, and direction. Armed with this knowledge, an herbalist could identify which plants were most useful for a particular illness.

The Four Natures or Temperatures

Chinese herbalism divides herbs into warm, hot, cool, and cold. A cooling or cold plant is suitable for a "yang" (congested, full, toxic) hot disease, and a hot or warm herb is given for a "yin" (dissipating energy, debilitated, chilly) cold disease. Some herbs are considered "neutral" and can be given for both cold and hot conditions.

The Five Flavors

Plants are also classified according to flavor: sour, bitter, sweet, spicy, and salty.

Sour-tasting herbs are known to stop secretions, contract tissue, and promote digestion and liver function. Examples are Lemon (*Citrus limon*), Rose hips (*Rosa* spp.), Hawthorn berries (*Crataegus* spp.), and Chinese Dogwood (*Cornus officinalis*).

Bitter-tasting herbs are cooling, anti-inflammatory, and antiviral, and they help clear parasites from the body. They improve stomach function, clean the blood via the liver, clear cholesterol from the venous system, and help the heart. Examples include Goldenseal (*Hydrastis canadensis*),* Gentian (*Gentiana lutea*), Centaury (*Centaurium umbellatum, Erythraea centaurium*), and Mugwort (*Artemisia vulgaris*).

Sweet-tasting herbs are building and nourishing. Foods and herbs that contain complex carbohydrates, proteins, and sugars are found to be nutritive and building to the body. Examples are Ginseng (*Panax quinquefolius*), Rehmannia root (*Rehmannia glutinosa*), Date (*Phoenix dactylifera*), and Barley malt (*Hordeum vulgare* L.).

Spicy herbs and foods are drying and warming to the body. They are useful for mucous congestion, arthritis, colds, flu, and menstrual cramps when taken internally; applied topically they relieve bruising and injuries. Examples are Red Pepper (*Capsicum annuum*), Cinnamon (*Cinnamomum verum, C. cassia*), Ginger (*Zingiber officinale*), and Prickly Ash (*Zanthoxylum clava-herculis, Z. americanum*).

Salty-tasting herbs are cooling and moistening to the body, because of the way they help the organs retain water. Seaweeds (marine algae) are a good example of this kind of plant.

Bland-tasting plants such as mushrooms are classified as mildly sweet and diuretic.

The Four Directions

In Chinese philosophy every substance in nature is understood to float, sink, rise, or descend, depending upon its inherent qualities. Seasons are also seen to have these characteristics: summer has floating energy, fall has descending energy, winter has sinking energy, and spring has ascending energy.

Leaves and flowers have ascending energy, making them useful for acute, surface-level diseases such as colds and flu. Barks, roots, seeds,

---

*Goldenseal root is tonic to the system when taken as no more than one-tenth part of a formula. Taken alone, Goldenseal becomes an antibiotic and must be treated with caution, as with any antibiotic. After a course of Goldenseal, take plain yogurt, sauerkraut, miso soup, raw apple cider, or any probiotic supplement to restore intestinal flora.

and berries have sinking energy and thus move deeper into the system to aid chronic conditions.

What's in a Name?

When you look at an herbal you will notice that a plant may have several common names. Pay attention to the folk names for herbs, because the old-timers named them that way for a reason.

Eyebright (*Euphrasia officinalis*) got its name because it helps the eyes. Liverwort (*Anemone hepatica*) is called that because it helps the liver (*wort* is an old word for "herb").

Mouthroot or Gold Thread (*Coptis greenlandica*) is good for ulcers and mouth sores. Heartsease (*Viola tricolor*) leaves are a tonic for the heart. Kidneywort (*Cotyledon umbilicus*) helps with inflammation and kidney stones. Lungmoss (*Lobaria pulmonaria*) helps with pulmonary problems. Skullcap (*Scutellaria lateriflora*) is for headaches.

Other examples are Cough Herb (*Tussilago farfara*), Puke Weed/ Asthma Weed/Indian Tobacco (*Lobelia inflata*), Heal-all (*Collinsonia canadensis*), Self-heal (*Prunella vulgaris*), Nosebleed (*Achillea millefolium*), Colic Root (*Dioscorea villosa*), Boneset (*Eupatorium perfoliatum*), Dysentery Bark (*Simaruba amara*), Feverwort (*Erythraea centaurium*), Pilewort (*Ranunculus ficaria*), Scabwort (*Inula helenium*), and many more. You get the idea.

CLASSIFICATION ACCORDING TO THE FOUR HUMORS

Until the seventeenth century, European herbalists relied on the classification system of Galen and the four elements as understood by ancient Greece and Rome. In this system people were said to be divided into four "humors," corresponding to the four elements: Earth, Air, Fire, and Water. This system classified plants and people as hot, cold, dry, or moist.

The Sanguine or "Air" type of person was hot and moist. Such persons were cheerful, with a ruddy complexion, but with a tendency to overindulge. They were prone to diseases of excess such as gout and diarrhea and had a tendency to develop inflammatory conditions. Cool and dry herbs such as Burdock (*Arctium lappa*) and Figwort (*Scrophularia nodosa*) helped to cleanse and restore these people.

The Energetics of Color

Many spiritual healing systems refer to the chakras, energy nodes that exist in specific areas of the body. The healthy functioning of each of these nodes and the circulation of energy between them can be enhanced by plants of the appropriate color.

Pink and red flowers and fruits benefit the heart, the fourth chakra.

Red-flowering plants such as Wild Ginger (*Asarum* spp.) will help move energy to the second chakra, the sexual node of the body.

Orange-flowered plants such as Calendula (*Calendula officinalis*) tend to spread cleansing energy over the whole body.

Yellow (solar) plants such as Dandelion (*Taraxacum officinale*) and Elecampane (*Inula helenium*) enhance the sense of personal power and the (universal) Self. Plants such as Chamomile flowers (*Matricaria recutita, Chamaemelum nobile*) also strengthen the stomach and solar plexus, or third chakra.

Plants that are mostly green such as Self-heal (*Prunella vulgaris*) are soothing to the eyes and to the entire bodily system

Blue flowers such as those of Mint (*Mentha* spp.) point to the throat chakra and communication.

Plants with flowers that are indigo, dark blue, or dark purple, such as Gentian (*Gentiana lutea*) and Skullcap (*Scutellaria lateriflora*), enhance the third eye (*ajna* in Sanskrit) and kill pain.

Violet plants such as Skullcap (*Scutellaria lateriflora*) are attuned to the crown chakra at the top of the skull, to the hormonal and nervous systems and the pineal and pituitary glands.

The Melancholic or "Earth" type was cold and dry, pale, and prone to constipation and depression. They could be visionaries but also suffered from mental or sexual disorders. Hot herbs such as Senna (*Cassia acutifolia*, *C. angustifolia*) and Hellebore (*Veratrum album*) were used restore balance to this type.

The Phlegmatic or "Water" person was cold and moist and sometimes a little slow or dull. They tended toward congestion, mucous accumulation, and rheumatic conditions. Warming and drying herbs such as Thyme (*Thymus serpyllum*, *Thymus vulgaris*) and Hyssop (*Hyssopus officinalis*) were recommended for these disorders.

The Choleric or "Fire" person was hot and dry, easily angered, and susceptible to liver disease, high blood pressure, rashes, fevers, and sunburn. Cool, moist plants such as Rhubarb (*Rheum palmatum*), Violets (*Viola* spp.), and Dandelion (*Taraxacum officinale*) were found to be helpful for them.

2

HERBS OF SPRING

A weed is a plant whose uses have yet to be appreciated.

I live in an oak forest in New England. There is very little light here for growing things, so I mostly rely on wildcrafted roots, barks, leaves, flowers, and berries, but I follow a few cautions before I pick.

- The first is expressed by an old Native American saying: "Walk by the first seven, leave the eighth for the animals, and you may take the ninth." Always leave enough plants behind to feed the wild creatures and to make seed for next year's crop.
- Gather plants at least one thousand feet from a roadway to avoid the pollutants that abound there, such as those from car exhaust and brake linings.
- Act fast, because Nature doesn't wait: there is usually just a short window of opportunity for gathering from the wild.
- Know your herbs: be sure you have a good guide or a teacher to point things out to you, and never pick endangered species in the wild.

Every season brings its own moment of opportunity. In the spring there are already an abundance of edibles and medicinals available in fields and forests, for those with the eyes to see and the determination to seek them out.

Bloodroot (*Sanguinaria canadensis*)

The delicate white flowers of Bloodroot are among the first flowers to appear in woodlands in spring. The root of the plant was once added to tinctures and syrups for lung conditions such as asthma, bronchitis, and fevers. As it is now considered a toxic irritant, a better way to deliver the medicine is to put the tincture or tea of Bloodroot into a vaporizer and inhale the mist. It helps open the capillaries in cases of COPD (chronic obstructive pulmonary disease) and other lung disorders. As it is an antiseptic, Bloodroot is still used in toothpastes and mouthwashes.

Cattail, Bulrush (*Typha* spp.)

Cattail is delicious in spring. Cut off the new green growth and peel back the outer layers to reveal the pale green center, which is something like heart of palm. Steam the tender center and serve with butter. The hardest part about gathering Cattails is finding a pond or a swamp that is not polluted by runoff from farms or roadways.

Chickweed or Starwort (*Stellaria media*)

Stellaria media thrives in cool weather. It can be cooked like spinach, added to healing salves, or made into a tea. Very high in vitamin C, it is a good food for invalids; use it in salads, sautéed, and in soups. The plant is also added to herbal salves for itchy skin conditions.

The tea can help ease constipation and bladder and bronchial problems. *To make the tea:* Steep one tablespoon per half cup of water for twenty minutes. Take up to one cup a day in quarter-cup amounts.

Chicory (*Chichorium intybus*)

Chichorium intybus is a familiar bright blue wayside flower. Gather the young leaves before the blossoms appear and add them raw to salads or cook them like spinach. The leaves are also used in poultices for inflammation. Later in the season you can sprinkle the open flowers onto salads, open-faced cream cheese sandwiches, and cakes. Try freezing them into ice cubes for festive occasions.

The roots can be gathered from March to May. Sauté the roots when fresh, or dry them, grind them, and add them to coffee. A tea made from the roots will aid the digestive tract. A tea can also be made of the leaves and flowers (don't pick after blooming); it will clear mucus, aid in passing gallstones, and improve digestion. Acne, liver problems, eczema, rheumatic complaints, and gout may also benefit from the tea. Tea made from the leaves can also be used as a mouthwash for gum conditions.

To make the tea: Simmer one teaspoon of chopped root per half cup of water for ten minutes, or steep one teaspoon of herb per half cup of water for twenty minutes. Take one tablespoon three times a day in separate doses, in water or milk.

Dandelion (*Taraxacum officinale*)

Dandelion greens are at their best in the early spring when they first appear. Then rinse the leaves and eat them mixed into a salad, or cook them like spinach with a little butter, sea salt, and lemon juice. You can also dust them with flour, salt, and pepper and then fry in butter. A classic way to cook Dandelion greens is to sauté them with onion and bacon.

The flowers are used to make Dandelion wine. Add the petals (but not the green sepals, which are too bitter) to salads for a calcium boost.

Dandelion root tea is used for acne and eczema and for liver issues. *To make the tea:* Simmer two teaspoons of root per half cup of water for about fifteen minutes. Take up to one cup a day in quarter-cup doses.

Daylily (*Hemerocallis fulva*)

The classic orange Daylily is found in many gardens, and every part of this plant (except maybe the stem) is edible. Gather the new leaves in the spring and cut them up into salads. Once the roots have been carefully cleaned, they can be sliced raw into salads or cooked like potatoes.

Later in summer, when the buds appear, you can sauté them with other vegetables. The open flowers are added to soups as a thickener.

> **Caution: There is considerable disagreement about whether other types of Daylilies are edible, so be sure to research other varieties carefully.**

Forsythia (*Forsythia* spp.)

Yellow Forsythia flowers are some of the first spring blooms. Add a few to your salad.

Ground Ivy, Creeping Charlie, Gill-over-the-Ground (*Glechoma hederacea*)

Ground Ivy starts to proliferate in spring and can be made into a tea for colds, diarrhea, bronchitis, sore throat, gout, gravel, stone, and liver problems. *To make the tea:* Steep one teaspoon of fresh leaves per half cup of water for twenty minutes. Take up to one cup a day in quarter-cup doses.

> **Caution: Do not take Ground Ivy in large amounts or for long periods.**

Hemlock (*Tsuga canadensis*)

Hemlock is probably the tastiest conifer to eat, although the new growth of most conifers can be munched right off the tree, added to salads, and simmered into teas. The twigs and needles can be used year-round to make a slightly antiseptic, vitamin C–rich cold remedy. (See chapter 15 for more ideas on how to use conifers.)

Japanese Knotweed (*Polygonum cuspidatum*)

Considered an invasive pest by many in the northeastern United States, the root of this plant has been shown to be useful in diseases such as Lyme. In fact, it has spread to exactly the areas where Lyme is proliferating (I think Mother Nature knows something we humans have yet to understand). Japanese Knotweed proves the old adage, "A weed is a plant whose uses have yet to be appreciated." I have noticed that this plant is a great favorite of the bees.

Gather the spears of new growth in the spring and use them in pies, in crumbles, and as a rhubarb substitute.

Lamb's-quarter, Wild Spinach (*Chenopodium album*)

Look for Lamb's-quarter in old farmyards. A relative of Quinoa, this plant should be eaten when it is young. Cook the greens just like spinach or eat them raw. The seeds can be ground into flour.

A cool tea of the leaves can be used as a fomentation for sunburn and headaches. *To make the tea:* Steep two teaspoons of fresh leaves or one teaspoon of dry leaves per cup of water for ten minutes. Apply cool or cold.

Locust (*Robinia* spp.)

The white flowers of Black Locust (*Robinia pseudoacacia*) can be used in fritters and made into tea. The flowers of Pink Locust (*Robinia neomexicana*) are also edible.

Caution: Avoid the Locust pods, which are poisonous.

Mallow (*Malva neglecta*)

Malva neglecta flower buds, flowers, roots, and very young leaves can be cooked and eaten in the spring. The fresh leaves make a nice poultice for burns, rashes, bites, and itchy skin conditions. The "cheeses" or seed pods can be eaten raw or pickled.

The buds, flowers, roots, and very young leaves can also be used to make a tea for coughs and sore throats. *To make the tea:* Steep two teaspoons of herb per half cup of water for twenty minutes or longer. Take one quarter cup four times a day on an empty stomach.

Milkweed (*Asclepias syriaca*)

Look for the unopened flower buds of Milkweed and cook them like broccoli. The opened flowers can be made into fritters.

Caution: Avoid the leaves and stems, which are poisonous.

Nettles (*Urtica* spp.)

Nettles are antihistaminic and a nice alternative to allergy medications. Fresh Nettles should be gathered while wearing rubber gloves. Rinse for a few seconds under cold water in the sink and all traces of the "sting" will disappear.

Caution: Do not eat Nettles raw.

Nettles can be added to soups, sautéed with other vegetables, folded into omelets, and so on. Try baking Nettles into a pie or adding them to quiche. Delicious!

Nettles can be made into a warming tea. ***To make the tea:*** Steep three tablespoons of chopped Nettles in a cup of freshly boiled water for three to ten minutes. Take one quarter cup four times a day on an empty stomach.

The following Nettle bread recipe from Irish chef Kenneth Culhane can be served as a green bread roll for Saint Patrick's Day.*

Nettle Bread

½ cup organic whole milk

½ cup nettle tips

2 cups plus 2½ teaspoons organic flour

⅓ cup white sugar

1½ tablespoons fresh yeast

2½ teaspoons Cornish sea salt

6 organic, free-range eggs

½ cup unsalted organic butter, softened

Egg yolk, for glaze

Warm the milk with the nettle leaves and blitz in a blender; leave to cool.

Mix all the dry ingredients together in a bread mixer or in an ordinary dough mixer. Add the milk and nettle mix and beat gently with the paddle for six minutes. Add the eggs one by one. When the eggs are fully incorporated, beat the butter into the dough mixture on a fast speed. Place in the fridge to rest for 5–6 hours.

Shape the dough into small balls and leave to rise in the warmth of the kitchen for approximately 30 minutes. Brush the rolls with egg yolk and bake for 8–10 minutes in a preheated oven at 375 degrees. Makes between 12 and 15 rolls.

---

*Adapted from www.irishpost.co.uk/spd/recipe-kenneth-culhanes-delicious-foraged -nettle-milk-bread-for-st-patricks-day.

Norway Maple (*Acer platanoides*)

Add the flowers of Norway Maple to salads.

Ostrich Fern (*Matteuccia struthiopteris*)

Ubiquitous in Chinese markets in spring, the fiddleheads of Ostrich Fern can be sautéed with butter and a little sea salt.

Plantain (*Plantago* spp.)

Gather the new leaves of Plantain and add them to herbal salves; the fresh leaves can also be used to poultice cuts, stings, bites, and inflammations. For gingivitis, chew and pack the fresh leaves into the buccal area. The very smallest leaves can also be added to salads.

Poke (*Phytolacca americana*)

"Happy as a pig in the poke" is an old saying that expresses the joy of finding a stand of young Poke shoots. Gather the leaves when the plant is no more than six inches high and cook like spinach (pour off the water and simmer twice).

Early American settlers kept the roots in their "root cellars" and clipped off the new growth all winter for fresh greens.

> **Caution: Do not eat Poke if the plant is more than six inches tall; after that it becomes poisonous!**

Purslane (*Portulaca oleracea*)

Portulaca oleracea is another garden "weed" whose uses have yet to be appreciated. It is high in omega-3 fatty acids and thus protective of the heart and immune system. It also benefits the liver. Add it to soups and sautés.

> **Caution: Pregnant women and those with weak digestion should avoid Purslane.**

Redbud (*Cercis canadensis*)

The flowers of *Cercis canadensis* can be sprinkled on a salad and the unripe pods can be sautéed.

Sassafras (*Sassafras albidum, S. variifolium*)

I like to dig up a Sassafras root each spring to make homemade birch beer. See page 178 for instructions on how to make this classic spring tonic.

Shagbark Hickory (*Carya ovata*)

Carya ovata can be made into syrup!

 ## Shagbark Hickory Syrup

> 2 pounds shagbark hickory bark
>
> 2 cups granulated organic sugar

Preheat the oven to 325 degrees.

Scrub the bark thoroughly in clean water to remove debris. Break the bark into roughly 8-inch pieces and place on a baking sheet. Toast it until it is slightly brown and toasty smelling, about 25 minutes.

Place the toasted bark in a large pot and add enough water to cover by 1 inch. Bring to a simmer and simmer for 30 minutes. (Do not boil.)

Remove the bark and discard.

Add sugar to the liquid. Bring to a boil and reduce until it thickens to the consistency of warm syrup. It will take about an hour.

Cool the syrup, then store in an airtight container in the refrigerator for up to 3 months. Makes about 2 cups of syrup.

Spicebush (*Lindera benzoin*)

Native American healers used a decoction of the inner bark for colds and fevers, rheumatic complaints and as a blood cleanser. They made a tea of the berries for cramps, coughs, measles, and delayed menstruation. Early settlers used the inner bark tea for worms, gas, and colic and the berry tea for gas and colic. The aromatic leaves can be added to sachets to repel insects. You can grind the fresh berries in a coffee grinder and freeze them for later. Add the berries to marmalades or use when cooking meats. The berries can also be used to make ice cream.

To make the tea: Loosely pack the fresh leaves in a jar of cold water to make a sun tea in the summer. In winter, break the twigs into one to two inch sections and steep two tablespoons of twigs per cup of freshly boiled water for fifteen minutes.

Strawberry (*Fragaria ananassa,* or if wild, *Fragraria virginiana*)

Eat the flowers on a salad. According to Native American tradition, the whole plant—leaves, berries, and roots—can be taken as a springtime blood-cleansing tea, which is both laxative and diuretic. Strawberry leaves and fruits are a good food during pregnancy and menstruation. Modern studies are showing that strawberries help clear cholesterol from the blood.

Sycamore (*Platanus occidentalis*)

Sycamore sap flows on warm winter days—days during the January thaw and days during the maple syrup season that are too warm for maple sap to flow (when daytime temperatures are greater than 50—and even 60—degrees Fahrenheit).

The sap can be tapped from the tree and drunk fresh or boiled down just like maple syrup. It can also be made into sugar by heating the syrup. First rim your pot with butter at the top to keep the syrup from boiling over. Then heat to 255 degrees, stirring continuously with a wooden spoon so that the syrup doesn't burn. Be very careful of boiling over.

The liquid will eventually start to foam, and at that point you should turn the heat to low and keep stirring until sugar granules appear. Then transfer the syrup to a room-temperature roasting pan with high walls, off the stove, and keep stirring and working it for about ten minutes to break up lumps.

One gallon of syrup makes about eight pounds of sugar.

Tulip (*Tulipa* spp.)

The flower petals are edible and can be used as colorful cups for tuna salad, chicken salad, and dips.

Violets (*Viola* spp.)

The young leaves and flowers of *Viola odorata* can be eaten raw in salads, as can the flowers of Johnny-jump-up (*Viola tricolor*), Majestic Giant (*Viola wittrockiana*), Skippy XL Plum-Gold (*Viola cornuta*), and Yesterday, Today, and Tomorrow (*Viola hybrida*). Or stir the flowers into raw local honey with fresh lemon juice. Eat immediately or freeze for later use.

Violet tea is taken for cough, fever, and bronchitis and to ease depression, nervousness, and anger. ***To make the tea:*** Steep one teaspoon of flowers and leaves per half cup of water for twenty minutes. Or simmer roots gathered in the fall: one tablespoon of chopped root per half cup of water. Take one quarter cup four times a day on an empty stomach.

Violet, Rose, or Dandelion Jelly

Fill a glass jar with one of the following:

- dandelion flowers (*Taraxacum officinale*)—remove the stems and green sepals from the dandelion flowers or the jelly will be bitter
- fragrant old-fashioned tea-style rose petals (*Rosa* spp.)—please do not use the genetically engineered scentless varieties
- blue violets (*Viola odorata*)

Pour enough boiling water over the flowers to fill the jar. Allow the jar to sit overnight.

Strain out the flowers and reserve the liquid.

For every 2 cups of liquid, add the juice of 1 lemon and a package of powdered pectin or liquid pectin.

Place the liquid in a non-aluminum pot and bring to a boil.

Add a tiny piece of butter (to prevent froth) and 4 cups of organic cane sugar and bring to a boil again.

Boil hard for 1 minute; pour into clean jars and refrigerate or process in boiling water to preserve.

Wild Onion (*Allium* spp.)

Look for Wild Onions in grassy areas. Chop the greens and float them on soups or add them to herb butters. Use the bulbs in cooking, just like the store-bought varieties.

Wisteria (*Wisteria* spp.)

The raw flowers of *Wisteria* spp. can be sprinkled onto a cream cheese–covered cracker or sandwich.

> **Caution: Avoid Wisteria seeds and pods, which can be toxic.**

Wood Sorrel (*Oxalis* spp.)

Wood Sorrel and Sheep Sorrel (*Rumex* spp.) are used the same way—to make lemony-tasting sauces and soups.

> **Caution: Wood Sorrel and Sheep Sorrel are high in oxalic acid, so it's best to avoid them if you have kidney issues.**

Yarrow (*Achillea millefolium*)

Tiny new Yarrow leaves can be added to salads and also to wound salves for their styptic properties.

Yellow Dock, Curly Dock (*Rumex crispus*)

In very early spring the newest leaves of *Rumex crispus* are edible. Bring to a simmer and pour off the water twice before consuming.

> **Caution: Do not eat large amounts of Yellow Dock, as it can irritate the kidneys.**

3

HERBS OF SUMMER

As I write this, it is Lughnasad ("Loo-nah-sah"), the old Celtic festival of the first fruits of the harvest that takes place during the first two weeks of August. In Christian times the feast was renamed Lammas or Loaf-Mass, when everyone brought the first loaf of bread made from the year's new grain to church to be placed on the altar and blessed.

Late summer is an especially rich time to harvest from nature. Here are a few of nature's abundant offerings.

Berries (*Vaccinium* spp., *Rubus* spp.)

Berries are the signature wild fruit of the season. Syrups are a nice way to make use of the extra berries you find. Blueberries, Saskatoon berries, Raspberries, Huckleberries, Blackberries, and even wild purple Grapes can be made into syrups.

Wild Berry Syrup*

1 organic lemon

5 cups berries

1 cup water

1 cup organic sugar or ½ cup raw local honey

Slice two or three ½-inch strips of peel from the lemon and set aside. Juice the lemon and set the juice aside.

---

*Recipe adapted from "How to Make Your Own Blueberry Syrup," Simple Bites, www.simplebites.net/how-to-make-your-own-blueberry-syrup/.

Put the berries into a non-aluminum pot and crush with a potato masher. Add the water to the berries and bring to a boil, then lower to a simmer. Simmer for 15 minutes, stirring occasionally.

Ladle the berries into a fine-mesh sieve placed over a bowl and mash with a large spoon to press out all the juice (save the residue to eat over yogurt, ice cream, pancakes, granola, etc.).

Pour the juice back into the pot, add the lemon peel (you can also add lavender flowers or cinnamon at this point for flavor) and sugar, and bring to a boil, then simmer for 10 minutes until slightly thickened.

Add just 2 tablespoons of the lemon juice and stir it in.

Boil for another 1–2 minutes. (No more! Do not overcook or you might end up with jelly.) Then remove the lemon peels.

Pour into very clean glass jars or bottles, cap tightly, and keep in the refrigerator for up to 3 months (or in the freezer for up to 9 months). Makes 3 cups of syrup.

Cranesbill, Storksbill (*Erodium cicutarium*)

Erodium cicutarium tastes a bit like parsley and can be added to salads. The whole plant is used as a tea to stop excessive bleeding from the uterus.

Caution: Small doses of Cranesbill may raise blood pressure and larger doses may lower it.

Elder (*Sambucus nigra, S. canadensis*)

Elder has been called "Elder Mother" because her berries and flowers are healing for children and adults. Elderflower tea is beneficial for chest colds such as bronchitis, flu, and rheumatic conditions. *To make the tea:* Steep two tablespoons of the fresh or dried flowers in a cup of freshly boiled water for twenty minutes; take three times a day. Add a little sweetener and fresh lemon for better taste. Add Elderflower tea to washes and baths for the skin.

Elderberries can be made into healing elixirs (see page 54 for two recipes). Another way to keep the berries is to steep them in apple cider vinegar for about a week, and then strain and bottle, to add to salads.

Fennel (*Foeniculum vulgare*)

A friend of mine has a nice patch of Fennel growing wild around her house, and she lets me pick a few stalks each year in the fall to make Fennel liqueur. It is a great hit at Yuletide for gifts. I use just the Fennel flowers and leaves.

 ## Fennel Liqueur

I have also made liqueur with Thai basil, rosemary, lemon balm, thyme, bee balm, raspberries with echinacea, pears with ginger, organic orange with Saint-John's-wort flowers, and blackberries with Concord grapes. But everyone seems to like the fennel best.

2 cups fresh fennel (or another herb or fruit)

1½ cups vodka (or enough to barely cover the herbs or fruit)

1½ cups organic sugar or ¾ cup honey (I use less)

¾ cup water

Combine the fennel (or herb or fruit) and vodka in a clean glass jar with a tight lid. Let stand for 6 weeks in a cool, dark place. Shake every few days.

Combine the sugar and water in a pan. Heat until the sugar melts completely. Allow to cool.

Strain the herbs (or fruit) from the vodka using cheesecloth or a strainer. Combine with the sugar-water mixture, bottle, and keep for up to 1 year. I use only organic sugar, organic fruits and herbs, and well water. This is a medieval recipe; in the old days they would have used honey.

Goldenrod (*Solidago* spp.)

I like to make Goldenrod vinegar; using it in salads is a nice way to build your immune system. It is also said to benefit the kidneys and help with arthritis. There are a number of different Goldenrod species that flourish in my area and I use them all. In late summer I strip the fully opened flowers off the stem, stuff them into a jar, and cover them with apple cider vinegar. I let them steep for about a month, and then I strain and bottle the vinegar for use in salads all winter.

Poison Ivy Wash

One of the drawbacks to exploring the woods can be the impact of certain plants such as Poison Ivy, which can cause a very uncomfortable rash. But the woods themselves provide the remedy, too.

Take Sweet Fern (*Comptonia peregrina*), a woody-stemmed fragrant herb that grows in wild places at the edges of fields and forests. Place the leaves in a clean glass jar until the jar is two-thirds full. Add Plantain leaves (*Plantago* spp.) and Jewelweed (*Impatiens aurea*) until the jar is packed full. Pour vodka over the herbs to the level of the top of the jar. Cover with a tight lid and allow the tincture to sit for about three days, or until the plant matter starts to break down. When the herbs begin to wilt and the liquid is brown, strain out the herbs and reserve the liquid. Store the jar in a cool dark place. Apply locally to Poison Ivy rash with a cotton ball, four times a day.

SOME WOODLAND HERBS

If you are fortunate enough to live in or near the woods, here are some useful woodland plants.

English Ivy (*Hedera helix*)

A tea of this shade-loving plant can be used to remove phlegm from the body in conditions such as bronchitis and whooping cough, and for fevers, gout, and rheumatism.

To make the tea: Steep one teaspoon of crushed leaf per cup of cold water for eight hours. Take a quarter cup, four times a day.

> **Caution: An overdose of English Ivy can cause diarrhea, vomiting, and even coma. Not for long-term use.**

The leaf tea is bactericidal and parasiticidal and—made stronger— can be used externally as a wash for sores, cuts, burns, and dandruff. The tea can be used as a douche for vaginal infections.

The twigs and leaves of English Ivy are added to sunburn salves and used to poultice injuries to the nerves and sinews. The leaf poultice is also applied to ulcers, glandular swellings, painful rheumatic parts, boils, and abscesses.

Horsetail (*Equisetum hyemale*)

This plant is found in shady, wet areas near streams. High in silica, this plant can help strengthen organ linings. The root was given to teething babies by Native American healers. The juice of this plant helps with anemia and promotes coagulation of blood. For this reason it can help bleeding stomach ulcers. Take one teaspoon of fresh juice in water, three or four times a day. Externally, it has been used as a hemostatic poultice for wounds.

A tea of the fresh or dried aboveground parts has been used to benefit the bladder, the kidneys, gout, gonorrhea, and stomach problems, to help with constipation, and as a diuretic. The tea has been used for lung conditions such as tuberculosis. The tea is also a douche for vaginal infections and makes a wash for skin lesions and mouth sores.

To make the tea: Steep four tablespoons of plant matter per cup of freshly boiled water for twenty minutes. Take a quarter cup, four times a day. For internal bleeding, take two cups a day in tablespoon doses. For external use make a stronger tea by steeping for forty minutes.

> **Caution: Horsetail tea may interfere with thiamine metabolism, so it's not for long-term use.**

Jack-in-the-Pulpit, American Wake Robin, Indian Turnip (*Arisaema triphyllum*)

> **Caution: Use extreme care with this plant. The roots are very irritating if misused; never eat the roots raw. The berries are poisonous too.**

The dried and aged root (sliced very thin and dried for at least three months) was used by Native American healers for whooping cough, bronchitis, and asthma and to make a person sterile. Externally, the boiled and beaten root poultice was used for snakebite, rheumatism, swellings, and boils.

Purple Loosestrife, Willowherb (*Lythrum salicaria*)

Although regarded as invasive in the United States, this marsh-loving perennial was brought over by European settlers who could not imagine life without it. We Americans need to appreciate its virtues and come to accept this new immigrant. The challenge is to find it growing in clean waters and bogs.

The tea is used for diarrhea, dysentery, and typhoid fever, including diarrhea in babies. It also helps stop internal bleeding. The tea can also be used as a gargle for sore throat, as a douche, and as a wound wash.

To make the tea: Use the whole plant, fresh or dried; steep one ounce per cup of water for twenty minutes. Take a quarter cup, three times a day.

Purslane (*Portulaca oleracea*)

Portulaca oleracea is known as Verdolagas to Spanish speakers. Another example of a weed whose uses have yet to be fully appreciated, it is high in omega-3s and iron. Eat it raw in sandwiches and salads or sauté with other vegetables.

Red Raspberry (*Rubus idaeus*)

Raspberry is a blood-building fruit that is rich in iron, phosphorus, potassium, and magnesium. The leaf tea is used in pregnancy to prevent nausea, assist contractions, and keep hemorrhages in check during childbirth. After the birth this plant helps increase breast milk. The leaf tea is also taken to normalize menstruation.

To make the tea: Steep one tablespoon of fresh or dried leaf per cup of freshly boiled water for about fifteen minutes. Take a quarter cup four times a day. Add mint, lemon, honey, and so on for taste. Combine the Raspberry tea with Slippery Elm (*Ulmus fulva*) to make a douche for leukorrhea or vaginitis.

Shepherd's Purse (*Capsella bursa-pastoris*)

Capsella bursa-pastoris seed pods and leaves can be eaten cooked or raw, but be sure to gather them before the flower stalks appear. The roots can be used as a Ginger substitute. Dried and powdered, this plant is a styptic (stops bleeding when applied to wounds and cuts).

Thistle (*Cirsium* spp.)

Thistles are misunderstood biennial "weeds" that can be eaten in their first year of growth. Peel and cook the roots like carrots. In the first year the plant is a rosette low on the ground. In the second year it sends up stalks and produces flowers. By then the roots are too tough to tackle.

White Sarsaparilla, Spikenard (*Aralia nudicaulis*)

The roots are dried and made into a tea for fevers and coughs and to benefit kidney and bladder conditions. Native American healers used the tea as a blood cleanser and as a general tonic. ***To make the tea:*** Simmer two ounces of the dried roots per pint of water for twenty minutes, take three tablespoonsful, four times a day.

Externally, the root poultice can be applied to sores, burns, ulcers, boils, wounds, swellings, rheumatic parts, and infections.

EAT AND
WEAR THE FLOWERS

Summer is a wonderful time to enjoy flowers. In northern latitudes the time of blooming is all too brief. Everyone should learn to appreciate the wild and domesticated blooms that are available, and not just for their visual beauty and fragrance. The flowers of many plants can be eaten or made into tea or wearable fragrances.

 Flower Tea

This magical and delicious tea is also a love potion. Share it with your intended on a full moon night.

Equal parts fresh or dried:

- chamomile flowers (*Matricaria recutita, Chamaemelum nobile*)
- lemon balm (*Melissa officinalis*) leaf
- rose buds (*Rosa* spp.)

¼ part lavender blossoms (*Lavandula vera, L. angustifolia*)

Infuse two tablespoons of the mixture per cup of water in a pot of freshly boiled water. Cover tightly and steep no more than ten minutes or the delicate flowery aroma will be lost. Serve immediately with a touch of honey.

Nasturtium Flower Sandwiches

Use thick slices of crusty whole-grain bread. Slather on thick coats of natural cream cheese, soft goat cheese, or Neufchâtel. Place peppery nasturtium flowers (*Tropaeolum* spp.) on top of the cheese and serve the sandwiches open-faced.

The fresh young leaves are a nice peppery addition to salads of all kinds, and the flower petals can be strewn over grilled fish.

Red Clover Blossom Tea Sandwiches

Cut the crusts off white bread slices. Spread with real butter and then place fresh red clover (*Trifolium pratense*) blossoms on top of each slice. Cover with watercress leaves and top with another slice of buttered bread. Serve this with organic black or green tea in the garden.

Daylily Sides

Unopened Daylily (*Hemerocallis fulva*) buds can be sautéed and served as a vegetable side dish. The roots and leaves can be chopped and eaten raw in salads. The roots can also be steamed like baby potatoes and served with butter. (Be sure to clean the roots carefully by removing the dirt and then soaking them in water with a few tablespoons of vinegar or sea salt for about twenty minutes, to remove parasites.)

Flower Cake

Make the batter for a delicate yellow layer cake. Before you pour the batter into the cake pans, put five fresh leaves of rose geranium (*Pelargonium graveolens, Geranium terebinthinaceum* Cav., *Pelargonium terebinthinaceum*) in the bottom of each pan.

Once the cake is baked and cooled, frost it with a thick white frosting (you can add a few drops of rose or rose geranium oil to the frosting).

Press rose petals or entire roses (*Rosa* spp.), fresh daylily blossoms (*Hemerocallis fulva*), daisies (*Bellis perennis, Leucanthemum vulgare*), zucchini blossoms (*Cucurbita pepo*), elderflowers (*Sambucus nigra*), johnny-jump-up (*Viola tricolor*) or violet flowers (*Viola odorata*), bee balm (*Monarda* spp.), calendula (*Calendula officinalis*), hollyhock (*Alcea* spp.), or fresh lavender (*Lavandula vera, L. angustifolia*) blossoms into the frosted surface of the cake.

Place a ring of fresh mint (*Mentha* spp.) leaves around the base.

Eat the whole thing.

Flower Salad

To a salad of fresh mixed lettuces add fresh rose petals (*Rosa* spp.), johnny-jump-up blossoms (*Viola tricolor*), violet flowers and young leaves (*Viola odorata*), dandelion petals (remove the green sepals—they are too bitter) and baby leaves (*Taraxacum officinale*), red clover blossoms (*Trifolium pratense*), and young leaves of oxeye daisies (*Leucanthemum vulgare*). Sprinkle with freshly grated carrot and thinly sliced spring onion. Use a delicate lemon juice and olive oil dressing. Top with a pinch of sea salt.

Queen of Hungary Rosemary Cologne

This garden cologne makes a cooling facial spray for the heat of summer or a gentleman's aftershave for any time of year.

Fresh rosemary needles (*Rosmarinus officinalis*)

Fresh lavender blossoms (*Lavandula vera, L. angustifolia*)

Lemon balm leaves (*Melissa officinalis*)

A fragrant rose or two (*Rosa* spp.; make sure the roses have a strong scent—some genetically engineered varieties are scentless)

A little lemon zest

Gin or equal parts vodka and witch hazel

Fill a brown or blue glass jar with rosemary and add small amounts of lavender, lemon balm, rose, and lemon zest. Just barely cover the herbs with gin (gin is flavored with juniper berries, which have their own fresh scent) or a mixture of half vodka and half witch hazel. Seal tightly with a lid.

Let the mixture sit for two weeks, then strain and bottle.

Make Your Own Rosewater

This makes a nice skin toner or after-bath body splash. However, it will only work if you use the petals of non-GMO, old-fashioned roses.

1 cup strongly scented fresh rose petals (*Rosa* spp.), with the leaves and stems removed
2 cups boiling water

Put the petals into a ceramic or glass bowl. Pour in the boiling water, cover the bowl with a plate or lid, and allow the petals to steep until the water cools.

Strain and store in a glass container with a tight lid.

4

HERBS OF FALL

It is early October as I pen this chapter. Farm stands and store shelves are groaning with local produce: glowing pumpkins of all sizes and colors, varieties of apples, apple cider and pies, jams and jellies made from local fruits and berries, broccoli, garlic, fennel, grapes, Brussels sprouts, cabbages, beets, cauliflower, chard, celery, kale, leeks, lettuce, mushrooms of all kinds, onions, parsley, pears, potatoes, peas, and turnips. Local fruits and vegetables are displayed in rows like rough jewels to be taken home to be cut, refined, and processed.

But the bounty does not appear in farm stands and supermarkets alone. Nature continues to bestow her bounty in fields and forests, to those who have an eye to see the wealth.

Fall is the time to gather nuts and roots. When harvesting roots from the ground, be sure to scrub off the dirt, then soak them in water with vinegar or sea salt for about twenty minutes, to remove parasites, before you rinse and chop.

Burdock (*Arctium lappa*)

Burdock is one of those "weeds whose uses have yet to be appreciated." In Japan the root is grown as a vegetable called Gobo. Burdock is a biennial, meaning that the flowers and seeds appear in the second year. Dig out the root of a first-year plant in the fall, or a second-year plant in the early spring; by the time the flowers appear it is too late to take the root. After soaking in salt water or vinegar water, soak again in fresh, clear water for about ten minutes to improve the taste. Then chop and sauté the roots.

Burdock is considered a gentle blood and liver cleanser. Think of it for skin eruptions such as acne. The fresh leaf tea can be used as an external wash for sores, acne, poison ivy rash, and poison oak rash. *To make the tea:* Simmer one teaspoon of root per cup of water for about twenty minutes, or grate the fresh root, add half as much water as you have of root, squeeze out the liquid, and drink up to one cup a day in teaspoon doses.

In my experience Burdock root tea or capsules (two capsules three times a day for a 150-pound adult) should be taken for about a week to relieve poison ivy rash, which is actually a systemic condition. Burdock helps clear the poison ivy toxins from the blood via the liver.

Cattail, Bulrush (*Typha* spp.)

These pond dwellers have been termed "the supermarket of the swamp" due to their availability for food and medicine all year. In spring cut the new shoots and peel them open. The center reveals a delicate pale green vegetable that, when steamed, resembles hearts of palm. In the early summer the young flower heads are boiled and eaten like corn on the cob. When the pollen appears in the summer it can be collected and added to flour. Native Americans used the fuzz to diaper babies (packed into a buckskin diaper), to line moccasins, and to stuff pillows.

In the fall when the plants have started to brown and die back, it is time to gather the roots. One difficulty is that you must find cattails growing in nonpolluted water, which may require hiking away from roads. The roots can be simmered to make a diuretic tea or cooked until soft, then mashed and cooled and applied to wounds, sores, burns, and other skin eruptions. You can also add the softened roots to poultices for skin healing.

False Solomon's Seal, False Spikenard (*Maianthemum racemosum, Smilacina racemosa, Vagnera racemosa*)

This plant can be easily distinguished from True Solomon's Seal (*Polygonatum multiflorum*), as the "true" variety has a line of bell-shaped flowers all along the stalk, while the "false" has a cluster of flowers at the end of the stalk. True Solomon's Seal root is used in poultices for bruises and wounds, but it is an endangered species so I do not recommend wildcrafting this plant.

The mashed roots of False Solomon's Seal can be applied to swellings and boils and used to relieve itching and stop bleeding. They are anti-inflammatory and can be chopped and simmered in honey to make a syrup for coughs and sore throats. *To make the syrup:* Use one part root to four parts honey, simmer gently until the roots are very soft, then strain.

Native Americans used the root tea for conditions such as constipation, rheumatism, stomach problems, menstrual issues, and coughs.

Caution: False Solomon's Seal tea can be a strong laxative for some people. Try a small amount and see how it affects you first!

Goldenrod (*Solidago odora, S. virgaurea,* and others)

Goldenrod is still available in the early fall. Add the flowers to muffins, pancakes, soups, and vegetable stir-fries. The leaves have been used in salves for insect stings. Taken in herbal teas, the flowers and leaves can benefit skin conditions such as eczema as well as arthritis, colds and flu, hemorrhoids, and urinary tract infections. Externally, the tea can be applied to cuts and insect bites.

The leaves of Sweet Goldenrod (*Solidago odora*) in particular make a nice-tasting beverage tea; add them to other medicinal teas to improve taste. The leaf tea helps with fevers, stomach cramps, colds, coughs, diarrhea, and measles. It makes an external wash for rheumatic conditions and can be used in compresses for headaches. It is diuretic and emmenagogue.

To make the tea: Steep a teaspoon of flowers per cup of freshly boiled water for about ten minutes. Adults can take up to two cups a day.

Caution: Be careful to gather leaves without signs of fungus or mold.

Once the cold autumn air has caused the plant to die back, the sap returns to the roots, which can be washed, dried, and eaten in soups or ground into bread mixes. The powdered dried root is applied to wounds. The roots (and flowers) are also used to make salves and poultices for burns, sore joints, and old sores.

> **Caution: Goldenrod may help milder kidney conditions, but those with severe kidney problems or who might be pregnant should avoid this herb.**

Marshmallow Root (*Althaea officinalis*)

In the fall the roots of *Althaea officinalis* are gathered for their demulcent (tissue-soothing) properties. Add the roots to poultices and salves for skin irritations, burns, and wounds. You can also grate the cleaned fresh roots, mix with honey, and spread on a cloth. Apply to minor burns, wounds, and skin irritations for about an hour and then discard. The roots are helpful for sore throat and coughs, and the root tea can also be used in douches, as a soothing eye wash, and for colitis and stomach ulcers.

To make the root tea: Peel the roots, then simmer one teaspoon of root per cup of water for twenty minutes. (Be sure to simmer for twenty minutes or more and then strain through an organic coffee filter if you plan to use it in your eyes.) Take one quarter cup four times a day on an empty stomach.

To make the flower and leaf tea: Steep two teaspoons of flower and leaf per cup of freshly boiled water for about five minutes. Gargle as needed to soothe a sore throat.

Skunk Cabbage (*Symplocarpus foetidus*)

Seek the roots of Skunk Cabbage in very late fall or very early spring. A denizen of swamps, streams, and boggy grounds, these roots (in tea or tincture preparations) are a classic remedy for wet lung conditions such as asthma, bronchitis, and whooping cough. The roots are also used for nervous problems, depression, rheumatic conditions, and swellings. The roots have pain-relieving qualities and cause relaxation of tissues.

To make the tea: Steep one teaspoon of roots per cup of freshly boiled water for about twenty minutes. Take up to one cup a day in tablespoon doses.

To make the tincture: Chop the roots and pour enough vodka over them to just barely cover the plant matter (you may have to add a little more as the root material expands). Allow to extract for about a week in a dark place, shaking once a day to redistribute the herbal mass. Strain and put into a green, blue, or brown glass bottle. Keep on hand for asthma and coughs; take three to fifteen drops in water.

> **Caution: This plant can be easily confused with False Hellebore (*Veratrum viride*), which is poisonous. Use your nose—False Hellebore does not have the wonderfully stinky smell of Skunk Cabbage!**

The roots can also be simmered in oil to make a salve for ringworm, sores, and swellings.

The tender leaves of this plant are actually quite tasty and very edible if gathered in early spring when they first appear (when they are six inches long or less). Simmer and pour off the water twice, simmer again, then serve with butter.

Yellow Dock (*Rumex crispus*)

The young leaves of *Rumex crispus* can be eaten in a salad or cooked. However, as they are high in oxalic acid, this should be done with caution. The seeds can be ground and added to flour, but first remove the chaff by rubbing the seeds between your hands. The roots of this herb are cleansing to the blood and liver, meaning they will help clear skin problems such as acne. The roots are also said to relieve constipation, anemia, and jaundice. The root tea is a gentle, iron-rich laxative, suitable for pregnant women.

To make the root tea: Simmer one teaspoon of root per cup of water for twenty minutes. Adults can take up to two cups a day.

The roots can be added to healing salves or dried and powdered and applied to cuts. The fresh leaf is used to poultice rashes and stings.

WE ARE ALL A LITTLE NUTS

And here is why: many of us are surrounded by an amazing free food source that our ancestors relied on for millennia and which we often completely ignore. Wheat was introduced into the human diet only about ten thousand years ago. Before that we humans relied on nuts for carbohydrates. And all we had to do was sit and wait for the crop to fall from the trees! The way I see it, Mother Nature does everything she can to feed her children, and capitalism just doesn't enter into it.

Acorns

Acorns are a good source of carbohydrates, protein, and fiber as well as phosphorus, niacin, potassium, calcium, and magnesium. The tastiest ones are of the White Oak variety (*Quercus alba*), but all species of acorns can be made palatable by leaching. In ancient times the leaching process was accomplished by putting whole acorns into covered baskets in a running stream. The baskets were topped with rocks to deter critters and left in the running water for a few weeks. Cold leaching is the method that preserves most of the nutrients. (If you do this make sure the stream is not polluted.)

◖ Leaching Acorns for Acorn Flour

A quicker method of leaching is to boil the nuts. First put the nuts in water and remove any that float. Then spread the rest on a cookie sheet and bake for 15 minutes at 150 degrees. This step makes the nuts easier to shell.

Shell the nuts; while you are doing that, bring two pots of water to a boil on the stove. Put the nuts into one pot and boil until the water turns dark. Strain out the nuts, put them in the second pot, and boil until the water becomes colored. Reheat the first pot with fresh water, bring to a boil, and transfer the nuts. Keep transferring the nuts between pots of boiling water until the water runs clear. Do not put the acorns into cold water as you do this; it will make them bitter (bitterness can sometimes be corrected by soaking the acorns in milk).

Keep the colored acorn water from the leaching and freeze it in ice cubes for later use. It is antiviral and antiseptic and can be used as a wound wash or as a wash for poison ivy rash and other wet, weepy skin conditions.

When the water runs clear, bake the acorns at 325 degrees for about an hour and then grind into flour. The flour can be kept for months in an airtight container in the refrigerator. Dried whole acorns can be kept for up to a year.

Acorn Bread*

2 cups acorn flour

2 cups organic white flour

3 teaspoons baking powder

½ cup milk

⅓ cup maple syrup or raw honey

1 egg

3 tablespoons olive oil

Bake in an oiled and floured pan for 30 minutes or until done at 400 degrees.

(**Note:** You can use any flour you like: wheat, rice, corn, oat; the more acorn flour you add, the denser your bread will turn out.)

Acorn Cake†

1 cup acorn flour

1 cup other organic flour

1 teaspoon baking powder

1 teaspoon baking soda

½ teaspoon salt

½ teaspoon ground cardamom

½ teaspoon ground cinnamon

¼ teaspoon ground allspice

¼ teaspoon ground nutmeg

6 eggs

---

*Adapted from Green Deane, "Acorns: The Inside Story," www.eattheweeds.com/acorns -the-inside-story/.

†Adapted from Danielle Prohom Olson, "Let Us Eat Acorn Cake! A Lazy Cook's Guide," gathervictoria.com/2014/11/04/let-us-eat-acorn-cake-a-lazy-cooks-guide/.

1 cup olive or coconut oil

1 cup raw honey

½ cup applesauce

1 cup organic sugar

Confectioners' sugar to dust on top

Grease and flour a Bundt pan. Preheat the oven to 350 degrees.

Mix the dry ingredients and spices in a bowl.

Beat the wet ingredients together in a separate bowl.

Combine the wet and dry mixtures and pour into the Bundt pan. Bake 30–40 minutes, or until a knife inserted in the center comes out clean. Let cool in the pan for 15 minutes, and then turn out onto a rack.

Once the cake is completely cooled, dust lightly with confectioners' sugar.

Acorn Muffins*

3 tablespoons raw honey

2 tablespoons melted butter

2 tablespoons organic sugar

1 egg

½ cup milk

1 cup acorn flour

1 cup whole-grain flour

1 teaspoon baking powder

½ teaspoon baking soda

½ teaspoon sea salt

½ teaspoon apple pie spice

Mix together the honey, butter, sugar, and egg. Gradually stir in the milk and acorn flour.

Mix together the whole-grain flour, baking powder, baking soda, sea salt, and apple pie spice in a separate bowl.

Combine the wet and dry ingredients and mix well.

---

*Adapted from "Acorn to Acorn Muffins in 1 Day!" www.instructables.com/id/Acorns -to-Acorn-Muffins-in-1-Day.

Pour into greased muffin tins or cupcake papers and bake at 350 degrees for 15–20 minutes.

Hickory Nuts

Shagbark Hickory (*Carya ovata*) and Shellbark Hickory (*Carya laciniosa*) are probably the best hickory trees for eating, and Mockernut (*Carya tomentosa*) can also be used. Avoid Bitternut (*Carya cordiformis*). In ancient times Native Americans would pound the nuts and shells to a paste and then boil them. Eventually they would strain the liquid out and use it as a type of oil or milk for cooking corn bread and hominy grits. You can do this too.

 ### Hickory Nut Oil/Milk

First put the nuts into water and discard the ones that float. Rinse the good ones. Bake at 350 degrees for 15 minutes and then cool. This facilitates cracking.

Break each nut open with a hammer or sledgehammer on a hard surface like a rock. (Cover the nut with a piece of cloth so the pieces don't go flying.) Try hitting the nut with repeated light hits until it cracks, then finish with one hard blow. You can also use a vise or a nutcracker to crack the nuts.

Reserve the shells and discard any dark-colored nutmeats, as they may be rotten.

Toast the nuts again at 350 degrees for 15 minutes to sweeten and sterilize them.

Put the shells and nut pieces into a pot and barely cover them with fresh water. Boil for about 15 minutes to an hour, until the water turns brown. The longer you boil, the sweeter the "milk" will turn out.

Strain out the colored water, put the nuts back into the pan, cover with fresh water, and boil again. Repeat three to five times, each time reserving the liquid. When you are done, add a lot of water to the pot one more time and the nuts will rise as the shells sink. Strain out the nut pieces (do not rinse or you will wash away the flavor) and dry, toast, and eat them. You can also blend them with water to make "nut milk"; use some of the reserved liquid from the boiling for added flavor.

Pour the milk onto cereal or oatmeal, use it in soups or baked goods, or just drink it. Try adding a bit of salt for improved taste. Serve the milk hot, spiced with cinnamon, honey or maple syrup, cardamom, salt, cloves, nutmeg, and so on.

If the milk is left to stand, a layer of oil forms at the top, which can be used in cooking or to soften the hands. Use it to stir-fry vegetables, add it to salad dressings, and so on.

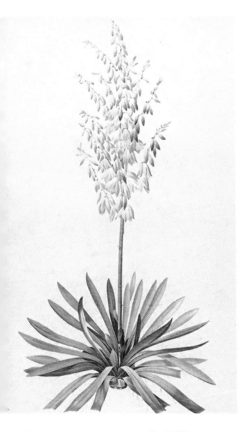

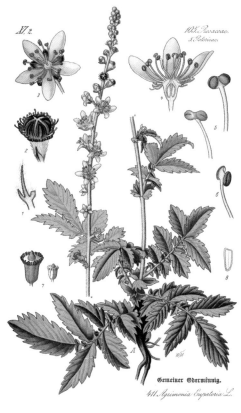

Plate 1 (left). Adam's Needle (*Yucca filamentosa*)

Plate 2 (right). Agrimony (*Agrimonia eupatoria*)

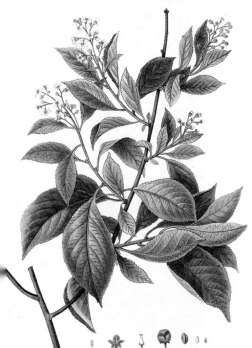

Plate 3. American Bittersweet, Bittersweet Vine (*Celastrus scandens*)

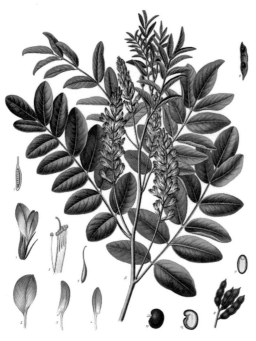

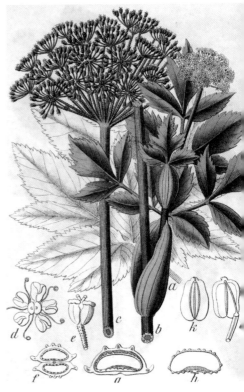

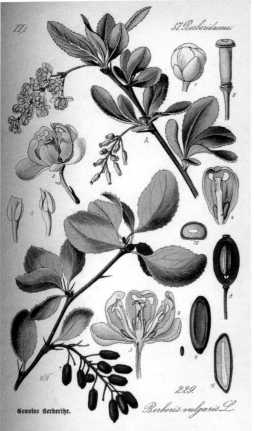

Plate 4 (left). American Licorice (*Glycyrrhiza lepidota*)

Plate 5 (right). Angelica (*Angelica atropurpurea*)

Plate 6. Barberry (*Berberis vulgaris*)

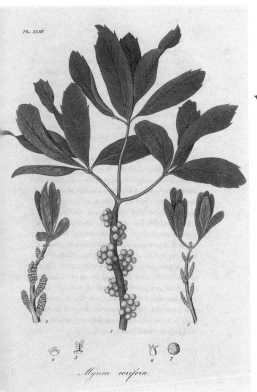

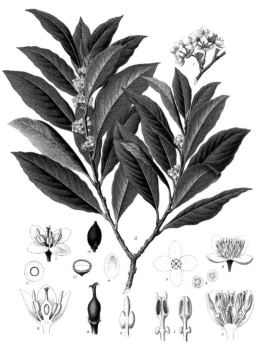

Plate 7 (left). Bayberry, Wax Myrtle (*Myrica cerifera*)

Plate 8 (right). Bay Laurel (*Laurus nobilis*)

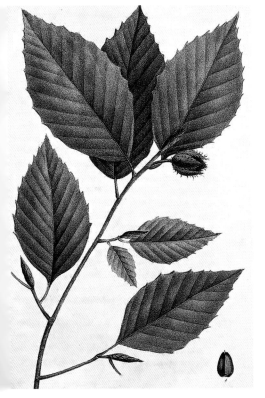

Plate 9. Beech, American Beech (*Fagus grandifolia*)

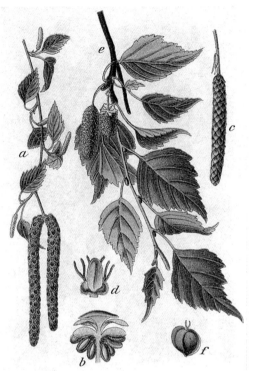

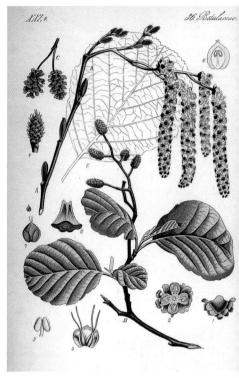

Plate 10 (left). Birch (*Betula pendula*)

Plate 11 (right). Black Alder (*Alnus glutinosa*)

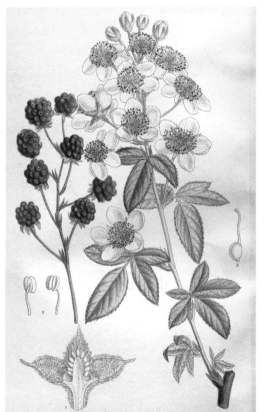

Plate 12. Blackberry (*Rubus villosus*)

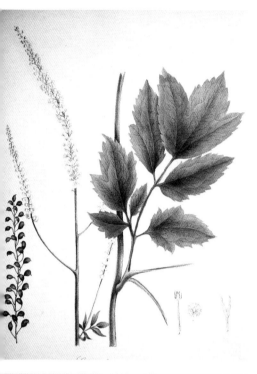

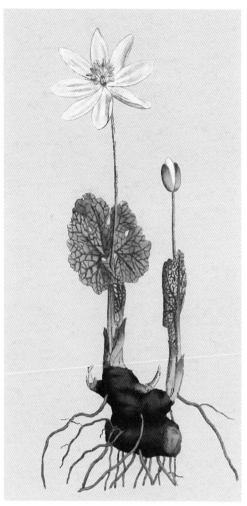

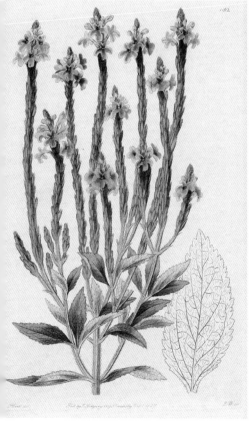

Plate 13 (left). Black Cohosh, Black Snake Root, Rattle Root, Black Bugbane (*Cimicifuga racemosa*)

Plate 14 (right). Bloodroot (*Sanguinaria canadensis*)

Plate 15. Blue Vervain, Swamp Verbena (*Verbena hastata*)

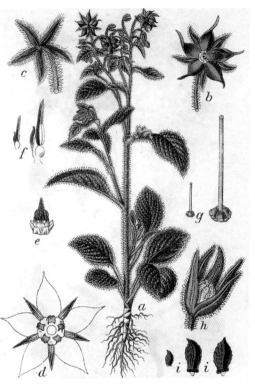

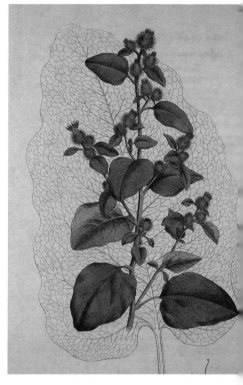

Plate 16 (left). Borage (*Borago officinalis*)

Plate 17 (right). Burdock (*Arctium lappa*)

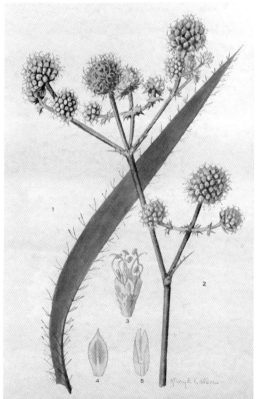

Plate 18. Button Eryngo (*Eryngium yuccifolium* var. *synchaetum*)

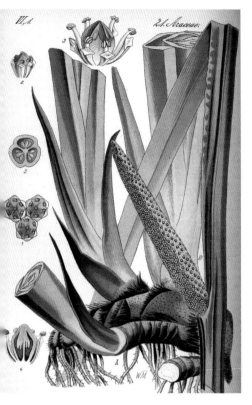

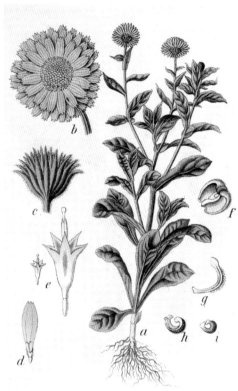

Plate 19 (left). Calamus, Sweet Flag (*Acorus calamus*)

Plate 20 (right). Calendula (*Calendula officinalis*)

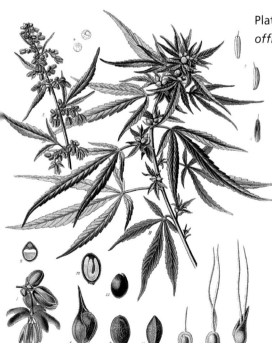

Plate 21. Cannabis, Da Ma (*Cannabis sativa*)

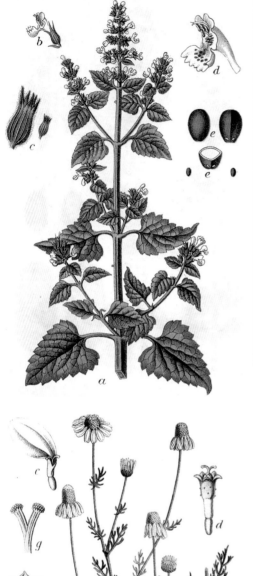

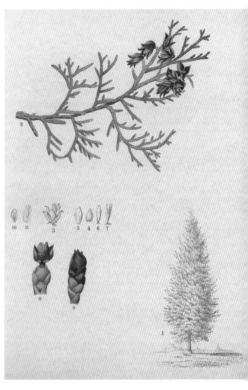

Plate 22 (left). Catnip (*Nepeta cataria*)

Plate 23 (right). Cedar, Arborvitae, Thuja (*Thuja occidentalis*)

Plate 24. Chamomile (*Matricaria recutita, Chamaemelum nobile*)

5

WINTER COLD AND FLU CARE, NATURALLY!

Temperatures are plummeting and winter has set in as I write. A flock of wild turkeys has stopped by on their daily morning forage under the bird feeders and a freezing rain has everyone wishing they were inside, safe from the bone-chilling winds. This is the time to have plenty of winter remedies on hand to ward off flu and chill, and to help heal from their effects.

Here is one recipe for a general tonic that will help boost your immune system.

◗ Fire Cider*

A friend passed this recipe along to me and he swears he hasn't had a cold in four years. Take a few tablespoons of this remedy at the first sign of a cold. Please use only the finest organic ingredients.

½ cup grated ginger root (*Zingiber officinale*)
½ cup grated horseradish root (*Armoracia rusticana*)
1 medium onion (*Allium cepa*), chopped
12 cloves garlic (*Allium sativum, A. canadense*), chopped
2 hot peppers (chili peppers, *Capsicum annuum*), chopped
Zest and juice from 1 lemon (*Citrus limon*)

---

*Adapted from *The Mountain Rose Blog*, "Craft Your Own Fire Cider!" http://mountainroseblog.com/fire-cider/.

Zest from 1 small orange (*Citrus sinensis*)

1 tablespoon turmeric powder (*Curcuma longa*)

½ teaspoon whole black peppercorns (*Piper nigrum*)

¼ teaspoon ground cayenne (*Capsicum annuum*)

Other herbs to consider: thyme (*Thymus vulgaris*), rose hips (*Rosa* spp.), ginseng (*Panax quinquefolius*), grapefruit zest (*Citrus paradisi*), astragalus (*Astragalus membranaceus*), schizandra berries (*Schisandra chinensis*), parsley (*Petroselinum crispum*), burdock root (*Arctium lappa*), oregano (*Origanum vulgare*), basil (*Ocimum basilicum*), Siberian ginseng (*Eleutherococcus senticosus*)

Organic apple cider vinegar

¼ cup raw organic honey

Put all the spices and herbs in a glass jar and barely cover with apple cider vinegar. Cap tightly and store in a cool, dark place. Shake the jar regularly. After about a month you can strain out the vinegar and reserve it in another very clean glass jar. Add the honey and stir until well blended.

You can use the strained-out spices and herbs in a stir-fry with cabbage and carrots when everything is finished.

HERBAL MEDICINES FOR COLDS AND FLU

Certain herbs, foods, vitamins, and minerals are particularly helpful in the prevention and treatment of colds and flu. Here are some of those I recommend:

Andrographis (*Andrographis paniculata*)

Andrographis is a Chinese and Ayurvedic (traditional Indian medicine) herb that shortens the duration of an illness. The usual dose is about 400 mg three times a day.

Ashwagandha (*Withania somnifera*)

Ashwagandha is an Ayurvedic plant used to ward off disease. About a quarter cup of the tea per day is helpful in preventing illness. It is also available in tincture and capsules.

Astragalus (*Astragalus membranaceus*)

Astragalus root (tincture, capsules, or tea) builds white blood cells and the immune system. The yellower the root, the better the quality. However, Astragalus should not be taken once flu symptoms appear. Also, this herb should be avoided by those who do not sweat easily. As a form of prevention, try adding it to soups. The usual dose is about 250 to 500 mg of root extract, three or four times a day, or simmer six to twelve grams of dried root in twelve ounces of water for about twenty minutes and divide into three or four doses throughout the day.

Chrysanthemum (*Chrysanthemum morifolium, C. indicum*)

In Chinese medicine the flowers of *Chrysanthemum morifolium* or *C. indicum* are used as a tea for colds, fever, flu, sore throat, and skin conditions such as acne. The tea is drunk as a "pick me up" and is said to benefit the liver and the eyes and to help with coronary heart disease and hypertension. The tea is also used externally as a compress for varicose veins and atherosclerosis.

To make the tea: Pour four cups freshly boiled water over one cup of yellow or white dried flowers and allow to steep for five minutes. Sweeten to taste. When the teapot is empty, boiled water can be poured over the flowers again to make a second pot.

Echinacea (*Echinacea* spp.)

Taken at the first onset of illness, this herb can shorten the duration of a cold or even stop it entirely. Take about a quarter cup of the tea of the root (*E. angustifolia*) or the leaf and flower (*E. purpurea*) every two hours. You can also take the tincture, about twenty drops four times a day in water, not with meals. The best way to take this herb is in hot water, to inhibit virus replication.

Elder (*Sambucus nigra, S. canadensis*)

Elderberries are proven immune enhancers and antiviral as well. For the best effect, take as a tea (simmer one teaspoon of the berries per cup of water for twenty minutes) or tincture added to hot water three or four times a day. Hot liquids stop viruses in the throat from multiplying. I find that fresh Elderberries make the very best elixir/tincture, but dried berries can be purchased if necessary. There are two ways of making them into an elixir or tincture, an excellent remedy for sore throats, coughs, and colds.

Alcohol-Based Elderberry Elixir/Tincture

The simplest way to make an elderberry elixir is to fill a jar with the berries, then barely cover them with vodka (or any alcohol that is 80 proof or above). I like vodka because it is basically tasteless and the flavor of the berries comes through. Let the jar steep for a few weeks, shaking every few days to distribute the liquid. When the berries begin to break down, strain the liquid through cheesecloth into a glass jar, and store in a dark cupboard or in an amber or blue glass bottle. Because of the alcohol, no refrigeration is needed; the tincture keeps for about five years in a cool, dark place.

To further enhance the potency, add echinacea root (*Echinacea angustifolia*), fresh or dried, or echinacea leaf and flower (*Echinacea purpurea*) to the jar. You can get even fancier by adding astragalus root (*Astragalus membranaceus*), rosehips (*Rosa* spp.), Siberian ginseng (*Eleutherococcus senticosus*), or elecampane root (*Inula helenium*).

The elixir/tincture can be taken 20–40 drops at a time in hot water when you are sick, three or four times a day, or added to a warm cup of tea.

Cooked Elderberry Elixir

Another method is to cook the herbs. First make a decoction of the roots and berries.

7 cups water

1 cup elderberries (*Sambucus nigra, S. canadensis*)

1 ounce Siberian ginseng (*Eleutherococcus senticosus*), which builds stamina and the immune system, especially when taken for 3 months or longer

1 ounce rosehips (*Rosa* spp.), which provide bioflavonoids and vitamin C

A few inches of fresh ginger root (*Zingiber officinale*), sliced, which moves internal secretions and helps break down mucus while warming the body

1 ounce elecampane root (*Inula helenium*), which dries up wet lung
  conditions

½ ounce nettles (*Urtica dioica*), which are very warming to the system and
  provide trace minerals

½ ounce elderflowers (*Sambucus* spp.), which help lower a fever

¼ ounce mint leaves (*Mentha* spp.), which lower fever and improve taste

Honey

Simmer (never boil!) all of the ingredients (leaving out nettles, elderflowers,
and mint leaves) for about 20 minutes in a pot with a tight lid.

Remove from the flame. Now you can add leaves and flowers such as the
nettles, elderflowers, and mint leaves.

Steep in the pot for about half an hour, strain, and while still warm, add
honey to taste. Keep for two months in the refrigerator in a glass jar with a
tight lid.

Take this as a daily tonic all winter (about 2 teaspoons a day); in the event
of illness an adult dose is about ¼ cup, three or four times a day.

Eleuthero, Siberian Ginseng (*Eleutherococcus senticosus*)

Siberian Ginseng (*Eleutherococcus senticosus*) root is immune-enhancing,
antiviral, and a builder of T cells and killer cells. I like to add it to
large batches of green and black teas (*Camellia sinensis*), which can be
stored in the refrigerator for about a week. To do this, simmer the herb
in water for about twenty minutes in a pot with a tight lid. Take the
pot off the stove, add the green and black teas, and steep for five to ten
minutes. Strain into a large glass jar with a tight lid.

Other herbs to add to tea are Rose hips (*Rosa* spp.), Osha (*Ligusticum
filicinum, L. porteri*), Astragalus (*Astragalus membranaceus*), Pau D'Arco
or Taheebo Tea (*Tabebuia impetiginosa, Tabebuia avellanedae*), and Goji
berries or Wolf berries (*Lycium barbarum, Lycium chinense*). Use a small
amount of each herb, about two tablespoons for a large pot of water.

> **Caution: Goji berries have shown significant interactions
> with warfarin and other medications for hypertension
> and diabetes. Large amounts of Pau D'Arco may interfere
> with blood-thinning medications.**

Garlic (*Allium sativum*)

This herb should be used daily in cooking, salads, and so on. It is antibacterial and antiviral, but it has to be taken raw (take it with a meal to avoid stomach upset). Before penicillin was discovered, Garlic was the best remedy for infection.

> **Caution: Avoid Garlic for two weeks before surgery and also if you are taking any blood thinners.**

Ginseng (*Panax quinquefolius*)

Taken over time this herb can build resistance to and shorten the duration of colds. The usual amount is 400 mg a day.

Green Tea (*Camellia sinensis*)

Green tea strengthens immunity, reduces the duration of a cold, and is antioxidant. Taken over time, it can ward off colds altogether.

Mushrooms (*Lentinula edodes*, *Grifola frondosa,* and others)

Mushrooms such as shiitake (*Lentinula edodes*) and maitake (*Grifola frondosa*) can be added to stir-fries and soups to build the immune system.

Reishi (*Ganoderma lucidum*, *G. tsugae*, *G. sichuanense*) also enhances immunity and is a good antiviral, including for conditions such as herpes. It is taken as a powder or tincture and is not a good mushroom to cook with. About one gram a day of the powder or one milliliter a day of the tincture is the dose.

Slippery Elm (*Ulmus fulva*)

The inner bark of this tree is very helpful for sore throats when taken as tea. See the "Elm" entry on page 170 for additional healing uses and recipes.

South African Geranium (*Pelargonium sidoides*)

Pelargonium sidoides is a good herb to treat colds and bronchitis. The usual dose is thirty drops of tincture three times per day.

Vitamin C

To be effective this vitamin needs to be taken in 2,000 mg doses (1,000 mg taken twice a day).

Zinc

This mineral actually lessens symptoms and shortens the duration of colds. Zinc lozenges are taken every one to three hours for three to fourteen days or until symptoms subside.

 Chicken Soup

Your grandmother was right—chicken soup boosts immunity and reduces throat-cell inflammation, especially when garlic and onions are added. Every cook needs to have a good chicken soup recipe. Here is mine:

1 free-range organic chicken
½ cup organic apple cider vinegar
4 large carrots
1 bunch celery with leaves
2 cups chopped asparagus
1 large onion
4 cloves garlic, chopped
3 tablespoons chopped parsley
1 tablespoon chopped dill
Sea salt
Freshly ground black pepper
Celery salt

Skin the chicken and discard the skin.

Remove the liver, kidneys, and giblets; mince and sauté them in a little water for the cat or the dog.

Place the "naked" bird into the pot and just barely cover with cold water.

Add the vinegar and bring to a slow boil, then simmer for about 2 hours (the vinegar leaches the minerals out of the bones). Keep a tight lid on the pot.

As the fowl cooks, you can chop up the carrots, celery, asparagus, onion, garlic, parsley, and dill.

Gently remove the bird from the soup stock and place it in a colander over a large pot (to catch the drippings). When the bird is cool enough to handle, remove the bones and then put the meat back into the original pot along with any drippings.

Put the veggies into the pot and simmer for another half an hour (with a tight lid on the pot to hold in the steam).

Season to taste with sea salt, pepper, and celery salt.

HERBAL SUPPORT FOR FLU

In the initial phase of flu look for warming herbs that build the immune system such as Turmeric (*Curcuma longa*), Ginger (*Zingiber officinale*), and Garlic (*Allium sativum, A. canadense*). Avoid heavy foods and take liquids as much as possible.

When cough sets in, look for cooling herbs that help lower fever such as Peppermint (*Mentha piperita, M. balsamea* Willd.), which is mildly antiviral and helps cool a fever; Elderflower (*Sambucus* spp.); King of Bitters (*Andrographis paniculata*), which is antiviral and does well when combined with Siberian Ginseng (*Eleutherococcus senticosus*); and Boneset (*Eupatorium perfoliatum*) and Honeysuckle flower (*Lonicera* spp.). Catnip (*Nepeta cataria*) is especially useful as a calming antiviral for children; add Ginger (*Zingiber officinale*) or Licorice (*Glycyrrhiza glabra*) for taste.

Baikal Skullcap root (*Scutellaria baicalensis*) helps deal with flu symptoms (avoid if there is diarrhea). Asian Red Sage (*Salvia miltiorrhiza*) can be taken as a cooling tea (avoid this plant if you are on blood thinners). Hyssop (*Hyssopus officinalis*) is antiviral and also supports the lungs.

Finally, as a restorative tonic, follow with demulcents such as Licorice (*Glycyrrhiza glabra*), which is antiviral and loosens dry cough; Slippery Elm (*Ulmus fulva*), which is particularly helpful to soothe a sore throat; and Pleurisy Root (*Asclepias tuberosa*), which is an expectorant.

**Caution: Licorice is not for diabetics; it is sweeter than
sugar. It should also be avoided by persons
with high blood pressure.**

Warming Winter Brandy for Grownups

This drink can help with sleep, chills, and stiff joints.

3 tablespoons dried or 8 tablespoons fresh or frozen cherries

2 tablespoons elderberries (*Sambucus nigra, S. canadensis*)

2 tablespoons chopped ginseng root (*Panax quinquefolius*)

½ tablespoon elecampane root (*Inula helenium*)

½ tablespoon wild cherry bark (*Prunus serotina, P. virginiana*)

¼ tablespoon gentian root (*Gentiana lutea*)

2-inch piece cinnamon bark (*Cinnamomum verum, C. cassia*)

1-inch piece ginger root, chopped (*Zingiber officinale*)

10 whole black peppercorns (*Piper nigrum*)

6 crushed cardamom pods (*Elettaria cardamomum*)

3 tablespoons raw honey

Brandy

Combine all the herbs in a very clean glass jar with a tight lid. Add the honey. Pour brandy over the herbs until they are well covered. Place in a warm location and shake regularly. After a month strain out the herbs and bottle.

Cough Syrup

Steep 1 ounce dried horehound (*Marrubium vulgare*) leaf in 1 pint freshly boiled water for 10 minutes. Strain and add twice as much honey as tea. Blend well, then cool and bottle. Store in the refrigerator for up to 2 months. Use 1 teaspoon four times a day.

Other herbs can be added such as 1 ounce hyssop (*Hyssopus officinalis*), 2 ounces peppermint (*Mentha piperita, M. balsamea* Willd.), or ½ ounce thyme (*Thymus serpyllum, T. vulgaris*).

Plain raw honey taken in teaspoon doses can be an effective cough remedy for children but:

Caution: Do not give honey to a child less than one year of age.

Antibiotic Tea for Kids

½ teaspoon echinacea root (*Echinacea angustifolia*) or leaf and flower
(*E. purpurea*), depending on the species which stimulates immune cells
½ teaspoon licorice root (*Glycyrrhiza glabra*) (but see caution, page 59)
½ teaspoon Oregon grape root (*Mahonia repens*) or barberry root bark
(*Berberis vulgaris* L.)
2 cups water

Combine the echinacea, licorice, and grape root with the water in a non-aluminum pot with a tight lid. Simmer for 20 minutes, then strain and bottle. A 50-pound child can take ¼ cup four times a day. Infants can take the herb through their mother's breast milk. The tea can also be added to juice.

Make Your Own Vicks VapoRub Salve*

1 cup coconut oil
¾ cup chopped or grated beeswax
½ cup olive oil
35 drops or more eucalyptus (*Eucalyptus* spp.) essential oil
30 drops or more peppermint (*Mentha piperita, M. balsamea* Willd.)
essential oil
15 drops lavender (*Lavandula vera, L. angustifolia*) essential oil
15 drops rosemary (*Rosmarinus officinalis*) essential oil
10 drops camphor (*Cinnamomum camphora*) essential oil

In a double boiler melt the coconut oil, beeswax, and olive oil. Stir in the eucalyptus, peppermint, lavender, rosemary, and camphor essential oils. Pour into containers and allow to set before capping. Rub under your nose, on your chest, and on your feet when you have a cold.

---

*Recipe adapted from "All Natural Vapor Rub Recipe," Garden Therapy, gardentherapy .ca/vicks-vapo-rub-recipe/.

STOMACH FLU

A classic triangle of herbs for stomach flu is Yarrow (*Achillea millefolium*), Elderflower (*Sambucus* spp.), and Peppermint (*Mentha piperita, M. balsamea* Willd.). They can be easily ingested as a tea.

To make the tea: Use equal parts of these herbs, one teaspoon of each per one cup of water; steep in freshly boiled water for about twenty minutes. Add honey and lemon to taste. Take a quarter cup four times a day.

GENERAL PREVENTION STRATEGIES

To ward off colds and flu, make sure you are getting enough sleep and eating a fiber-rich, plant-based diet. Have your vitamin D levels tested and then try to get twenty minutes of sunlight daily, to keep up your vitamin D levels. If you are surrounded by others who are sick at work or at school, wash your hands frequently and avoid touching your nose and eyes.

Stress seems to be a leading factor in loss of immune function. Meditation twice a day, soothing music, and gentle exercise such as yoga and walks in nature help manage stress. Aerobic exercisers experience far fewer colds than others.

Making love to your partner at least once a week actually increases immunoglobulin A (IgA), a natural defense against colds.

6

BUG STUFF

Plants to Repel Mosquitoes, Ticks, and Fleas

Fans of wildcrafting and of just being outdoors will want to know how to make natural bug repellents. Here are some suggestions for human use. But be *very careful* before you apply any of these to your pets. A cat of mine actually went into convulsions and nearly died after I applied an "all natural" herbal oil combination that I bought at a pet store to her fur.

Some practical measures that will keep bugs in the house at bay include vacuuming the house frequently, washing pet bedding regularly (avoid shaking out flea-infested bedding as it will only spread the eggs), and rinsing your pets and their bedding with water and a bit of apple cider vinegar (because fleas dislike the smell).

If you live in an area where plants like Eucalyptus and Rosemary are prolific, hang bunches around the patio and the porch and place the crushed fresh leaves in open glass jars and muslin sacks around the house and yard.

PLANTS IN YOUR GARDEN THAT REPEL FLEAS AND TICKS

If you have animals that wander around the garden (like dogs and cats) or if you have children who like to play in the dirt and grass, these plants can help keep down the pest population without the use of poisons. Use them as a border around the house and garden, but pay attention to the "**Cautions.**"

First some commonsense measures. Ticks dislike dry, sunny spaces, so keep the yard around the house trimmed. Put leaf piles far away from trafficked areas because ticks multiply in the damp conditions found under leaf piles. Use wood chips or gravel to make a natural barrier between house and forest; the barrier should ideally be about three feet wide.

Do not place dishes under your potted outdoor plants and make sure there are no containers in the landscape that will hold tiny pools of water, a breeding ground for mosquitoes. Change the water in your birdbath frequently to avoid mosquito breeding. If you have a pond or a homemade waterfall and pond, stock it with fish such as Koi, which eat mosquito larvae.

Chrysanthemum (*Chrysanthemum cinerariaefolium*)

Lovely to look at, this variety of Chrysanthemum flower also discourages ticks and fleas. Work these plants into your anti-bug border. As an added bonus, other pests such as cockroaches, bedbugs, silverfish, and lice also dislike this plant. Pyrethrum is derived from this variety of Chrysanthemum. The dried and powdered flowers were once spread on vegetables and other plants to repel bugs (don't breathe the dust if you try this).

Fleabane (*Erigeron speciosus*)

Erigeron speciosus is a daisy that repels fleas, ticks, flies, gnats, and mosquitoes. Grow it around the edges of the garden or lawn (and place a wire fence between this herb and any cats or dogs, if they are likely to nibble on it!).

> **Caution: Butterflies love Fleabane, but it is toxic to cows, horses, goats, dogs, and cats.**

Some birds will line their nests with Fleabane to repel mites, and it was once added to mattress stuffings such as Bedstraw or Cleavers

(*Galium aparine*) to discourage insects. Try stuffing it into a dog bed or a cat pillow where it won't get eaten.

Garlic (*Allium sativum*)

Try making a hedge of Garlic around the borders of your garden or lawn to repel ticks. Adding crushed bulbs of fresh garlic to the soil along the perimeter of your garden will strengthen the protective barrier.

> **Caution: Garlic is toxic to cats. Don't apply crushed Garlic to your lawn or garden if you have a cat!**

Harvest Garlic bulbs in the fall, eat some, and replant the rest. Garlic scapes (flower stalks) can be eaten in spring. Pick them when they are still tender (don't worry, your Garlic bulbs will continue to grow underground) and chop them up as an addition to a salad, sprinkle them on soups or on fish, use them in sandwiches, grill them, or sauté with other vegetables.

Mint (*Mentha* spp.)

This is another plant to add to your protective barrier. It will provide you with fresh leaves for summer drinks and with dried leaves for stomach-soothing winter teas. Gather the fresh leaves and stalks and hang them in cloth bags around the porch and patio.

Rosemary (*Rosmarinus officinalis*)

Fleas and ticks dislike this herb. Plant it around the perimeter of the yard and dry the leaves for bug-repelling sachets. Dried Rosemary leaves can also be sprinkled in the grass and around the edges of the garden. Rosemary is a nice herb to sprinkle on fish, chicken, and lamb dishes.

ESSENTIAL OILS FOR PEST CONTROL

The following essential oils have shown tick-repelling properties and can be safely sprayed on humans and pets: Geranium, Lavender, Lemongrass, Sage, and Thyme.

Other oils can be put into spray bottles and used on humans:

Eucalyptus, Rosemary, Tansy, Citronella, Clove, and Basil. Pennyroyal can also be sprayed on humans but definitely not on pets.

> **Caution: Do not spray Pennyroyal on your pet as it can cause seizures or even death.**

 ## Tick and Mosquito Repellent

Try spraying this on clothing and hair every few hours.

Essential oil of clove
Essential oil of eucalyptus
Essential oil of lemongrass
Essential oil of peppermint

Combine 5 drops of each oil per 1 ounce of water in a spray bottle. Shake and apply.

 ## Lemon Flea Spray for Pets*

Use this daily on pets and stuffed furniture (test your fabric first to see if the lemon bleaches out any color).

Cut six lemons in half and boil them in one quart of water for 5 minutes.

Allow the lemons to steep in the water overnight, keeping a tight lid on the pot.

Pour the liquid into a spray bottle and, when not being used, refrigerate (it will keep for up to seven days).

Give your pet a flea bath and then spray them with the lemon mixture. (Cats don't like the scent of lemon but at least it's non-toxic!) Avoid getting any spray into your pet's eyes, as it will burn. Wash your pet's bedding then spray it with the lemon spray.

 ## A Lemon "Flea Collar"

Place a few drops of lemon essential oil on your pet's collar. Wash your hands immediately to avoid getting the oil in your eyes.

---

*Adapted from Kathy Adams, "Homemade Lemon Spray for Flea Control," http://homeguides.sfgate.com/homemade-lemon-spray-flea-control-75930.html.

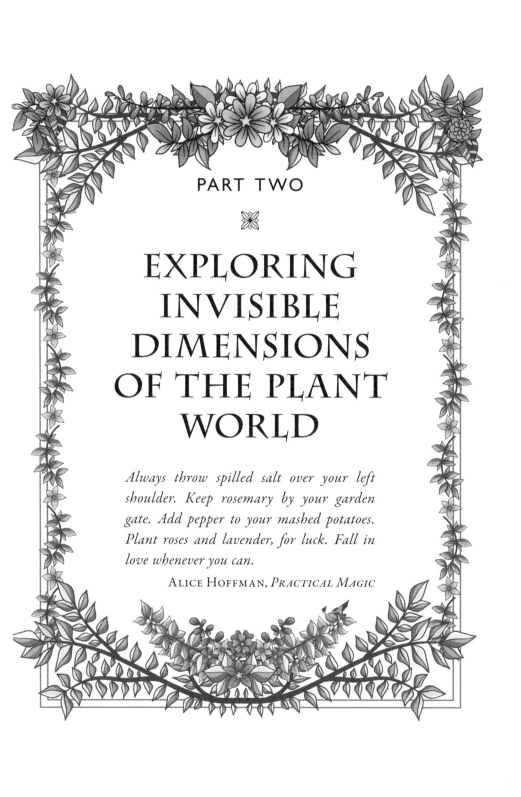

PART TWO

EXPLORING INVISIBLE DIMENSIONS OF THE PLANT WORLD

Always throw spilled salt over your left shoulder. Keep rosemary by your garden gate. Add pepper to your mashed potatoes. Plant roses and lavender, for luck. Fall in love whenever you can.

ALICE HOFFMAN, *PRACTICAL MAGIC*

7

MAGIC OF THE DRAGON AND THE HAG

Dracaena* and Mullein

Plants evoke wonder, not only because of their beauty and ingenious ways of survival, but because they offer humans such a multitude of uses. This wonder has led certain plants to be cherished as sacred or magical, and their uses have been passed down in stories and rituals for generations.

DRAGON'S BLOOD—A MAGICAL AID

Dracaena is one of the oldest living trees on Earth and was a sacred tree of the Guanches of Tenerife in the Canaries, who once used it to embalm dead bodies. Dracaena trees have a distinctive shape: a large base, then a pulled-together middle. In the upper reaches of the tree the branches spread out again to form an umbrella-shaped top. The plant is struggling in its native habitat and is an endangered species.

Dragon's Blood is the resin of the tree *Dracaena draco,* which was once reputed to contain the blood of elephants and dragons. Dracaena resin is used as medicine, varnish, incense, and a dye, and in alchemy and magic. According to Maude Grieve's book, *A Modern Herbal,* the

---

*A version of the section on Dracaena originally appeared in *The Witches' Almanac* 34 (2015–2016).

resin was once used to treat syphilis. Dragon's Blood has also been used for internal injuries such as trauma, postpartum bleeding, and menstrual problems. In magic, Dragon's Blood is said to quicken spells and add potency to any working. As incense, Dragon's Blood is said to clear negativity. A woman may burn it while sitting near an open window at night to draw back a straying lover. Place the herb near the bed to cure impotence in a man. The powdered resin may be strewn under carpets, in entranceways, on windowsills, and anywhere you want protection from ill wishes or negative energies.

Caution: Do not do sprinkle the resin in living spaces if there are infants or pets that might be harmed by its strength. Note that adulterants, unrelated plants, and even synthetic substitutes—any of which may be poisonous— are commonly sold as "Dragon's Blood."

Dragon's Blood belongs to Mars and is of the Fire element. It is sacred to the Hindu god Shiva and appropriate to use in a ritual to honor him.

The ancient Romans, Greeks, and Arabs used *Dracaena cinnabari* (Cinnabar) as a dye and in paints, as a remedy for lung and gastrointestinal problems, diarrhea, and skin problems such as eczema, and for wound healing.

Dracaena terminalis is the variety used in China to make red lacquer. The roots can be made into a sugary syrup and also an intoxicating drink. This variety has been used to treat fevers and diarrhea.

Croton draco is the Mexican variety (Sangre del Drago) that has been used as a wound herb.

🖋 Make Dragon's Blood Ink*

You can use Dragon's Blood ink to write in your own Book of Shadows (a secret book wherein you record all the little practices and inspirations that have helped you achieve your magical ideals). The ink is also used in fire spells, where you write your wish on a

---

*Adapted from "Ancient Ink Formula Recipe: How to Make and How to Use Dragon's Blook Ink," www.magicalrecipesonline.com/2012/04/ancient-ink-formula-recipe -dragons.html.

***piece of paper or a light-colored tree bark, such as birch, and give
it to the fire.***

1 part powdered resin from true *Dracaena draco*

1 part gum arabic

13 parts alcohol

Mix the resin with the gum arabic, then very slowly blend in the alcohol, until
everything is fully dissolved. Filter through cheesecloth and bottle. For best
results, do this under the waxing moon.

In African-American hoodoo and New Orleans voodoo, the herb is
used to make a trick bag, gri-gri, wanga, nation sack, mojo hand, or root
bag to attract luck, money, or love.

◗ Making a Mojo Bag*

To make the bag use an appropriate color, such as red flannel for love mojo,
green flannel for money mojo, white flannel for a baby blessing, light blue
flannel for a home blessing or for spiritual peace, or orange to incite change.
Mojo bags may also be made of leather or cotton cloth.

The bag should contain at least three symbols of your need, such as a
petition paper with your wish written upon it (write it in Dragon's Blood
ink for greatest effect), a seal or sigil (best drawn with Dragon's Blood ink),
coins, crystals, stones, herbs, and roots. The total number of ingredients
should equal an odd number: 3, 5, 7, 9, 11, or 13. Add Dragon's Blood resin to
strengthen your bag.

After it is made, you must "fix" your bag. Smoke it with incense or in the
smoke of a candle, or breathe on it to bring it to life. Make a petition to your
patron god or goddess for aid, then tie, wrap, or sew the bag shut. This step
is called "tying the mojo," and most practitioners use a miller's knot for this
purpose.

Now "feed" your bag by sprinkling it with alcohol such as whisky, Florida
water, or perfume (use your own bodily fluid for a sex magic bag). A tiny
dab will do. You must keep feeding your bag periodically to keep it alive.

---

*Adapted from Catherine Yronwode, "Mojo Hand and Root Bag," Hoodoo in Theory
and Practice, www.luckymojo.com/mojo.html.

The mojo bag is worn hidden from sight. It may also be hidden somewhere in the house. Hiding is important because if someone else touches the bag, that could kill its spirit.

MULLEIN, HAG'S TAPERS

Mullein (*Verbascum* spp.) is an invaluable plant with many healing properties. When I first moved into the house I live in, there was no Mullein in the yard, so I went outside and called it in, singing of my need. Within a year it started to appear. However, Mullein refuses to grow where I scatter the seeds. It prefers to pop up in the most unpredictable places, usually from cracks in the cement patio.

Mullein has many other names: Aaron's Rod, Blanket-leaf, Candle-wick, Feltwort, Jacob's Staff, Old Man's Flannel, Shepherd's Club, Velvet Dock, Velvet Plant, Punchón, Gordolobo, Wild Ice Leaf, Our Lady's Flannel, Hedge Taper, Torches, Candelaria, and Quaker's Rouge. Many of these names refer to the use of Mullein as a torch or a wound herb. Quaker's Rouge refers to the custom of young ladies rubbing their faces with the slightly irritating leaves to make their cheeks glow.

A few centuries ago, before there were flashlights, our ancestors carried torches or lanterns. Those who lived in country areas also made use of Mullein, a common wayside plant, to light their way on dark nights. I like to imagine the old women of the village winding down a dark country road, maybe on their way to a witches' coven, leaning on their walking sticks and trying hard not to stumble on roots and stones. Being poor, they are dressed in the simplest black, and they carry hag's tapers to light their way.

Making Hag's Tapers

To make hag's tapers you must seek out old mullein stalks. The plant likes to grow in disturbed ground, so they will often be found near roadways and train tracks. Cut the tall stalk at the base and dry it upside down in an old paper bag.*

---

*The stalks are dried this way because, as they desiccate, they release their seeds. The seeds can be planted in the fall (by scattering lightly on the ground) in a sunny garden area. However, the herb is biennial, so the tall stalk won't appear until the second year.

Once the stalks are dry, soak the heads in a mixture that is half hot melted wax and half hot oil, melted lard, or suet (I like to save old beeswax candles and melt them down for this purpose). Lift the heads out of the oil and wax mixture and allow them to dry slightly, then dip again. Repeat a few times.

When the flower heads are fully waxed and dry, you can light the tip of your hag's taper, and use it as a torch in a religious procession or any time you want to take a walk in the dark. Through experimentation I have found that the tapers yield five minutes of light per inch of flower head burned.

Mullein and Magic

The wise old women that I referred to would no doubt have been aware of Mullein's magical gifts. With its bright yellow flowers and torch-making properties, Mullein is said to drive away evil spirits and to protect a person from ill-intentioned sorcery. The root is an aid in grounding a person and can be carried on your person or worn as a charm, or the tincture can be rubbed onto your body.

According to Frazer in *The Golden Bough*, Mullein was once passed through the Midsummer fire to make a charm to protect the herds. The powdered leaf can be used as a substitute for graveyard dust, according to ancient grimoires.

Mullein for Coughs and Other Lung Conditions

Think of Mullein leaf when there is a tight cough, especially if there is stubborn "stuck phlegm" that is hard to budge. A tea made from Mullein leaf alone or combined with soothing Marshmallow root (*Althaea officinalis*) or Lungwort (*Pulmonaria officinalis*) is a great expectorant, especially if there is dry cough and congestion.

To make the tea: Steep one teaspoon of leaf in one cup freshly boiled water for about half an hour. Take a quarter cup at a time, every few hours, up to two cups a day.

> **Caution: Some people may be sensitive to the hairs on Mullein leaves. Filter the tea through an organic coffee filter to prevent further irritation of a sore throat.**

Mullein leaf can be combined with Elderberry (*Sambucus nigra,*

S. canadensis) in tinctures as a lung tonic to help with bronchitis, coughs, and other respiratory conditions.

Dry asthma and chronic lung conditions may be helped by the leaf tea and also by inhaling the smoke. Mullein leaf is a good emergency medicine for those having a severe asthma attack. Set the dried leaves on a hot plate and inhale the smoke to calm respiratory spasms.

 ## Mullein Flower Oil for Ear Infections*

An oil made from mullein flowers is excellent for bacterial infections in the ear, "swimmer's ear," and so on. The flower oil can also be used to treat ear mites in animals and to help soften accumulations of earwax in humans.

Mullein flowers tend to open individually along the stalk, so you will need to revisit your plant daily and gather the blossoms as they pop open.

Fill a brown or blue glass jar with the flowers and just barely cover with good-quality oil (I like cold-pressed olive oil). Screw the lid on the jar tightly and leave it outside in the hot sun for twenty-one days. The flowers will rot inside the jar, forming their own alcohol as a preservative.

After twenty-one days or so, strain the contents of the jar through cheesecloth, and bottle the oil.

To apply the oil: Warm *slightly* in a pan or by holding a tablespoonful over a candle flame for a few seconds, then use a dropper to put the oil into the ear and pack with cotton. Leave in overnight. Try adding a few drops of garlic oil for severe infections.

> **Caution: If the eardrum is ruptured,
> do not place the oil into the ear!**

Mullein for Swollen Lymph Glands

Dry Mullein leaves can be simmered slightly in hot water until soft, cooled, and then applied to a swollen lymph gland, or the fresh leaves

---

*In the case of severe or chronic ear infections, it will be helpful to eat fresh garlic and take Echinacea (*Echinacea purpurea, E. angustifolia*) internally. Also try eliminating dairy from the diet for two weeks and then follow with probiotic supplements and foods.

can be bruised slightly and laid on the area. Swollen glands in the throat will be helped if Echinacea (*Echinacea purpurea, E. angustifolia*) is taken internally at the same time.

A poultice of Mullein combined with one-quarter part Lobelia (*Lobelia inflata*) is very helpful for swollen glands. Make a fomentation by steeping Mullein leaves alone or with a little Lobelia, then soak a cloth in the tea. Fill the soaked cloth with the plant matter, fold, and apply to a swollen gland.

Drink the tea or take the tincture of the root or flower concurrently for greatest effect.

Caution: Some people may experience contact dermatitis from handling Mullein leaves.

Mullein for Healing and Soothing Pain in Muscles and Bones

My teacher, William LeSassier, taught me to use Mullein for sore muscles and traumatic injury where there is pain and swelling, such as whiplash. He would combine Mullein root, flower, or leaf with Chamomile (*Matricaria recutita, Chamaemelum nobile*) leaves and flowers and Sage (*Salvia officinalis*) to make a poultice. Slipped disks, old fractures that are still painful, pain in the hips, small broken bones in the hands and feet, problems with spine alignment, arthritic pain, sprains, and joint pains can all also be helped by a Mullein poultice. Take a few drops of the root tincture concurrently, several times a day.

◊ Mullein Poultice

If you're using fresh herbs, just put them in the blender with a little water and grind them up coarsely. If you're using dried herbs pour a little boiled water over them to soften them.

When the leaves are soft enough, pour them into a bowl and add a handful of powdered slippery elm bark (*Ulmus fulva, U. rubra*). (If you don't have slippery elm on hand use spelt or buckwheat flour.). Then mix with your fingers until you have a "pie dough" consistency.

Form into a ball and roll onto a clean cloth with a rolling pin (if you don't have a rolling pin use a glass bottle).

Apply to the affected area for one hour, then discard the poultice.

The flowers can be taken as tea or tincture for recent injuries. Old chronic injuries, resulting in sharp pains in the joints, neck, or spine, arthritis pain, sciatica, nerve damage, and broken bones may benefit from the root tincture taken internally (about fifteen drops in water every few hours).

Herbalist David Winston has used Mullein for facial nerve pain, combined with nervines such as Saint-John's-Wort (*Hypericum perforatum*) and Jamaican Dogwood (*Piscidia piscipula*).

Mullein and Your Skin

Steep the leaves in vinegar and hot water, then cool and apply to skin inflammations and hemorrhoids.

Mullein and Your Bladder

Mullein is mildly astringent and can reduce inflammation in the bladder. Think of it in cases of recurring bladder infections, cystitis, or benign prostatic hypertrophy. The root may help tone the bladder when there is weakness such as bedwetting, adult incontinence, or prostate inflammation (provided the condition is not related to sexual abuse or emotional trauma). Take half a teaspoon of the tincture in a quarter cup of water or a quarter cup of the root tea before bed.

8

ANIMAL SPIRIT
MEDICINES

I will tell you a little story. Some years ago I was doing regular sweats with a local Native American group. They had invited two elders to come here to New England from the Rosebud reservation in South Dakota, and I invited them to the forest where I live to do a full-moon pipe ceremony.

On the morning of the full moon a dense fog came up and everyone got lost trying to find the house. The elders got pretty upset about that, thinking it was "bad spirits." Someone in the car had previously told the elders I was a "witch" (I am not and have never been a witch). Witches are very serious business on Native American reservations because they sometimes hurt and even kill people.

When they all got here the elders set everyone to work making tobacco ties in the ritual space as a form of protection. Tobacco ties are small cloth bags filled with tobacco. The elders said to make about a hundred of them, in four colors. They tied twenty-five red ones to a tree, twenty-five black ones to another tree, and twenty-five white ones and twenty-five yellow ones to two others, to mark the four directions: North, East, South, and West.

The elders told me that I was not allowed to touch ANYTHING. Not the tobacco, not the firewood, nothing. In fact they said I was not allowed to leave the house until the moment of the ceremony. It was all very surreal, and it reminded me of my days in a Sufi ashram when the guru made me stay indoors for three months as a type of ritual purification. Anyway, all I was allowed to do was sit in the kitchen.

Finally the time of the ritual arrived and guests from near and far started showing up for the pipe ceremony. I was allowed to troop out to the woods with the rest, and after it was done everyone went back to the house for snacks. One of the elders said he would remain in the ritual circle after we finished, doing some things, though I didn't know what. Gradually the guests left. Soon there was no one left but me, the two elders, their driver, and another member of my then shamanic lodge whom I had invited.

The elder who had stayed back at the circle for a while returned to the house and then sat down before me with tears in his eyes. I did not know what was upsetting him so. He said the Little People had spoken to him in the forest after the ceremony, and he said they had told him that I was the priestess of that area and that he owed me a big apology. He was crying. I accepted his apology of course.

That was when I was given my name: Willow (Red Willow, a type of Red Osier). When the other elder, who was a Lakota grandmother, said my name was Willow, I asked her what the name meant. She said: "The Willow helps the Tobacco to get to heaven because you put the Willow into the pipe with the Tobacco. Tobacco is masculine and Willow is feminine."

The elder who had spoken with the Little People added that I should put my ritual fire in the East, not in the center of the circle where it had been built. He said he had been shown that by a shaft of moonlight illuminating the eastern direction.

The whole incident led me to the serious investigation of Native American herbs, starting with Red Osier, and I have been learning about Native plants ever since.

I am indebted to several authors and teachers for the contents of this chapter, particularly herbalist Matthew Wood, author of *The Book of Herbal Wisdom: Using Plants as Medicine* (North Atlantic Books), who has been a personal friend and colleague for many years, and Daniel E. Moerman, author of *Native American Medicinal Plants: An Ethnobotanical Dictionary* (Timber Press), whose books have enabled me to understand the connections between the Spirits of plants and animals.

I have had Moerman's book for several decades at least. I bought the original two-volume set when it was still the old University of Michigan Museum of Anthropology Technical Report Number 19. It's now out as a compact paperback and I highly recommend that book for an understanding of how specific tribes used plants for healing.

Another important source is Jamie Sams and David Carson's classic book *Medicine Cards: The Discovery of Power through the Ways of Animals* (Bear and Company), which has also been long recommended by Native American teachers as an authentic guide. I use the book frequently to interpret "day signs" (when a special animal appears in front of me during the day, at night, or in a dream).

I have also had the privilege of spending time with a number of Native American medicine people over the years, including Lillian Pitawanakwat (Ojibwa-Potawatomi of the Thunderbird Clan), with whom I was able to participate in sweat lodges and healing ceremonies. Through their teachings, and through time spent at the Maniwaki reservation in Canada, I gained respect for the deep and wide river that is the indigenous American healing tradition.

One traditional medicine society is called Midewiwin; it is an initiatory society of healers for whom the turtle is a sacred animal. The turtle is an image of the entire landmass of North America, also called "Turtle Island," and represents healing derived from nature, the land, and the Earth Spirits.

Jugleurs or *djasakee* are medicine people of the Anishnabe (the Odawa, Ojibwa, and Algonquin peoples) who are able to move objects using their mind. They know how to travel to the Spirit World to retrieve the soul of a sick person to effect healing. The Wabeno Society communicates with and receives guidance from medicine people who have passed over. (This is very similar to the Christian and Islamic practice of praying to saints, knowledgeable healers, and ancient wise persons who have passed over, for guidance, support, and healing.)

There are many other medicine societies and most of them are secret. They work with Spirits, both live humans and the dead, to cause change in individuals. Animal Spirits are also worked with to receive their power or guidance. As with human nations, each animal nation has a leader that those of their kind follow and obey. It is important to understand that for First Nations peoples, animals are actually closer to the Creator than we humans are, with cleaner souls and purer hearts. We humans are the newest creatures to have arrived on this planet, making the Earth, Air, Fire, Water, rocks, herbs, trees, animals, birds, and fish our elder relations from whom we can learn much. Understanding animal medicines is a sacred task.

Below is a sampling of some of the animal medicines used by Native American healers over the millennia.

Teas and Poultices in Animal Spirit Medicines

The preparations included in this chapter are based on the following methods.

To make a tea: Use about two teaspoons of plant material per cup of water. Roots, barks, and berries are simmered (not boiled) for twenty minutes in a tightly covered pot. Leaves and flowers are steeped for about half an hour in freshly boiled water.

The usual dose for teas is a quarter cup taken four times a day, not with meals. (This assumes a 150-pound adult is taking the brew. Adjust according to body weight. Infants can get the tea via their mother's breast milk.)

To make a poultice: Blend the fresh plant with enough water to make a paste (or pound in a mortar and pestle to make a paste). Spread the paste on a clean cloth and apply to the affected body part. If dried plant material is used, then add just enough boiling hot water to soften the plant material, blend, and spread on a clean cloth.

Caution: Always check for drug and herb interactions and contraindications if you are on pharmaceutical medicines.

BEAR SPIRIT AND USING BEAR MEDICINE PLANTS

The Midewiwin teach that every plant and tree on the Earth has a use, and for the Anishnabe, herbalism is called "the bear path." To follow the bear path means knowing how to get to the root of things; bears delve deep into the soil with their claws and pull out medicines and foods by their roots. A person destined to be an herbalist may dream of bears. Someone on the bear path will work with all aspects of a person—body, mind, spirit—to get to the root of his or her disease. There is tremendous power in bears to heal others, and that power can hit like a tidal wave. It is extremely important to be attentive to the natural order and timing in a healing, as some people must get sick, suffer, and even die.

Bears walk upright just like humans, and indigenous peoples studied their habits to learn herbalism. Bears are particularly fond of cherries, acorns, and Juneberries, pointing to these plants as potent plant allies and important additions to medicinal compounds. They eat Osha root (*Ligusticum filicinum, L. porteri*) before and after hibernation, indicating that herb as a strong ally for digestion. Bears also load up on berries and acorns before their winter sleep.

When I undertook a traditional four-day fast (no food or water) with traditional Ojibwa-Potawatomi elder Lillian Pitawanakwat (Thunderbird Eagle Woman—Ninkii BinessMijissi Kwe of the Thunderbird Clan), we began and ended with a tea of Osha roots and we finished with a celebratory drink made of mashed berries.

According to Spirit medicine, people who need bear medicines are large, powerful, introspective types who like to sleep and dream but will act decisively once they are awakened by some urgent calling. Bear teaches us how to dream into solutions, to go deep into the dark to find an answer, reemerge with a vision, and then act powerfully.

Bear medicines strengthen the adrenal cortex and add strength and bulk to the body. These plants often have oily, furry brown roots. If they are berries they may be sedative and cooling to the body.

American Licorice (*Glycyrrhiza lepidota*)

The root was chewed by singers to soothe their throats, and it was chewed in the sweat lodge and at the sun dance ceremony as a cooling agent. The root was also chewed and kept in the mouth for toothache.

The root tea was taken for sore throat, chest coughs and pains, diarrhea, stomachache, and children's fevers. Taken in larger amounts, the root tea was used as a cathartic. Externally, the root tea was used as a wash for swellings.

The leaf tea was placed in the ear and a leaf poultice applied to the ear for earache. The leaf poultice was applied to horses' sores. Leaves were put in the shoes to absorb moisture.

American Spikenard (*Aralia racemosa*)

The root tea was taken as a spring tonic and for diabetes, tuberculosis, coughs, menstrual pain, rheumatism, whooping cough, sore throat, tiredness, and stomachaches. The roots were also abortifacient. The root tea was used externally to wash deep wounds and was applied to a woman's head during childbirth.

A tea of the roots and berries was taken for fever, as an expectorant, and for lung diseases and asthma. The berry and root tea was given to children for colic and grippe. A tea of the root mixed with Angelica root (*Angelica atropurpurea*) was taken for colds and coughs. The tea of the root and inner bark was taken as a blood cleanser and for kidney and liver diseases, for calf and shin swellings, and for prolapse of the uterus.

The sap of the mashed roots was applied to burns, wounds, and cuts, and a hot pounded-root poultice was applied to sprains, boils, strained muscles, and bone fractures. The plant was chewed to pass tapeworms.

The roots were dried and smoked with Red Osier Dogwood (Red Willow, *Cornus sericea*) for headaches.

Arrowleaf Balsam Root (*Balsamorhiza sagittata*)

The root was chewed for sore throat or mouth and toothache and to allay hunger. The chewed root was applied to sores and blisters, and a root poultice was applied to deep wounds, insect bites, and swellings.

The smoke of the burning root was inhaled for body aches and used to purify a sick room. The powdered dried root was applied to syphilitic sores.

The root tea was taken by women at the start of labor and was also taken for rheumatic pain. The root tea was rubbed into the scalp to make the hair grow and was used as an eyewash. The steam of the tea was inhaled for headache.

The tea of the leaf, root, and stem was taken for headache, fever, colds, stomach pain, tuberculosis, whooping cough, and venereal diseases. The leaf tea was used as a wash for sores and poison ivy rash. The leaf poultice was applied to burns.

The young shoots were eaten for insomnia. The seeds were eaten to stop diarrhea and dysentery.

Fernleaf Biscuitroot
(*Lomatium dissectum*)

The raw root was chewed for sore throat. The root oil was used as eye drops for trachoma and gonorrheal eye infections. The root sap or oil was used to salve cuts and sores. The powdered root was used in burn salves and sprinkled on wounds and sores in horses and people. The powdered root was smoked for colds and flu and burned as incense to be inhaled for asthma and bronchitis. The root smoke was given to horses with distemper.

The powdered root or a root poultice was applied to an infant's severed umbilical cord. A poultice of the roots was applied to wounds, cuts, bruising, infections, sore limbs, and compound fractures and placed on horses' sores. The root poultice or a hot tea of the root was applied as a wash to rheumatic swellings, rashes, and sprains.

The root tea was applied externally as a wash for wounds, sores, and dandruff and as a general wash for the sick. It was also taken internally for stomach problems and added to tonics to strengthen the weak and for colds, coughs, flu, hay fever, sore throat, bronchitis, pneumonia, tuberculosis, and venereal diseases. The root tea was used as an herbal steam for lung and nasal congestion.

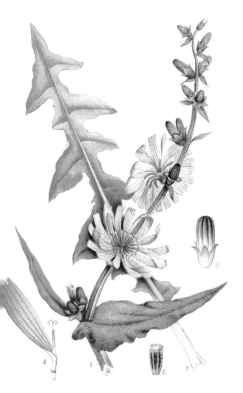

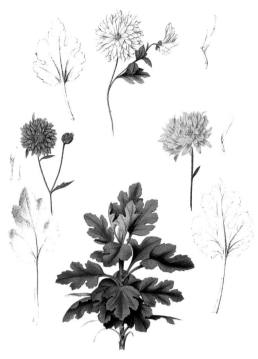

Plate 25 (left). Chicory (*Chichorium intybus*)

Plate 26 (right). Chrysanthemum
(*Chrysanthemum morifolium,*
C. indicum)

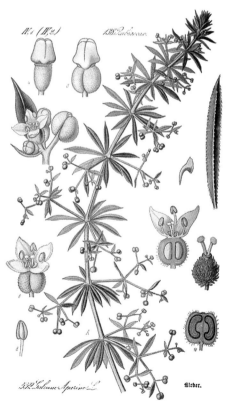

Plate 27. Cleavers, Bedstraw
(*Galium aparine*)

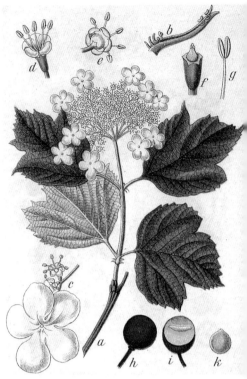

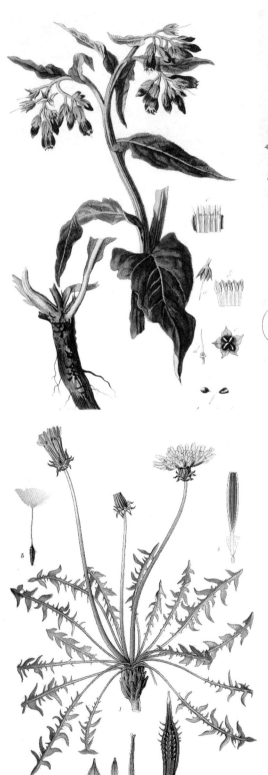

Plate 28 (left). Comfrey (*Symphytum officinale*)

Plate 29 (right). Cramp Bark (*Viburnum opulus*)

Plate 30. Dandelion (*Taraxacum officinale*)

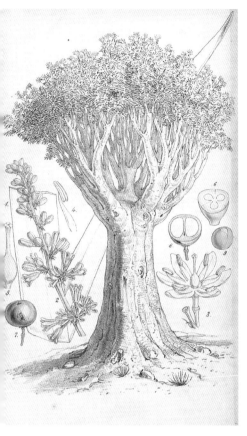

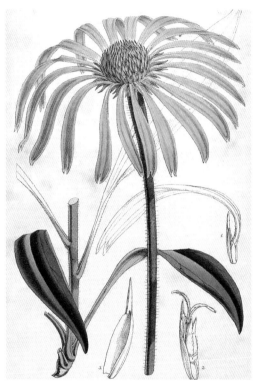

Plate 31 (left). Dragon's Blood (*Dracaena draco*)

Plate 32 (right). Echinacea (*Echinacea purpurea*)

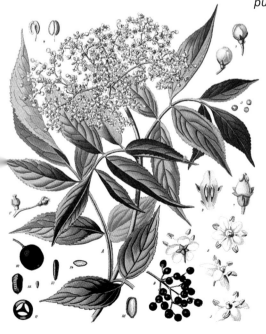

Plate 33. Elder (*Sambucus nigra, S. canadensis*)

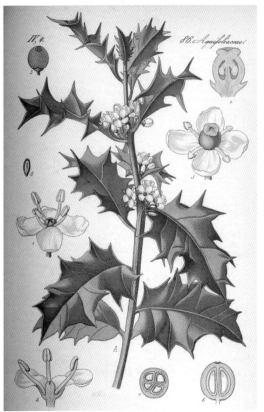

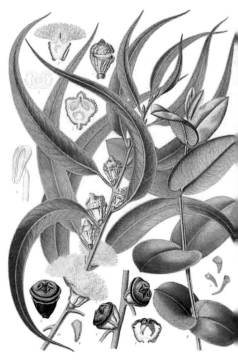

Plate 34 (left). English Holly (*Ilex aquifolium*)

Plate 35 (right). Eucalyptus (*Eucalyptus globulus*)

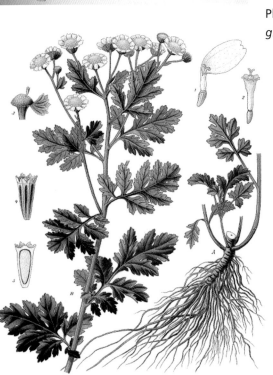

Plate 36. Feverfew (*Tanacetum parthenium*)

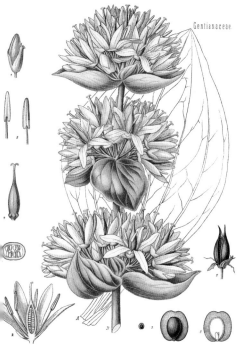

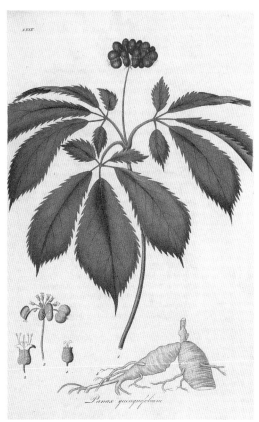

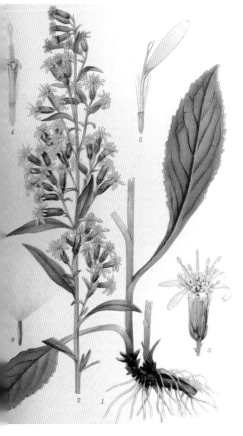

Plate 37 (left). Gentian (*Gentiana lutea, G. officinalis*)

Plate 38 (right). Ginseng (*Panax quinquefolius*)

Plate 39. Goldenrod (*Solidago vigaurea*)

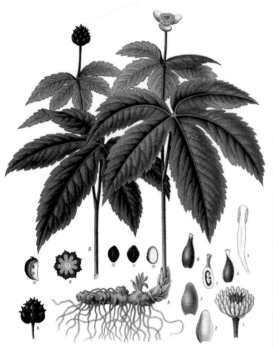

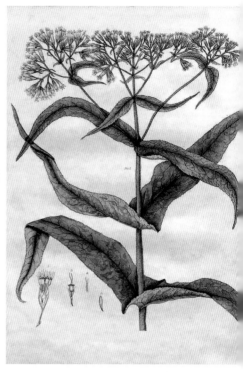

Plate 40 (left). Goldenseal (*Hydrastis canadensis*)

Plate 41 (right). Gravel Root, Sweet-Scente Joe Pye Weed, Queen of the Meadow (*Eupatorium purpureum*)

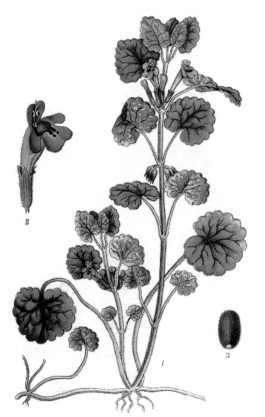

Plate 42. Ground Ivy, Creeping Charlie, Gil over-the-Ground (*Glechoma hederacea*)

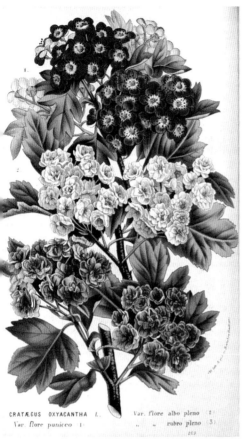

CRATÆGUS OXYACANTHA L.   Var. flore albo pleno 2
Var. flore puniceo 1   „   „   rubro pleno 3
                                               109

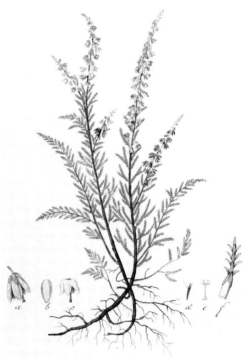

Plate 43 (left). Hawthorn (*Crataegus oxyacantha*)

Plate 44 (right). Heather (*Calluna vulgaris*)

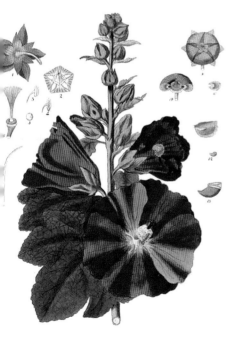

Plate 45. Hollyhock (*Althaea rosea*)

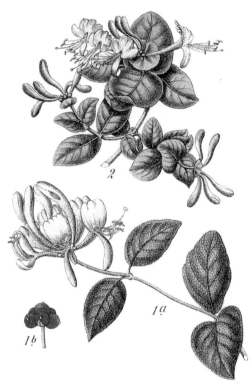

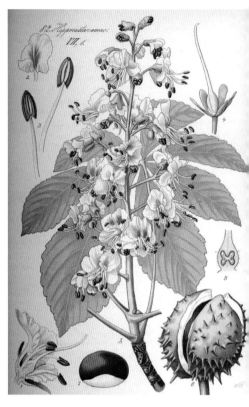

Plate 46 (left). Honeysuckle (*Lonicera periclymenum*)

Plate 47 (right). Horse Chestnut (*Aesculus hippocastanum*)

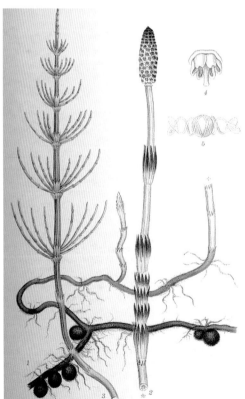

Plate 48. Horsetail (*Equisetum arvense*)

A tea of the dried, powdered stems, leaves, and root (or just the dried root alone) was taken for stomach pain. The above ground portion of the plant was smoked for the treatment of coughs, colds, hay fever, bronchitis, asthma, influenza, pneumonia, and tuberculosis.

Osha, Fernleaf Licorice Root
(*Ligusticum porteri, L. filicinum*)

The root was considered a panacea and in particular was used as a lung-strengthening tea for coughs. The root tea was taken for catarrh, colds, bronchial pneumonia, flu, and other respiratory infections. It was also used to treat fever, diarrhea, gastrointestinal disorders, hangover, sore throats, and rheumatism. The root was chewed by medicine men during ceremonies.

Purplestem Angelica (*Angelica atropurpurea*)

The root tea was used to "bring on the menses"; for gas, colic, and other stomach problems; for colds, flu, pneumonia, and fevers; as a blood cleanser; and to calm the nerves. It was also used as a gargle for sore throat or sore mouth.

A poultice of the cooked, pounded roots was applied to swellings, painful areas, and broken bones.

Burdocks

Greater Burdock (*Arctium lappa*)

A tea of the root or seeds was taken to clean the blood, for gravel in the urine, and for venereal diseases. The buds and roots were applied to sores and chancres. A boiled leaf poultice was applied to scrofulous sores on the neck.

Lesser Burdock (*Arctium minus*)

The root tea was taken for rheumatism, fevers, grippe, pleurisy, and whooping cough and as a blood purifier and stimulant. A warm mashed root poultice was applied to boils and abscesses. A leaf poultice was applied to the head for headache and used widely for pain, rheumatism, and boils.

Sunflowers

Annual Sunflower (*Helianthus annuus*)

The fresh or dried root was chewed by a medicine person before sucking venom out of a snakebite and a root poultice was applied to snakebites. The root tea was used externally as a warm wash for rheumatism.

The leaf tea was taken for fever and used as a wash for horses affected by screwworms. The crushed herb was applied to snakebites, spider bites, and cuts. The flower tea was taken for chest pains and lung problems.

The pith was burned as moxa on warts to remove them. A salve of the powdered seed and root was applied to injuries. The powdered leaves were used in salves for sores and swellings. The hardened sap was chewed by elders to prevent thirst. The seed oil was applied to the face and body for ceremonies, and the dried, powdered seed was eaten by warriors to prevent fatigue. The seeds were eaten to increase appetite.

Cusick's Sunflower (*Helianthus cusickii*)

The root tea was taken for heart problems, gas, and tuberculosis. The root poultice was applied to swellings and placed on the body for chills and fever. The root was burned in the home after a death or a long sickness with fever and chills, and to keep away disease.

Fewleaf Sunflower (*Helianthus occidentalis*)

A poultice of the crushed root was applied to bruises and sores.

Nuttall's Sunflower (*Helianthus nuttallii*)

A tea of the dried leaf was taken for stomach problems.

Paleleaf Woodland Sunflower (*Helianthus strumosus*)

A tea of the root was taken for worms in both children and adults, and for lung problems.

Prairie Sunflower (*Helianthus petiolaris*)

A cold tea of the whole plant was regarded as a cure-all. The powdered leaf was applied alone or used in salves for sores and swellings.

Sawtooth Sunflower (*Helianthus grosseserratus*)

A poultice of the flowers was applied to burns.

Showy Sunflower (*Helianthus niveus* ssp. *canescens*)

The stem sap was applied to bleeding wounds.

Thinleaf Sunflower (*Helianthus decapetalus*)

A root poultice was placed on old sores.

Western Sunflower (*Helianthus anomalus*)

The plant was used externally as a spider bite medicine.

Yuccas

Adam's Needle (*Yucca filamentosa*)

The roots were rubbed on the skin and used in salves for sores and as a poultice for sprains. The root tea was taken internally for skin diseases and for diabetes.

Aloe Yucca (*Yucca aloifolia*)

The boiled and mashed root was used in salves.

Banana Yucca (*Yucca baccata*)

A tea of the pulverized leaf was taken for vomiting and heartburn. The root suds were used in ceremonial purification baths. The juice was used to lubricate a midwife's hands. The fruits were eaten raw as a cathartic and to promote labor.

Narrowleaf Yucca (*Yucca angustissima*)

The crushed root was used as a shampoo to grow hair. The root tea was taken as a laxative.

Small Soapweed (*Yucca glauca*)

The smashed roots were applied as a tea or a powder to sores, scabs, and skin conditions. A tea of the grated root was applied to sprains and saddle sores. The powdered root tea was taken for stomach problems. The fresh root tea was taken cold to hasten the delivery of a baby or placenta. A tea of the dried root was used as a hair wash for dandruff and the hair was soaked with the root tea to kill vermin and promote hair growth. The root poultice was applied to bleeding or infected cuts.

A tea of the whole plant was taken as a laxative.

Soapweed Yucca (*Yucca glauca* var. *glauca*)

The root was used as a soap and hair wash.

BADGER SPIRIT AND USING BADGER MEDICINE PLANTS

Badger is sometimes called the "little bear." These incredibly fierce diggers are one of the very few animals that will attack and kill a grizzly bear; they do this by burrowing into the bear's belly with their powerful claws. Badger claws are the badge of a warrior; people who were ready to do battle would wear a badger claw necklace.

In a spiritual sense badger people respond instantly to life challenges from their gut. They may wound others with their words or their fists, but they are also the most loyal of friends. Badger is also the spiritual keeper of medicinal roots, the ones that hang down from the ceiling of their underground home. Badger knows how to aggressively go after disease. Badger medicine people have powerful stomachs and powerful gut instincts and appetites.

In Oriental medicine traditions, the abdomen is the *hara* or the center of the *chi* (life force). Badger medicine plants are often yellow tonic laxatives, oriented to the bowels and stomach.

American Ginseng (*Panax quinquefolius*)

The root was chewed to ease colic. It was also added to blood-cleansing and spring tonic mixes and used by women to promote fertility and to correct womb weakness.

The root tea was taken for convulsions, palsy, headache, nervous afflictions, vertigo, fevers, and short-windedness. The root tea was also taken for the vomiting of cholera or of gall, for lack of appetite, as a blood cleanser for boils, as an expectorant, for night fevers, and as a tonic to sharpen mental powers. It was used as a throat gargle for thrush and as general tonic and cure-all when other remedies failed. The root tea was used externally as a wash for sores and for children's sore eyes. The root tea was rubbed on the body and used in steam for joint swellings.

The dried root was smoked as a panacea for fainting spells. A poultice of the pounded roots was applied for earache and to boils and carbuncles. The plant poultice was applied to bleeding cuts.

False Rhubarb (*Rheum rhaponticum*)

The plant infusion was taken for constipation and used as an astringent wash for skin problems.

Goldenseal (*Hydrastis canadensis*)

The tea of the root was taken for cancers, for upset stomach and to improve appetite, and for whooping cough, diarrhea, tuberculosis, fever, and scrofula. The tea was taken with whiskey for heart ailments. A tea of the powdered root was taken for gas, liver troubles, and sour stomach. The root tea was used externally as a wash for inflammations and used on chapped and sore lips.

Poke (*Phytolacca americana*)

Caution: The roots, mature leaves, and seeds of Poke are highly toxic and should only be used in tiny amounts. The seeds should be swallowed whole and never chewed.

The roots were used in salves for ulcerous sores, old sores, and glandular swellings. A crushed root poultice was applied to bruises, sprains, swollen joints, and warts. The dried, powdered root was sprinkled on old sores. A tea of the powdered root was taken to help the kidneys. The root tea was taken for eczema. A tea of the berries was taken for arthritis (do not chew the seeds) and for dysentery. A tea of the roots and berries or the berry wine was taken for rheumatism.

The cooked greens were used to build blood.

> **Caution: Poke greens can be eaten only in the early spring when they are six inches or less in height. After that they are toxic.**

The roots and twigs were used in steams for rheumatism, and the stalks were cooked and eaten for rheumatism. A tea of the stems was used for chest colds. The raw berries were rubbed on skin lumps and a poultice of the mashed berries was applied to sore breasts.

Yellow Dock, Curly Dock (*Rumex crispus*)

The peeled root was eaten for stomach disorders. The mashed root was used on sores, swellings, and abrasions and for rheumatic pains, sprains, burns, and bruises. The fresh or cooked root was placed on the gums or a tooth for toothache. The dried, powdered root was applied for chafing on babies' skin.

A poultice of the pounded and moistened dried root was applied to wounds and sores, including saddle sores on horses, cuts, itching, ulcers, and swellings. A powdered root poultice was used on sores, rashes, and skin infections.

The root tea was taken for dysentery, as a kidney aid, as a laxative, for lung hemorrhage, for jaundice and other liver conditions, to increase appetite, for stomach flu, cramps, abdominal pain, and upset stomach, for venereal diseases, for coughs, and as a sore throat gargle. The root tea was drunk and a poultice applied for yellow fever, as a tonic to induce pregnancy, and to strengthen the muscles of athletes and runners. The root tea was used as a wash and the powdered root was applied for gonorrhea. The root tea was applied to athlete's foot.

The juice of the plant and the root tea were used as skin salves. The leaves were rubbed in the mouth for sore throat and a cold leaf tea was applied to mouth sores. A poultice of the crushed green leaf was used on boils to draw pus. The cooked leaves were eaten to benefit the stomach and to purify the blood. The powdered leaf was dusted on sores.

The seeds were boiled and taken for diarrhea. The dried seeds were smoked with Bearberry (*Arctostaphylos uva-ursi*) in kinnickinnic mixtures.

SNAKE SPIRIT AND
USING SNAKE MEDICINE PLANTS

Snake teaches us to shed our skin and renew ourselves, even after suffering many bites, poisons, and traumas. When we let go and allow the universe to re-create us, we transmute our suffering into divine power.

Snake medicine plants were used for snakebites, insect stings, infections, and poisoning. These herbs clean the blood by strengthening the liver, the organ that clears poisons from the bloodstream. They also help foster a strong metabolism.

Black Cohosh, Black Snake Root, Rattle Root, Black Bugbane (*Cimicifuga racemosa*)

The root tea was taken to "promote menstruation," for colds and coughs, for tuberculosis, for constipation, for hives, as a blood purifier, as a kidney aid, to promote breast milk, and for rheumatism. It was used as a sedative to help infants sleep and was considered a general tonic; sometimes it was mixed with Elecampane root (*Inula helenium*) and Stone Root (*Collinsonia canadensis*) to make a tonic.

The roots were infused in alcoholic spirits for rheumatic pain, and a tea of the roots and plant was used in steam and as a bath for rheumatism. A leaf poultice was applied to a baby's sore back.

Canada Snakeroot, Wild Ginger (*Asarum canadense*)

The root was cooked with food to improve digestion and cooked with spoiled meat to prevent poisoning. The cooked root was placed in the ear for earache. The root poultice was applied to inflammations, bruises, fractured bones, and contusions.

The root tea was taken for fevers, convulsions in infants, worms, coughs, colds, typhus, scarlet fever, ague, cramps, and urine stoppage, and also as a stomachic and an abortifacient. The cold root tea was taken for children's fevers, headache, convulsions, coughs, measles, asthma, and lack of appetite, and also by the elderly as a spring tonic. The tea was taken and the hands and face were washed with it to stop dreams of dead people.

A tea of the leaf and root was used as a wash for sore breasts. A tea of the root, leaf, and blossom was taken for nervous debility. The fresh leaf was used on wounds and in salves for sores.

Common Boneset (*Eupatorium perfoliatum*)

The root tea was taken to heal the kidneys and to stop the craving for alcohol, and also for typhoid, pneumonia, pleurisy, and snakebite. The root tea was used externally as a wash and a poultice on syphilitic sores. The root and leaf tea was taken for fever and chills.

The tea of the dried leaves, picked before the plant flowered, was taken as a general tonic. The leaf tea was applied as a poultice for broken bones. The tea of the leaves and flowers was taken for colds and fevers, as a diuretic, as an emetic, for ague and sore throat, as a laxative, and for worms. The stem and leaf tea was taken at the onset of a cold. A tea of the whole plant was fed to horses with a fever.

A poultice of the cooked plant tops was applied to rheumatic parts and to headaches. A poultice of the chewed plant was placed on rattlesnake bites.

Common Viper's Bugloss (*Echium vulgare*)

A tea of the leaf and root was taken to benefit the kidneys.

Virginia Snakeroot (*Aristolochia serpentaria*)

The root was chewed or a tea was made of the roots for colds, coughs, fevers, typhus, and ague, as a gargle for sore throat, and as a diuretic. The root was chewed and applied to snakebite or spider bite, or the whole plant was pounded and applied to snakebite and spider bite. The root was used by itself or mixed with Wintergreen (*Gaultheria procumbens*) as a general tonic. The root tea was used as an antiseptic wash. The leaf tea was taken for chills.

Baptisias

Blue Wild Indigo (*Baptisia australis*)

A hot tea of the root or the beaten root was held against the teeth for toothache.

Horsefly Weed (*Baptisia tinctoria*)

The root tea was taken for the spitting of blood and for kidney troubles. A tea of the roots was used to clean out ulcers, wounds, bruises, and cuts and was also used by women as a douche. The root tea was rubbed on the stomach, arms, and legs for cramps. A hot tea of the root or the beaten root was held against the teeth for toothache.

Largeleaf Wild Indigo (*Baptisia alba* var. *macrophylla*)

The root tea was taken for rheumatism and catarrh. The root and leaf were used to poultice swellings, old sores, wounds, hemorrhoids, and rattlesnake bites.

Longbract Wild Indigo (*Baptisia bracteata*)

The powdered seeds were mixed with buffalo fat and applied to the abdomen for colic.

Echinaceas

Blacksamson Echinacea (*Echinacea angustifolia*)

The root was chewed and the juice applied to the teeth for toothaches. The root was also chewed for tonsillitis, coughs, and sore throat. The root tea was taken as an antidote to rattlesnake bites. The leaf and root tea was rubbed on the neck for neck pain, taken for sore throat, and used in the mouth for sore gums. The chewed root poultice was applied to wounds, swellings, scars, septic conditions, and stings. The juice was used as a wash for the pain of burns.

The plant was chewed to relieve stomachache and when a person was thirsty or sweating too much. A poultice of the whole plant was applied to enlarged glands and mumps.

Eastern Purple Coneflower (*Echinacea purpurea*)

The root was chewed or tinctured in alcohol and taken for coughs. The root tea was used for dyspepsia and gonorrhea. The root was mixed with Staghorn Sumac root (*Rhus typhina, R. hirta*) and taken for venereal diseases.

Pale Purple Coneflower (*Echinacea pallida*)

The root was chewed to allay thirst, for colds, and for toothache. The root tea was taken for colic, worms, and sore eyes. It was also used externally as a burn dressing and as a wash for fevers. A tea of the root and leaf was taken for rheumatism, arthritis, smallpox, mumps, measles, sore mouth and gums, and sore throat and as an antidote to snakebite, venomous bites, and stings. A poultice of the roots was applied to inflammations to stop burning pain.

Eryngos

Button Eryngo (*Eryngium yuccifolium*)

A cold tea of the roots was taken for kidney, spleen, and bladder problems, and neuralgia. The root tea was also taken as a blood cleanser as well as for snakebite, whooping cough, diarrhea, stomachache, headache, bloody stool, and gonorrhea and as an emetic and antidote to poisons. An infusion of the dried leaf was taken for dysentery. The stem and leaf were chewed for nosebleed. A cold tea of the whole plant was used as a wash for body aches, sores, itchy skin, and foot swellings.

Rattlesnake Master (*Eryngium aquaticum*)

The root tea was taken for snakebite and as a diuretic and expectorant. It was also taken for tapeworms, pinworms, and venereal diseases. The tea of the whole plant was used for gonorrhea.

Rattlesnake Plantains

Downy Rattlesnake Plantain (*Goodyera pubescens*)

The root tea was taken for rheumatism, by women after delivery of a child, and for pleurisy. The cold leaf tea was taken for colds, to increase appetite, and for kidney problems and held in the mouth for toothache. The leaf poultice was placed on burns and a mashed leaf poultice was used to wipe a baby's sore mouth.

Lesser Rattlesnake Plantain (*Goodyera repens*)

It was used in exactly the same way as Downy Rattlesnake Plantain (*Goodyera pubescens*) above, and the fresh juice was swallowed for snakebite.

Western Rattlesnake Plantain (*Goodyera oblongifolia*)

The leaf tea was added to bathwater as a liniment for sore muscles. The leaf poultice was used on sores and cuts. The plant was chewed by women before and during labor.

Saint-John's-Worts (Hypericum spp.)

Caution: *Hypericum* should be taken for long periods of time only in the winter months; its use should be stopped one month before sun exposure is likely to occur. Prolonged use can cause photosensitivity.

Coastalplain Saint-John's-Wort (*Hypericum brachyphyllum*)

The plant tea was taken as a cathartic.

Common Saint-John's-Wort (*Hypericum perforatum*)

The root was chewed, a portion eaten, and the rest used to poultice snakebite. The root tea was taken as a reproductive aid to increase fertility. The root tea was used externally as a wash to strengthen infants. A tea of the whole plant was taken for bloody diarrhea, fevers, and coughs and as an abortifacient. The crushed plant was sniffed for nosebleed.

Gold Wire (*Hypericum concinnum*)

A tea of the plant was used as a wash for running sores.

Great Saint-John's-Wort (*Hypericum ascyron*)

The root tea was added to herbal mixtures for weak lungs and tuberculosis. The powder of the dried boiled root was applied to snakebite.

Orangegrass (*Hypericum gentianoides*) and St. Andrew's Cross (*Hypericum hypericoides*)*

The root was chewed and swallowed and the rest applied as a poultice for snakebite. A tea of the roots was used for colic and for the pain of childbirth. The root tea was used externally as a wash to strengthen infants. A tea of the mashed roots was used as a bath for a child too weak to walk. A tea of the root and bark was taken for fever.

The tea of the plant was taken for dysentery, for a child unable to urinate, and as an abortifacient. The leaf tea was taken for rheumatism. The plant tea or a tea of the leaves was used as an eyewash for sore eyes. The bark was packed into a sore tooth.

Peelbark Saint-John's-Wort (*Hypericum fasciculatum*)

The root tea was taken for blocked urination and constipation.

Saint-Peter's-Wort (*Hypericum crux-andreae, Hypericum multicaule*)

The root tea was taken for colic. A tea of the whole plant was taken for dysentery. The leaf tea was used as a wash for sore eyes.

Scouler's Saint-John's-Wort (*Hypericum scouleri*)

A tea of the tops was taken for a long time for venereal diseases. A tea of the whole plant was used to bathe sore feet. The plant was used to poultice wounds, cuts, swellings, and sores.

Sanicles, Blacksnakeroots

Canadian Blacksnakeroot (*Sanicula canadensis*)

The tea of the powdered root was an abortifacient. The hot tea of the root was taken for heart problems.

---

*These two plants were used in identical ways.

Maryland Sanicle (*Sanicula marilandica*)

The root tea was taken by children and used as a wash for sore navels. The root tea was also an abortifacient and was used for menstrual pain, for slow delivery of a fetus, and for rheumatism, kidney problems, fevers, and snakebite. A poultice of the pounded root was applied to snakebites.

Pacific Blacksnakeroot (*Sanicula crassicaulis*)

A poultice of the leaf was used on rattlesnake bites and wounds.

Poison Sanicle (*Sanicula bipinnata*)

The boiled plant poultice was placed on snakebites.

Purple Sanicle (*Sanicula bipinnatifida*)

The leaf tea was used on snakebites.

Snakeweeds, Plantains

Blackseed Plantain (*Plantago rugelii* var. *asperula*)

The fresh leaf poultice was applied to burns, inflammations, and swellings.

Common Plantain (*Plantago major*)

The tea of the root was used for dysentery, for diarrhea in babies, as a laxative, and for fevers, colds, and pneumonia. A poultice of the chopped root and leaf was applied to snakebite.

The leaves were bound to burns, bruises, snakebites, and insect bites. The leaf was chewed and eaten to treat stomach ulcers and chewed and applied as a poultice for sores, carbuncles, and hemorrhoids. A crushed leaf poultice was applied to bruises and used to pull pus from wounds and infections. A crushed leaf poultice was also applied to painful and rheumatic parts and swellings, burns, contusions, headaches, sprains, blisters, ulcers, cuts, boils, sores, and stings. A hot leaf poultice was used to draw thorns and splinters.

The leaf tea was taken for poisonous bites, stings, snakebite, and bloody urine. It was also used as a wash for sore eyes and as a douche, and it was applied to earaches. A poultice of the cooked flower stems was applied to abscesses. The tea of the whole plant was used for coughs, for stomach problems, and as a laxative. The tea of the seeds was used to improve digestion and regulate the menses.

Desert Indianwheat (*Plantago ovata*)

A cold tea of the seeds was used for diarrhea.

Heartleaf Plantain (*Plantago cordata*)

The raw leaf was used in poultices and salves for cuts, sores, burns, and boils.

Largebracted Plantain (*Plantago aristata*)

The root tea was taken for dysentery. The leaf tea was taken for poisonous bites and stings, snakebite, bloody urine, and diarrhea; it was also given to children to strengthen them. The leaf tea was used externally as a wash for bites and stings and as a douche for vaginal discharges. The juice was applied to sore eyes.

Mexican Plantain (*Plantago australis* ssp. *hirtella*)

The leaf poultice was used on boils and cuts.

Narrowleaf Plantain (*Plantago lanceolata*)

The root tea was used for dysentery and babies' diarrhea. The tea of the leaf was taken for poisonous bites, stings, snakebite, and earache. The leaf poultice or a tea of the leaf was applied to headaches, snakebites, burns, blisters, ulcers, and insect stings. The leaf tea was used as a douche for vaginal discharge.

Seashore Plantain (*Plantago macrocarpa*)

The tea of the roots was used as a general tonic.

Woolly Plantain (*Plantago patagonica*)

A poultice of the mashed leaf was applied to sores. The tea of the whole plant was taken for headache and for diarrhea, including bloody diarrhea. A cold tea of the whole plant was taken to curb appetite. The seed tea was used for babies' colic and for constipation.

ELK SPIRIT AND USING ELK MEDICINE PLANTS

Elk are animals that spend most of their time in same-sex social groups. Elk teaches us to value the wisdom and experience of our same-sex friends and teachers.

Spiritually, Elk medicine is connected to sexually attractive, charismatic, shamanic individuals who are recognized as social leaders. Elk medicine people are well proportioned and good looking.

Elk medicine plants act on the kidneys and build stamina and endurance.

Blue Vervain, Swamp Verbena (*Verbena hastata*)

The root tea was used for stomach flu and for cloudy urine. A tea of the leaves, seeds, and roots was taken for fever, dysentery, and diarrhea, as an abortifacient, and for "summer complaint" (acute diarrhea, especially in children, which often happened in summer). The leaf tea was taken for upset stomach.

Staghorn Sumac (*Rhus hirta*)

A poultice of the roots was applied to boils. The tea of the roots or berries was taken as a blood cleanser. The roots were decocted with Echinacea root (*Echinacea angustifolia*) for venereal diseases.

A tea of the leaf was used as a gargle for sore throat and was taken for tonsillitis and erysipelas (cellulitis caused by a strep infection). The flower tea was taken for stomach pain. A tea of the bark and flowers was used to prevent water from breaking too soon in pregnancy. The tea of the berries was taken to increase appetite, for vomiting, for bedwetting, for diarrhea, as a cough medicine, for fever, and in mixtures for tuberculosis. The tea of the berries was applied externally to sunburn blisters.

Angelicas

Brewer's Angelica (*Angelica breweri*)

The root was chewed for colds, headaches, coughs, and sore throat. A salve of the mashed root was applied to cuts and sores.

The root tea was taken for colds, chest conditions, kidney problems, tuberculosis, and whooping cough and used externally as a wash for venereal diseases. A tea of the scraped dried root was taken for flu and bronchitis. The dried root was smoked for head colds. The root poultice was applied to rheumatic pains and swellings and for pneumonia.

Hairy Angelica (*Angelica venenosa*)

A poultice of the plant was applied to twisted joints and sore muscles.

Henderson's Angelica (*Angelica tomentosa* var. *hendersonii*)

The plant tea was taken for poisoning from spoiled mussels.

Purplestem Angelica (*Angelica atropurpurea*)

The root tea was used as an abortifacient, for gas, colds, fevers, pneumonia, flu, ague, and stomach complaints, for nervous conditions, and as a gargle for sore mouth or throat. A tea of the dried root was taken to clean the blood. A poultice of the roots was applied to broken bones and a cooked root poultice was placed on swellings and painful areas. A tea of the whole plant was used in the sweat lodge for rheumatism (probably by pouring on the hot rocks) and for frostbite and exposure.

Wild Celery (*Angelica lucida*)

The leaf tea was taken for colds and sore throat and was used in the sweat lodge (probably by pouring on the hot rocks) for disease. The leaf poultice was applied for internal and external pains. The dried stems were burned to purify the home, inside and out.

Woodland Angelica (*Angelica sylvestris*)

The root tea was taken for coughs and sore throat and was mixed with Spikenard (*Aralia racemosa*) for colds and coughs.

Woolly Angelica (*Angelica tomentosa*)

The roots were chewed to prevent bad breath, for sore throat and hoarseness, and to preserve the throats of singers. The root tea was taken for colds and headaches, for diarrhea and stomachache, to ease menstrual cramps, and for menopausal symptoms, and it was used as an external wash for sores. A poultice of the roots or a fomentation of the root tea was applied externally for headaches.

Monardas

Mintleaf Bee Balm (*Monarda fistulosa* var. *menthifolia*)

The pulverized plant was rubbed on the head for headache. The dried plant or leaves were rubbed on the body and the infusion taken for fever or sore throat. The dried leaves were used to perfume horses, bodies, and clothing.

Oswego Tea (*Monarda fistulosa* var. *mollis*)

A tea of the flowers and root was taken for worms. The leaf tea was drunk by women after giving birth. The flower tea was used as an eyewash for inflamed eyes. The tea of the flower and leaf was used as a wash for children's eruptions. The moistened dried flowers and leaves were used to poultice burns and scalds.

Wild Bergamot, Bee Balm (*Monarda fistulosa*)

The root tea was taken for pain in the stomach and intestines. The tea of the leaf or root was drunk and wiped on the head for nosebleed. The chewed leaf was placed in the nose for headache. The hot leaf tea was taken for fever, measles, coughs, whooping cough, and fainting; the leaf tea was used in the bath for chills. The cold leaf tea was used as a wash for headaches, pimples, and other skin eruptions. The leaf fomentation was placed on sore eyes overnight.

A tea of the leaf and flower was used for catarrh. A tea of the leaf and plant top was taken for weak bowels and stomach and for abdominal pain. A tea of the plant top was used for colds. The flower tea was taken for colds. A tea of the stem and leaf was used as a strengthening bath for babies, and a tea of the whole plant was used as a bath for infant convulsions. A tea of the whole plant was taken for coughs and sore kidneys. The plant was boiled and the steam inhaled for catarrh and bronchial problems.

The leaf poultice was applied for headaches and to stop bleeding. A poultice of the flower heads was applied to burst boils. A poultice of the whole plant was used on cuts.

DEER SPIRIT AND USING DEER MEDICINE PLANTS

Deer teaches us to be gentle with ourselves and others, to bring about healing.

Deer medicines are very similar to Elk medicines and address many of the same conditions.

Wild Bergamot (*Monarda fistulosa*)

See uses listed for Elk medicine above.

Bedstraw, Cleavers

Fendler's Bedstraw (*Galium fendleri*)

The tea of the plant was taken for flu and applied externally to the head for headaches.

Fragrant Bedstraw (*Galium triflorum*)

The tea of the plant was taken for gallstones, kidney problems, and dropsy. A poultice of the plant was applied to the head to enhance hair growth, and the plant was rubbed on the chest as an analgesic for chest pain.

Licorice Bedstraw (*Galium circaezans*)

The tea of the plant was taken for coughs, asthma, and hoarseness.

Northern Bedstraw (*Galium boreale*)

The tea of the whole plant was used as a contraceptive, a diuretic, and a diaphoretic.

Oneflower Bedstraw (*Galium uniflorum*)

The tea of the whole plant was used as a diuretic and for fevers.

Rough Bedstraw (*Galium asprellum*)

The tea of the whole plant was taken as a diuretic, for fever, and for measles.

Shining Bedstraw (*Galium concinnum*)

The tea of the whole plant was taken for kidney problems, ague, and bladder troubles.

Stickywilly (*Galium aparine*)

The tea of the plant was taken as a laxative, as a diuretic, and for kidney problems, gravel in the urine, and urine stoppage. The cold tea was used to bathe skin conditions such as poison ivy rash and itching. Women would bathe in it as a magical aid to attract love. You can use this plant in chlorophyll-rich green juices; just blend with water and strain out the green liquid. Take one to two ounces a day, no more, or it will turn into a purgative.

Stiff Marsh Bedstraw (*Galium tinctorium*)

The tea of the whole plant was taken for lung conditions.

Threepetal Bedstraw (*Galium trifidum*)

The tea of the plant was taken for eczema, ringworm, and scrofula.

RABBIT SPIRIT AND USING RABBIT MEDICINE PLANTS

Rabbit is "deer's younger brother." Rabbit medicine is the next best thing when elk and deer medicines are not available.

Rabbit people are worn out from their constant fear of catastrophe and sickness. By dwelling on their fears, they eventually cause their own misfortune. The lesson of Rabbit is to recognize one's fear and to give it away to the Earth Mother and to the universe.

Rabbit medicines are helpful when a person is weak or malnourished and losing strength. Like rabbits, these people have become insecure; they are twitchy and nervous, with impaired immune systems, swollen glands, and a tendency to develop tuberculosis.

Bittersweet Vine, American Bittersweet
(*Celastrus scandens*)

The roots were chewed for coughs and used in salves for cancer and old sores. The root tea was drunk to clear up "liver spots" on the skin, for tuberculosis, to bring on the menses, and for stoppage of urine. The leaf tea was used as a wash for foul ulcers. A tea of the leaf and stems was taken as a diuretic, for fevers, for kidney problems after childbirth, and also for stoppage of urine. A tea of the stalks was applied to skin eruptions. The thorny branches were used to scratch rheumatic parts.

Rabbit Tobacco, Sweet Everlasting
(*Pseudognaphalium obtusifolium*)

The root tea was taken for chills. The leaf tea was taken to relieve vomiting and used as a throat wash for mumps, for fevers, and as a bath and beverage for children with fevers. The dried leaf tea was inhaled as steam for headache. A tea of the leaves and flowers was used for lung pain and for colds. A tea of the plant tops was used for insomnia and also as a beverage and wash for the aged and for people feeling they were pursued by ghosts or witches. The tea of the plant was taken for coughing, tuberculosis, and colds and was added to cough syrups. The warm tea was blown into the throat for diphtheria. A tea of the whole plant was used to wash the face in cases of insomnia or nervousness. The plant tea was massaged into scratches made over muscle cramps.

The plant was chewed for mouth sores and sore throat. A poultice of the leaves was applied to the throat during mumps. The dried stem and leaf were smoked to relieve asthma, and the smoke was blown into the nose of a person who had fainted. The leaves were burned as smudge to cause ghosts or witches to leave and to revive an unconscious person. The herb was used to flavor other medicinal formulas.

Nettles

California Nettle (*Urtica dioica* ssp. *gracilis*)

The root tea was used for dysentery, urine retention, and intermittent fever. Externally, the root tea was used as a hair wash. The root poultice was applied to swollen joints. A poultice of the leaves was used on heat rash and a hot leaf poultice was applied to rheumatic parts.

The tea of the leaves was taken for difficult labor and for colds, and it was used in the sweat lodge for rheumatic pain (probably by pouring on the hot rocks), tuberculosis, flu, and pneumonia. The powdered leaf was inhaled as a snuff for nosebleed.

The plant tips were chewed by women during labor. A tea of the whole plant was taken for bladder conditions. A tea of the stalks was used as a rub on sore and stiff body parts. A peeled bark tea was taken for headache and nosebleed.

The burning stems were used to cauterize sores and applied as moxa to swellings. The whole fresh plant was used as a whip for rheumatic parts and was used to sting paralyzed limbs to increase sensation.

Dwarf Nettle (*Urtica urens*)

The stem and root tea was used in the sweat lodge for rheumatism (most likely by pouring the tea over hot rocks).

Stinging Nettle (*Urtica dioica*)

The tea of the roots was given to pregnant women and taken for itching skin conditions and hives. The root tea was used externally as a hair tonic for long hair and as a fomentation for bleeding piles. A tea of the stem and root was used in the sweat lodge (probably by pouring on the hot rocks) for rheumatism.

The tea of the young leaves was taken for stomach upset and ague. The tea of the whole plant was taken to enhance blood flow after labor. The juice of the plant was taken for overdue pregnancy. The young shoots were eaten as a health tonic.

A leaf poultice was rubbed externally on headaches, backaches, sores, and general aches and pains as well as on the chest for pain and on the scalp to prevent hair loss. The fresh plant was whipped on arthritic and rheumatic parts and was used to whip the skin after the sweat lodge. A poultice of the steamed leaf and root was used on arthritic parts and applied to paralyzed limbs. The plant fiber was burned as a moxa to relieve headaches and swellings.

The leaf was rubbed on fishing lines to attract fish.

TURTLE SPIRIT AND USING TURTLE MEDICINE PLANTS

Some Native American indigenous cultures picture the Earth sitting on the back of a giant turtle, and the landmass of North America is called "Turtle Island." Like the Earth Mother herself, turtles have a hard outer shell, yet they are soft inside. Turtle represents the secrets of Mother Nature and her hidden ways. Turtle medicine is the oldest of medicines, the medicine of rocks and soil.

Turtle teaches us to stay grounded and connected to the Earth Mother and to view our predicaments and the foibles of others with motherly compassion. No matter how we treat the Earth, she always comes back with fresh greens and new growth for our benefit. When we ask the Earth Mother for help, she always provides.

Turtle medicines help remove gravel from the kidneys and will balance the proportion of liquids and solids in the body.

Calamus, Sweet Flag (*Acorus calamus*)
The peeled, chewed root was used for headache, diarrhea, colds, and sore throat, as a throat tonic for singers, by children with toothache, and as a styptic applied to bleeding piles. The root was carried to ward off illness, added to medicines to strengthen them, and added to an ailing horse's feed to fortify it.

The root tea was used for colds, bowel pain, menopausal symptoms, worms, convulsions, fever, gravel, kidney edema, children's colds, coughing of blood, upset stomach, gas and stomach cramps, teething, whooping cough, venereal diseases, colic, intestinal pain (with Sassafras), sore throat caused by singing, for high blood pressure, diabetes, cholera, smallpox, pneumonia, pleurisy, flu, and chills. It was also used after childbirth, as a laxative, as a sore throat gargle, and as an abortifacient. A tea made from the root and Chokecherry (*Prunus virginiana*) was used for coughs. The root tea was used externally for nettle rash and chills and in the ear for earache.

The ground root was mixed with tobacco and smoked for headaches and colds, and the smoke was sucked into a tooth for toothache. A snuff of the powdered root was taken for colds. A poultice of the roots and hot water was applied for cramps, sore chest, sore throat, sore muscles, rheumatic pains, cuts, earaches, limb swellings, lower back pain, facial paralysis, and toothache. The dried roots were cooked in sugar and eaten to sweeten the breath.

A tea of the plant was taken for colds, coughs, lung problems, fever, and gas and was given to fretful babies (infants can get the medicine via mother's breast milk).

Gravel Root, Sweet-Scented Joe Pye Weed, Queen of the Meadow (*Eupatorium purpureum*)

The root tea was taken for rheumatism, as a diuretic, as a pregnancy tonic, for dropsy and kidney problems, for gout, and as a laxative and was used as a strengthening wash for babies. The tea of the plant was taken as an antidote for poisons and for wounds. A poultice of the fresh leaves was used on burns. The hollow stems were used to spray medicines.

Richweed, Canada Horsebalm, Hardhack (*Collinsonia canadensis*)

The root tea was taken for bloody diarrhea, for kidney problems, for heart problems, and to strengthen children (as a beverage). The root tea was applied externally to rheumatic parts and boils and used as a wash to strengthen weak children. A tea of the plant was applied to sore breasts and taken as an emetic. The plant tea was used to wash horses with colic. The mashed leaf and flower were applied as a deodorant.

Oaks

In this section by "bark" I mean the inner bark, cambium, the thin green living layer underneath the dead outer bark. The best way to collect the inner bark is to scrape a branch or twig (never the trunk of a tree). When tree roots are used, the part you want is the bark of the root. These medicines are available year-round.

Blackjack Oak (*Quercus marilandica*)

A tea of the tree bark coal was taken to ease the cramps of childbirth and to release the placenta after childbirth.

Black Oak (*Quercus velutina*)

The bark tea was taken for chronic dysentery, as an emetic, after long intermittent fever, as a general tonic, and for indigestion, asthma, lost voice, milky urine, hoarseness, and lung problems. The bark tea was applied externally to sore, chapped skin, as an antiseptic, as a wash for fever and chills, and as a wash for sore eyes. The bark was chewed for mouth sores.

Blue Oak (*Quercus douglasii*)

A poultice of the ground galls and salt was applied to cuts, burns, and sores. The leaf was chewed for sore throat. (Deciduous tree leaves should only be chewed in the spring, before summer solstice. After that they will contain too many plant alkaloids.)

Burr Oak (*Quercus macrocarpa*)

A tea of the bark or root bark was taken for cramps, lung problems, heart trouble, and diarrhea, to expel pinworms, and as an abortive. The bark tea was applied externally as an astringent wash for the skin.

California Scrub Oak (*Quercus dumosa*)

A tea of the galls was used as an eyewash and as a wash for sores and wounds.

California White Oak (*Quercus lobata*)

The bark tea was taken for coughs and for diarrhea. A poultice of the ground galls and salt was placed on burns, cuts, and sores. The powdered bark was dusted on sores and placed on babies' sore umbilicus.

Cherrybark Oak (*Quercus pagoda*)
The bark tea was taken for dysentery. The bark and root bark tea was drunk for sore throats, for hoarseness, and as a general health tonic. A strong tea of the bark or root was used on swollen joints.

Chinkapin Oak (*Quercus muehlenbergii*)
A tea of the inner bark was taken as an antiemetic.

Gambel's Oak (*Quercus gambelii*)
A tea of the root bark was taken for postpartum pain, as a cathartic, and to expel the placenta.

Interior Live Oak (*Quercus wislizeni*)
The bark tea was taken for coughs and arthritis and applied as a burn dressing. The powdered bark was dusted on sores and babies' sore umbilicus.

Live Oak (*Quercus agrifolia, Quercus virginiana*)
The bark tea was taken for dysentery. The bark tea was used externally for pain and as a bath for aches and it was applied to sores, hemorrhoids, cuts, and back pain.

Northern Pin Oak (*Quercus ellipsoidalis*)
The inner bark was added to abortion compounds.

Northern Red Oak (*Quercus rubra*)
The bark and leaf tea was used as a form of bitters (however, the leaves can only be gathered before summer solstice). The tea of the root bark was taken for diarrhea. The tea of the bark was taken for chronic dysentery, after a long bout of intermittent fever, as a general tonic, and for indigestion, asthma, lost voice, hoarseness, milky urine, severe coughs, diarrhea (with fir buds or green cones added), and gonorrhea.

The bark tea was used externally for sore or chapped skin, as an antiseptic, to wash foul-smelling sores and itchy venereal diseases, as a wash to strengthen a weak child, and as a wash for chills and fever. The twig juice was taken for dysentery and used to help set loose teeth.

Oregon White Oak (*Quercus garryana*)

The bark tea was taken for tuberculosis. The pounded bark was rubbed on the belly and sides of a pregnant woman before her first labor.

Pin Oak (*Quercus palustris*)

The inner bark tea was taken for intestinal pains.

Post Oak (*Quercus stellata*)

The bark was chewed for mouth sores. The bark tea was taken for chronic dysentery, as an emetic, for indigestion, asthma, and lost voice, as a general tonic, for milky urine, and after long intermittent fever. The bark tea was applied to sore or chapped skin, as an antiseptic, and as a wash for fever and chills. The twig juice was taken for dysentery.

Shingle Oak (*Quercus imbricaria*)

The bark was chewed for mouth sores. The bark tea was taken for chronic dysentery, after intermittent fever, and for indigestion, asthma, lost voice, and milky urine. The bark tea was applied to sore or chapped skin and used as an antiseptic.

Southern Red Oak (*Quercus falcata*)

The bark was chewed for mouth sores. The bark tea was taken for chronic dysentery, as a general tonic, and for chills and fever, indigestion, asthma, lost voice, and milky urine. The bark tea was applied to sore and chapped skin.

Swamp White Oak (*Quercus bicolor*)

The bark tea was taken for cholera, broken bones, and tuberculosis. The dried leaves were smoked and exhaled through the nose for catarrh.

Wavyleaf Oak (*Quercus pauciloba*)

A tea of the root bark was taken for internal pain.

White Oak (*Quercus alba*)

The bark was chewed for mouth sores. The bark tea was taken for dysentery, as an emetic, to expel phlegm from the lungs, and for intermittent fevers, asthma, loss of voice, milky urine, coughs, sore throat, tuberculosis, diarrhea, and bleeding piles. It was also used as a disinfectant douche. The tea of the bark was applied to chapped skin and used to clean ulcers and as a liniment for muscle pain. The bark tea was given to horses with distemper and used as a liniment for horses.

Willow Oak (*Quercus phellos*)

A tea of the bark was used externally for pain, aches, sores, hemorrhoids, and cuts.

WOLF SPIRIT AND USING WOLF MEDICINE PLANTS

Wolves as animals are very conscious of their borders and boundaries, and they patrol their territory regularly. Wolf medicines relate to the conscious ego that sets firm rules and organizes life. At the same time Wolf represents the untamed wild and the unpredictable nature of wild creatures. Thus Wolf has the ability to change and transform as needed and as the moment dictates. Wolves jump at sharp right angles when chasing their prey. Wolf medicines have sharp right angles that represent this ability to change direction on a dime.

Wolves are strong individualists, yet they bond deeply with their mate and their pack. They pace the land at night, under the moon. Wolf people have strong intuitions and carry many secrets and powerful wisdom. For this reason they are the teachers who help explain the mysteries of life.

Wolves have ravenous appetites, swallowing their food very quickly in large bites. These medicines tend to act on digestion, specifically on the stomach and gallbladder.

Harvest Lice (*Agrimonia parviflora*)

The root tea was taken to build blood and to stop hunger in children. The bur tea was drunk for diarrhea and fever and to check gynecological discharge.

Spreading Dog Bane, Werewolf Root (*Apocynum androsaemifolium*)

Caution: This plant is poisonous to cattle and should not be taken in large amounts or for long periods of time by humans.

The root was chewed as a protection against sorcery. It was smoked for headache and used in poultices and teas for headache. A tea of the root was used in herbal steam; a very weak tea was given to infants with colds; the tea was also taken for heart palpitations, to increase breast milk, for stomach cramps, as a liver medicine, to expel the placenta after labor, for fever, as a diuretic, and as a urinary tract medicine. Taken once a week it was a contraceptive. A poultice of the root tea on cotton or of the mashed root was placed in the nose to stop bleeding. The dried, powdered root was used in different ways for insanity and for vertigo.

The dried leaf was smoked as an aphrodisiac. The milky sap was applied to warts. A tea of the green berries was used as a heart medicine and kidney aid.

Tall Hairy Agrimony (*Agrimonia gryposepala*)

A tea of the root was taken to build blood and for urinary complaints, and it was given to children to stop hunger. The plant tea was taken for diarrhea and vomiting. A tea of the burs was used for diarrhea and fever and to check gynecological discharge.

Solomon's Seals

Giant Solomon's Seal (*Polygonatum biflorum* var. *commutatum*)

The root tea was taken as a tonic to prevent measles and other illnesses. The root tea was inhaled as steam for headaches or sprinkled on hot stones in the sweat lodge for headaches.

Hairy Solomon's Seal (*Polygonatum pubescens*)

The tea of the root was used as an eyewash for eyes afflicted by snow blindness. The plant was used in teas for stomach gas and for spitting up of blood.

Solomon's Seal (*Polygonatum biflorum, P. multiflorum*)

The root tea was a tonic for lung conditions, for stomach problems, for profuse menstruation, and for coughs. The root was burned and the smoke inhaled to revive an unconscious person. A hot poultice of the bruised root was applied to swellings and pains.

9

HERBAL ASTROLOGY

Another invisible influence of plants is related to the astrological signs associated with them. These associations are a helpful guide to the alchemical properties and effects of the herbs. Here is a brief guide to plant alchemy.*

Plants have an affinity both to a sign of the zodiac and to the planets, Sun, and Moon of our solar system. The listing of plants below these associations shows which will help guide their effective use. As we have seen, herbs tend to direct their energies to unique organ systems and bodily functions. Some herbs will go to the lungs, others to the bowels, yet others to the skin, and so on. Planetary herbology is yet another system of plant classification where plants with specific affinities for certain emotional states, organs, and body parts are grouped together under a planetary ruler.

PROPERTIES INDICATED BY PLANETARY BODY†

Solar plants bestow positive ego strength, enhance personal will, and increase generosity, ambition, courage, dignity, and self-reliance.

---

*For more details on plant alchemy please see my book *A Druid's Herbal for the Sacred Earth Year* (Destiny Books, 1995).
†Uranus (discovered 1781) and Neptune (found in 1846) are not part of ancient astrological systems as they were unknown until modern times. Pluto, although it was not discovered until 1930 and some no longer view it as a planet, has come to be associated with sexual energies and plants that affect that sphere of life.

Managerial skills and personal authority are fostered, as is creativity.

Lunar plants facilitate past-life recall and channeling and help remove addictions and habits by relieving past-life traumas. They bring a resurgence of interest in the home and in domestic matters. They help you unwind and appreciate the simple gifts of life. They also help you be graceful and more sensitive and in tune with others. They will increase imagination.

Mercury-ruled plants enhance mental keenness, versatility, and wit and are especially helpful to writers and speakers. Mix these plants with solar and lunar herbs to increase psychic perception and the ability to manifest through the spoken word. When they are mixed with lunar herbs, psychic receptivity is increased. When mixed with solar herbs, telepathic sending is strengthened.

Venus-ruled plants increase personal magnetism and attractiveness and refine the senses. Venus promotes affection, friendship, and style. Those who seek to communicate with all types of people—musicians, actors, and artists—will find their effectiveness increased. Harmony and balance are fostered, as is communication with subtle Nature realms.

Mars-ruled plants stimulate the passions and make the user more gregarious and action-oriented. These plants can help develop the powers of telekinesis. Add them to formulas to liberate the potential of other plants. Combined with herbs of Mars, the Moon, and Mercury, they enhance the powers of manifestation.

Jupiter-ruled plants provide an expansive, affectionate mental outlook and promote an intuitive understanding of deep spirituality and of ritual. Healers, clergy, lawyers, and anyone working with pomp and circumstance will have their efforts enhanced. Jupiter is particularly allied with prosperity consciousness. Mixed with solar herbs, Jupiter-ruled plants increase an awareness of divine mercy. Mixed with Mercury-ruled plants, these herbs increase the understanding of philosophy and cosmic principles. The lighthearted, expansive joy of these herbs helps dispel depression and gloom.

Saturn-ruled plants bring sobriety and help one understand the karmic limitations of life. They bring steadying, solidifying, subtle, diplomatic, and patient energies. They are grounding to the user and will help a person focus on and finish projects. Add these herbs to any formula to ground plans and make their physical manifestation a reality.

Neptune-ruled plants are helpful in dream work and in bringing physical concepts to the next plane.

Uranus-ruled plants are often hybrids and easy to transplant, as Uranus is the planet of sudden changes. These are herbs that jump-start projects, energize, stimulate, and promote inspiration.

Pluto-ruled plants are helpful for enhancing sexuality and for harmonizing the physical and spiritual aspects of a personality.

Properties Indicated by Zodiac Affiliation

Plants of Aries deal with issues of the head, eyes, heat, headaches, and allergies.

Plants of Taurus deal with the neck, the throat, and overindulgence of food.

Plants of Gemini are for the arms and hands, nervous tension, pain, and the lungs.

Plants of Cancer benefit the stomach and the womb.

Plants of Leo help the heart, back, and spine.

Plants of Virgo are for the abdomen, intestines, and nerves.

Plants of Libra help the kidneys and issues of body weight.

Plants of Scorpio deal with the reproductive tract and stagnation in the body.

Plants of Sagittarius benefit the hips, thighs, and liver.

Plants of Capricorn help the knees, bones, and teeth.

Plants of Aquarius are for the lower legs and circulation.

Plants of Pisces benefit the feet and the lymph system.

ASTROLOGICAL NATURE OF SELECTED PLANTS

PLANT	PLANETARY BODY	ZODIAC AFFILIATION
Agrimony	Jupiter	Sagittarius
Alfalfa	Jupiter	Sagittarius
Aloe	Mars	Aries
Angelica	Sun	Leo
Arnica	Saturn	Capricorn
Ashwagandha root	Jupiter	Sagittarius
Astragalus	Jupiter	Sagittarius
Barberry root	Mars	Aries
Bayberry, Wax Myrtle	Sun	Leo
Black Alder, Buckthorn bark	Saturn	Capricorn
Blackberry	Venus	Taurus
Black Cohosh	Saturn	Capricorn
Black Haw	Saturn	Capricorn
Bladderwrack, Kelp	Moon	Cancer
Blessed Thistle	Mars	Aries
Blue Cohosh	Jupiter	Sagittarius
Blue Flag	Moon	Cancer
Borage	Jupiter	Sagittarius
Buchu	Jupiter	Sagittarius
Bugleweed	Venus	Taurus
Burdock root	Venus	Taurus
Butternut Tree, White Walnut	Sun	Leo
Calendula	Sun	Leo
Cannabis, Da Ma (Chinese)	Saturn	Capricorn
Cascara Sagrada	Mercury	Virgo, Gemini
Catnip	Mars	Aries
Cayenne	Sun	Leo
Cedar, Arborvitae, Thuja	Mercury	Virgo, Gemini
Celery seed	Mercury	Virgo, Gemini
Chamomile	Sun	Leo
Chasteberry	Moon	Capricorn
Cinnamon	Sun	Leo
Coltsfoot	Venus	Taurus

PLANT	PLANETARY BODY	ZODIAC AFFILIATION
Comfrey	Saturn	Capricorn
Coriander	Mars	Aries
Corn silk	Saturn	Capricorn
Cotton root	Mercury	Virgo, Gemini
Cramp Bark	Jupiter	Sagittarius
Damiana	Pluto	Scorpio
Dandelion	Jupiter	Sagittarius
Devil's Claw	Jupiter	Sagittarius
Dodder	Saturn	Capricorn
Dong Quai	Jupiter	Sagittarius
Dragon's Blood	Mars	Aries
Echinacea	Jupiter	Sagittarius
Elder	Venus	Taurus
Elecampane	Mercury	Virgo, Gemini
False Unicorn root	Jupiter	Sagittarius
Fennel	Mercury	Virgo, Taurus
Fenugreek	Mercury	Virgo, Gemini
Feverfew	Sun	Leo
Flax	Mercury	Virgo, Gemini
Garlic	Mars	Aries
Gentian	Mercury	Virgo
Ginger	Sun	Leo
Ginseng	Jupiter	Sagittarius
Goldenseal	Jupiter	Sagittarius
Gotu Kola	Jupiter	Sagittarius
Ground Ivy, Creeping Charlie	Venus	Taurus
Guaiacum	Venus	Taurus
Guarana	Mars	Aries
Hawthorn	Mars	Aries
Hops	Sun	Leo
Horsetail	Saturn	Capricorn
Hydrangea root	Jupiter	Sagittarius
Hyssop	Jupiter	Sagittarius
Juniper berry	Mars	Aries

PLANT	PLANETARY BODY	ZODIAC AFFILIATION
Lady's Slipper	Jupiter	Sagittarius
Lavender	Mercury	Virgo
Lemon Balm	Jupiter	Sagittarius
Licorice	Mercury	Virgo
Limeflower, Linden	Jupiter	Sagittarius
Lobelia	Venus	Taurus
Mandrake root	Mercury	Virgo, Gemini
Marshmallow root	Venus	Taurus
Milk Thistle	Jupiter	Sagittarius
Mistletoe (European)	Sun, Moon, Jupiter	Leo, Cancer, Sagittarius
Motherwort	Venus	Taurus
Mugwort	Moon	Cancer
Mullein	Saturn	Capricorn
Myrrh	Jupiter	Sagittarius
Nettles	Mars	Aries
Oak	Jupiter	Sagittarius
Orange peel	Sun	Leo
Oregon Grape root	Mars	Aries
Osha	Mercury	Virgo
Parsley	Mercury	Virgo, Gemini
Partridgeberry	Moon	Cancer
Passionflower	Moon	Cancer
Pennyroyal	Venus	Taurus
Peppermint	Venus	Taurus
Pine	Mars	Aries
Pipsissewa, Prince's Pine	Moon	Cancer
Plantain	Venus	Taurus
Pleurisy Root	Mercury	Virgo
Poke	Saturn	Capricorn
Prickly Ash	Mars	Aries
Psyllium seed	Venus	Taurus
Queen of the Meadow, Joe Pye Weed, Gravel Root	Saturn	Capricorn
Raspberry leaf	Venus	Taurus

PLANT	PLANETARY BODY	ZODIAC AFFILIATION
Red Clover	Mars	Aries
Redroot, New Jersey Tea	Moon	Capricorn
Rehmannia	Moon	Capricorn
Rhubarb root, Chinese Rhubarb root	Mars	Aries
Rose	Venus	Taurus
Rue	Sun	Leo
Sage	Venus	Taurus
Saint-John's-Wort	Sun	Leo
Sassafras	Mars	Aries
Saw Palmetto	Pluto	Scorpio
Scarlet Pimpernel	Sun	Leo
Shatavari root, Indian Asparagus	Moon	Cancer
Shepherd's Purse	Saturn	Capricorn
Siberian Ginseng	Pluto	Scorpio
Skullcap	Saturn	Capricorn
Slippery Elm	Saturn	Capricorn
Tansy	Venus	Taurus
Turmeric	Mars	Aries
Usnea	Jupiter	Sagittarius
Uva- Ursi	Venus	Taurus
Valerian	Mercury	Virgo, Gemini
Vervain	Venus	Taurus
Wahoo bark, Spindle Tree	Mercury	Virgo, Gemini
Watercress	Moon	Cancer
White Willow	Jupiter	Sagittarius
Wild Cherry bark	Venus	Taurus
Wild Lettuce, Prickly Lettuce	Moon	Cancer
Wild Yam	Jupiter	Sagittarius
Witch Hazel	Saturn	Capricorn
Yarrow	Venus	Taurus
Yellow Dock	Jupiter	Sagittarius
Yucca	Moon	Cancer

10

WORKING WITH PLANT SPIRITS

We are all flowers in the Great Spirit's garden. We share a common root, and the root is Mother Earth.

GRANDFATHER DAVID MONONGYE

As every gardener and lover of houseplants knows, plants have ways of communicating with us humans. It's obvious to us when they are "sick" or infested with some debilitating insect, and they let us know when they are thirsty or ready to mate, bloom, or bear fruit. We also know when our plants are vibrantly healthy and content.

We can interact with plants in ways that will make them happier and more fruitful. In some societies this is known as working with the elementals, gnomes, *devas* (Sanskrit, benevolent supernatural beings and forces), or fairies. Another way of looking at it is to realize that we are all connected at the quantum level and that thought and matter are part of a single continuum of Creation. An old magical maxim is: "Thoughts are things."

I have personally experienced being inside a giant Sequoia and receiving messages from the tree that came to me as a series of pictures. The tree told me that originally California had perennial green grasses and that the Wild Oat grass that has taken over in California, which turns yellow in the summer, is acting as a magnet for those who go there to find their purpose in life. It happens that Wild Oat is a Bach flower remedy for those who are seeking their true vocation, their soul's purpose.

The tree also told me that the function of the Sequoias on our planet is to act as a listening station for the stars. Each Sequoia is attuned to the stellar spheres, and when one is cut down the Earth loses a vital listening post and connection to those distant worlds, specifically the Pleiades.

It has been said by others that the best way to communicate with elementals and plant spirits is to send them a picture of your intent, mind to mind. Another essential aspect of this communication is love. I go out to the garden daily in all but the deepest snow of winter to admire the plants, see what they might need, remove bugs (by hand), and fertilize as necessary. Every good gardener will do the same, and the plants know and respond to those attentions. What is attention but love made visible? And the plants respond in kind.

I have had the experience of needing a particular plant for myself or for others. I live in a forest where there is little light and it is hard for me to grow medicinal plants, except in the fringe area around the house. Sometimes I will go outside and sing to the fairies and Plant Spirits, asking for a particular plant. Lo and behold, within a season or by the next year that plant has shown up in the garden.

Humans respond best to medicines that have been made from fresh ingredients grown or wildcrafted by a person in tune with the Plant Spirits. I teach my students to sing over or pray over each jar of medicine before they give it to a person or animal in need.

If diseases or other noxious influences are assaulting your garden or land, send love to the plants, waters, rocks, and soil to help them withstand the pressures. Bless the land, water, soil, and mycorrhizal fungi and they will respond in turn.

MAGICAL PLANT ENCOURAGEMENT

What some call "magic" is simply a ritual act that reinforces the will and intent of the practitioner. If our thoughts on a subject are strong enough, and our creative will and emotions become engaged, matter responds on the quantum level.

Here are a few practices that others have found to be successful ways to enhance our own divine creative power to manifest health and fertility for all beings.

- To increase seed germination and crop yield, try placing the seeds inside or on top of a copper pyramid before sowing. As the seeds grow, try giving them pyramid-treated water.
- Bury glass jars filled with vermiculite in a circle around your greenhouse to enhance germination.
- Water has its own intelligence, and traditional cultures have always blessed water with songs, prayers, seasonal well dressings, dances, and food offerings. Bless any water that you give to your plants. Similarly bless the food and drink that you give to your animals (and your family!).
- Create your own "love in a bottle" for your plants by putting plant food, fertilizer, seaweed, and compost—basically anything a plant would love—into a bottle with water. Bless the bottle and then add a few drops from the bottle to your watering can each time you give your plants a drink.
- Intentions are powerful. Take sections of plastic or clay pipe and fill them with crushed basalt. Write your intentions on paper and put them in the pipe sections, along with some compost and a map of your land, showing exactly what you want to effect. Plant the pipe sections in and around your land to radiate your intentions to the plant *devas*.

SINGING TO PLANTS

When gathering plants for medicine, sing to them before picking, or offer them a gift. Sing and pray as you make the brew, or charge your salves with prayer and good intent when they are finished. Singing to and praying with those who are sick is an extension of this practice.

Here are a few lovely examples. The Maha Mrityunjaya mantra, an ancient Sanskrit prayer to plants, is found in the Rig, Yajur, and Sama Vedas, ancient scriptural texts of India, and in Ayurvedic writings. In the Shiva Purana it is called *mrita sanjeevani vidya* (meaning "the knowledge that leads to everlasting life").

> I pray to the Divine Being who manifests in the form of fragrance in the flower of life and is the eternal nourisher of the plant of life. Like a skillful gardener, may the Lord of Life disentangle me from the binding forces of my physical, psychological, and spiritual foes. May the Lord of Immortality residing within me free me from death, decay, and sickness and unite me with immortality.

The following hymn to herbs is from the Rig Veda:

Oh, herbs! You are like our mothers. You are to be found in a thousand places. You have a thousand saplings. Many are the acts you are capable of performing. May you cure us of all ailments.

Oh, herbs, may you thrive and have flowers. May you look upon patients with favor. The diseases are like enemies, may you invade them like horses attacking foes. You free us from illnesses. You deliver us from disease. (Translation by Debroy and Debroy)

Here is one of many beautiful Navajo chants:

> The mountains, I become a part of it . . .
> The herbs, the fir tree, I become a part of it.
> The morning mists, the clouds, the gathering waters,
> I become a part of it.
> The wilderness, the dewdrops, the pollen . . .
> I become a part of it.

And a traditional Irish blessing:

> May the blessing of the rain be on you—
> the soft sweet rain.

May it fall upon your spirit
so that all the little flowers may spring up,
and shed their sweetness on the air.
May the blessing of the great rains be on you,
may they beat upon your spirit
and wash it fair and clean,
and leave there many a shining pool
where the blue of heaven shines,
and sometimes a star.

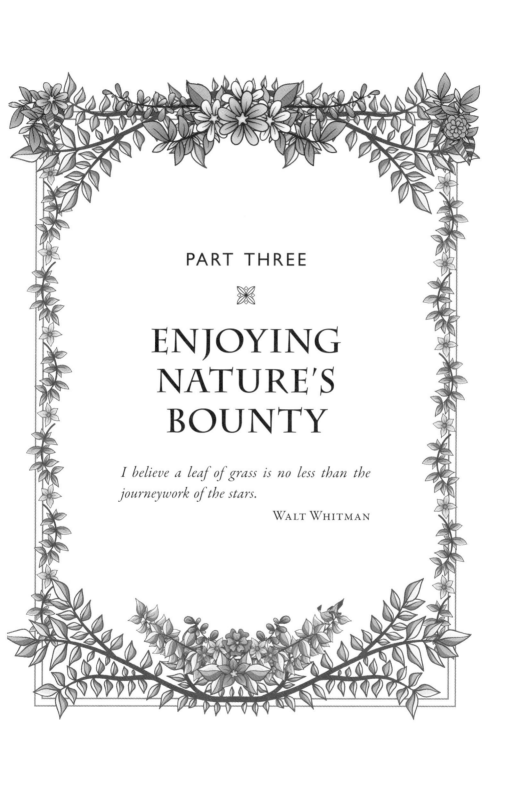

PART THREE

ENJOYING NATURE'S BOUNTY

I believe a leaf of grass is no less than the journeywork of the stars.

WALT WHITMAN

11

BEE MEDICINE

The Splendors of Honey

For thousands of years humanity has relied on bees to pollinate crops and on their honey for food and medicine. In a time when bees are threatened by the use of nicotine-based pesticides and fungicides, we need to learn all we can to protect them. Before you buy any plant make sure it has not been pretreated with bee-killing pesticides, and never spray poisons on your own garden!

Images of bees, of humans foraging for honey, and of beekeeping have come down to us from the Mesolithic. The Cuevas de la Arana (Spider Caves) in Valencia, Spain, have an eight-thousand-year-old painted image of a person climbing a vine to gather wild honey.

Ancient Egyptian images of bees and beehives appear on tombs, on obelisks (such as the obelisk of Luxor), on the Rosetta Stone, and on the pillars of the Temple of Karnak. The sarcophagi of Rameses II and other Egyptian nobles bear bee- and honey-related images.

HONEY AROUND THE WORLD THROUGH THE AGES

King Menes (4000–5000 BCE), the founder of the first Egyptian dynasty of kings, was called "the Beekeeper." The ancient Egyptians ate honey and drank a type of beer made with wheat, honey, and barley.

Egyptian papyri refer to bees, honey, and honey's medicinal powers. Jars of honey, cakes made with honey, and honeycombs were among the funeral gifts for the dead. Honey was also added to embalming fluids, and the tomb builders were once paid with honey.

Egyptian medicines were most often made with some combination of honey, wine, and milk. Egyptian healers applied honey to wounds and burns and prescribed it orally for stomach problems such as ulcers and as a general tonic to promote health.

Ancient Vedic texts describe honey as "nectar of the sun," a blend of the nectar of all flowers that represents the oneness of everything. Ayurvedic medicines have been made with honey for at least four thousand years. More than 634 Ayurvedic remedies are made with honey.

The Iron Age Celts ate salmon baked with herbs and honey. Honey was given as a thanks offering to the Earth when valuable medicinal plants were harvested. Honey mead was a favorite drink. Healing stones and stone circles were ritually purified by pouring a mixture of milk and honey over them at Lughnasad (the festival of the beginning of the harvest, usually observed in the first weeks of August). The Saxons (circa 1000 CE) used honey to treat wounds, sties, and amputations.

Ancient Georgians also placed honey in tombs around 4,700 to 5,500 years ago, to aid the deceased in their afterlife. The ancient Greeks believed that honey increased both virility and longevity. In ancient Rome honey was used to pay taxes. Cupid's arrows were said to be dipped in honey before being shot.

Traditional Chinese medicine regards honey as a cure for insomnia.

SACRED HONEY

In ancient Egypt, honey was regarded as a sacred substance—each bee was said to have been formed from the tears of the sun god Ra. As honey was considered a worthy sacrificial offering, Min, a fertility god, was given honey offerings. For Hindus honey (*madhu*) is an elixir of immortality that is poured over statues of gods and goddesses. For Buddhists, Madhu Purnima is a holy day commemorating the Buddha's retreat into the wilderness to preserve peace among his followers. While in the forest a monkey brought honey for him to eat.

In the Jewish religion honey is part of the Rosh Hashanah New Year's meal during which apple slices are dipped in honey. John the Baptist is a Christian figure said to have survived on wild honey and locusts. The Prophet Muhammad is said to have advised taking honey for health. The Qur'an mentions honey as a healing food.

Among the ancient Maya, honey was collected from stingless bees, which they regarded as sacred (and still do today).

Sacred Kyphi

Kyphi or *kapet* was an Egyptian temple incense and medicine sacred to the goddess Isis. The earliest mention of it is in the Pyramid Texts of the Old Kingdom (2400–2300 BCE). Recipes also appear in the Kyphi Ebers Papyrus (1500 BCE) and in the Papyrus Harris I. Plutarch mentions a first-century BCE text by Manetho (third century CE) called "Preparation of Kyphi-Recipes." Manetho states that the ingredients were added one at a time as magical chants were sung over them.

Kyphi was burned as incense by temple priests at dusk while Frankincense (*Boswellia* spp.) was burned at dawn and Myrrh (*Commiphora myrrha*) at midday. Dioscorides (100 CE) was the first Greek to mention kyphi, which he said was burned and also taken as a drink for asthma. In 200 CE a Syriac recipe for *kupar*, most likely a version of kyphi, was described as incense and also a remedy for liver disease, coughs, and other lung conditions.

◗ Ancient Method of Making Kyphi*

Egyptian healers prescribed kyphi as a drink to purify the body and to ease insomnia while also enhancing dreams. Several recipes for kyphi have been found, including references inscribed on the walls of the Edfu temple

---

*For a modern interpretation of kyphi and easy step-by-step instructions for how to make it, visit "Egyptian Temple Incense—Kyphi," http://magickwyrd.wordpress.com/how-to-topics/ritual-incense-recipes/egyptian-temple-incense-kyphi/.

and the Temple of Philae. Many of the recipes include some mixture of the
following plants.

- mastic (*Pistacia lentiscus*)
- pine (*Pinus* spp.) resin
- sweet flag (*Acorus calamus*)
- aspalathos (the species is not yet known; it could have been *Alhagi maurorum, Convolvulus scoparius, Calicotome villosa, Genista acanthoclada,* or *Capparis spinosa*)
- camel grass (*Cymbopogon schoenanthus*)
- mint (*Mentha* spp.)
- cinnamon (*Cinnamomum verum, C. cassia*)
- cyperus grass (papyrus grass, *Cyperus* spp.)
- juniper berries (*Juniperus phoenicea*)
- pine (*Pinus* spp.) kernels
- *peker* (an as yet unidentified species)

With a mortar and pestle grind the mastic, pine resin, sweet flag, aspalathos, camel grass, mint, and cinnamon. Grind to a powder and mix in the cyperus grass, juniper berries, pine kernels, and peker. Moisten the resulting paste with a little wine and soak overnight.

Add wine-soaked raisins and let the mixture sit again for another five days, then boil down until the liquid is reduced by one-fifth.

In a separate process, boil honey and frankincense (*Boswellia* spp.) until reduced by one-fifth. Then combine the two mixtures. Add ground myrrh (*Commiphora myrrha*) so the substance can be rolled into pellets and burned.

THE MAGICAL LORE OF HONEY

Those who have been there report that the fairy realm (Tir na n'Og, the Land of Youth) is a place of eternal spring, clear waters, sunshine, fruits, birds, flowers, and abundant honey.

Making an offering to the fairies is always a good idea because it will keep them on your side and out of mischief (one hopes). According to the lore, the fairies live underground, so offerings placed on or in the earth are always well received. Offerings of milk and honey can be poured directly on the earth or over a stone.

On the Celtic High Holy Days—Imbolc (February 2), Beltaine (May Day), Lughnasad (the first week of August), and Samhain (Halloween)—an offering can be left outside on a plate or on a fairy altar in the garden, or spilled on the ground or into a hole dug for the purpose.

Another traditional offering is a caudle. This custard-like mixture was traditionally poured into a hole in the ground. The first offering should always be given to the fairies, after which the humans may imbibe. Please note: it is useless to eat foods that have been left out as fairy offerings. Please discard any such foods after a few days because the fairies will have extracted the life-force and healing virtues from the food, rendering it unfit for humans.

To Make a Caudle

    1 pint milk

    2 tablespoons oatmeal

    ¼ tablespoon salt

    2 teaspoons honey

    ¼ teaspoon nutmeg

    Whisky or Heather Ale* to taste

Heat the milk in a pan with the oatmeal and salt. Bring to a boil while stirring, then remove from the flame and then let stand for 10 minutes.

Press the milk and oatmeal through a sieve into a clean pan and add the honey and nutmeg. Bring to a simmer, stirring well to prevent sticking.

Remove from the pan and add the whisky or Heather Ale.

A pinch of saffron can be added to give the caudle a yellow hue, symbolic of the sun.

A Different Method for Making a Caudle

Experimenting with your own variation of proportions, over a fire simmer eggs, oatmeal, butter, honey, milk, and pinch of saffron.

---

*See the recipe for Heather Ale on page 136.

MEDICINAL USES OF HONEY

> Caution: According to the FDA, children younger
> than two should not take allopathic cough and cold
> remedies. For coughs and colds, honey (1 teaspoon)
> can be safely given to children older than one.
> DO NOT GIVE HONEY TO A CHILD YOUNGER
> THAN ONE YEAR OF AGE. Honey contains
> spores of botulinum that could prove fatal.

> Caution: If bees forage on Rhododendron
> (*Rhododendron* spp.), the Tutu plant of New Zealand
> (*Coriaria* spp.), Sheep Laurel (*Kalmia angustifolia*),
> or Azaleas (subgenera of the genus *Rhododendron*),
> the honey could produce a type of intoxication or poisoning.
> (From what I have read this is only a problem if
> the bees feed exclusively on those plants.)

Honey can be used medicinally both internally and externally. When taken internally, it can help lower levels of insulin, C-reactive protein, and homocysteine. Taken alone in teaspoon doses, honey will soothe a sore throat while adding vitamins and minerals to your system. Ingesting local pollens and the pollens found in honey can build resistance to allergies over time. Make the effort to find a local beekeeper—these days they are even found in cities! Buy honey and bee pollen from the trees and flowers in your immediate area. The honey should be "raw"—that is, not heated or processed.

Honey has a highly acid pH and enzymes that create free radicals that kill off bacteria. Applied to an injury, honey creates an environment where bacteria cannot survive, as it helps the body simultaneously to dissolve dead tissue and to promote new cell growth. It creates an anaerobic seal over an injury, keeping out bacteria, viruses, and parasites. Honey thousands of years old found in Egyptian tombs was tested and was found to still have antibacterial qualities. Apply honey to skin ulcers and bedsores, burns, cuts, and abrasions.

◗ Garlic and Honey Wound Dressing

If you have a cut or a wound, wash it carefully, then apply mashed raw garlic to kill bacteria and viruses. Cover the garlic with a slather of honey and apply a clean bandage. The honey will keep the wound anaerobic (without oxygen) so bacteria will be unable to grow.

Medicinal Honey Syrups

Honey can be combined with many other herbs to make healing syrups and other preparations that are especially useful in the case of flu and other respiratory illnesses. Honey preparations can be kept for about two months when refrigerated.

To make a medicinal honey syrup: Simmer the fresh herb in water for about 20 minutes in a non-aluminum pot with a tight lid. Remove from the stove and add raw honey to taste. For a virus, use herbs such as Ginger root (*Zingiber officinale*) or Elderberries (*Sambucus nigra, S. canadensis*); for colds, use herbs such as Echinacea (*Echinacea purpurea, E. angustifolia, E. pallida*); for stomach complaints, use herbs such as Elderflower (*Sambucus* spp.), Yarrow (*Achillea millefolium*), and Mint (*Mentha* spp.); for fever, use herbs such as Willow bark (*Salix* spp.), Elderflower, and Mint.

A sore throat syrup can be made by simmering Rose petals and hips (*Rosa* spp.) in honey. To make the syrup you will need to gather very fragrant, old-fashioned red rose petals. The hips should be collected after the first frost when they are bright red. Split the hips open and remove the seeds and hairs before use.

◗ Honey Flu and Bronchitis Remedy

Slice a fresh ginger root (*Zingiber officinale*) and simmer in water, covered, for about 20 minutes (use about 3 cups of water per 6 inches of root). Remove from the stove and add a pinch of cayenne pepper (*Capsicum annuum*), raw honey to taste, and the juice of half a lemon. The ginger and cayenne help break up stubborn chest congestion and are warming to the body. The lemon adds a dose of vitamin C.

Golden Honey Immune Booster

Turmeric (Curcuma longa) is one of the strongest antioxidants known. It is also anti-inflammatory and anticarcinogenic. It builds the immune system while killing off bacteria and—unlike antibiotics, which interfere with the bacteria in your digestive tract—has a beneficial effect on intestinal flora and digestion.

For coughs, colds, and flu, mix 1 tablespoon powdered turmeric into 5 ounces of raw organic honey and store in a tightly capped glass container. For acute illness, take ½ teaspoon every hour. The next day, take it every 2 hours, and on the third day, take it three times, before meals. For chest conditions, try mixing Golden Honey into tea.

Caution: Avoid Turmeric if you have a diseased gallbladder, as it increases muscle contractions in that organ.

 Honey Throat Syrup

Blend a few peeled cloves of fresh old-fashioned (not genetically modified or "odorless") garlic with the juice of half a lemon until smooth. Add 1 cup raw honey and blend again. Take in teaspoon doses for a sore throat. (Strain any leftovers through a cheesecloth and bottle for later use.)

 Medicinal Onion Honey Syrup for Coughs

Put fresh onion slices into a jar and cover with honey. Let it sit for about 4 hours, then strain and refrigerate. Honey is a natural anti-inflammatory and the syrup may also be helpful to asthmatics.

 Old-Fashioned Remedy for Bronchitis
and Whooping Cough

Mix the juice of 1 lemon (or 1 tablespoon apple cider vinegar) with 2 tablespoons honey. Add 1 teaspoon cod liver oil and mix well. If the cod liver oil is rejected, just add more honey as a substitute. If the person taking this is elderly, add a teaspoon of whisky.

Violet Flower Syrup

The flowers of **Viola odorata** *and* **Viola canina** *are made into a syrup that is laxative and lowers a fever. It is also taken for epilepsy, insomnia, jaundice, sore throat, and headache.*

To make the syrup:

Pour freshly boiled water over an equal volume of flowers. Steep for 10 hours and then strain out the flowers.

Reheat the liquid, adding an equal portion of fresh flowers.

Let stand for 10 hours.

Do this several more times, then bring to a simmer, cool slightly, and add honey until a syrup consistency is reached.

SCOTTISH HIGHLAND REMEDIES USING HONEY

I am something of an expert in this area so I have chosen to include this small section. (If you want more details on Scottish Highland medicines, please see my book *Scottish Herbs and Fairy Lore.*) All these Highland plants grow in the northeastern United States, the area where I live.

Agrimony leaf tea: a tea made with *Agrimonia eupatoria*, sweetened with honey, is taken for liver ailments, fever, and ague.

Daisy cough remedy: *Leucanthemum vulgare*, Oxeye Daisy flowers, are simmered with honey and taken as an asthma tea and cough remedy.

Germander Speedwell for asthma and cough: *Veronica chamaedrys* is made into syrup with honey and taken for wet asthmatic conditions and wet coughs (ones that produce phlegm).

Ground Ivy cough and headache remedy: *Glechoma hederacea* is taken with tea for coughs and headaches.

Hazel nut cough remedy: *Corylus avellana* nuts are powdered and mixed with honey mead or honey water for chronic coughs.

Honeysuckle flowers for coughs and asthma: *Lonicera periclymenum* leaves and flowers are used in a honey syrup for asthma and coughs.

Houseleek for thrush: *Sempervivum tectorum* leaves and juice are mixed with honey and applied to thrush and mouth ulcers.

Maidenhair fern cough remedy: *Asplenium* spp. are infused and then honey is added to make a cough remedy.

Oats for cough, colds, and fever: *Avena sativa* is eaten as gruel with honey for coughs, colds, and fevers. The ancient Celts also mixed chopped Hazel nuts or Dandelion greens (*Taraxacum officinale*) into their oatmeal as a strengthening food for convalescents. The oatmeal was served with honey, butter, or cream.

Onion cough remedy: *Allium cepa* juice is mixed with honey for coughs.

Periwinkle laxative: *Vinca minor* flowers are simmered in honey to make a gentle laxative syrup.

Plantain for thrush: *Plantago* spp. seeds are simmered in water (one ounce of seeds per one and a half pints of water) until one pint of liquid remains, which is sweetened with honey and taken in tablespoon doses four times a day.

Wild Thyme tonic: *Thymus serpyllum* is taken as a tea with honey mixed in for coughs, heart troubles, painful menstruation, diarrhea, gastritis, anemia, headaches, and hangovers.

TRADITIONAL SCOTTISH DRINKS MADE WITH HONEY

Here are recipes for some Scottish drinks made with honey.

Hot Toddy

This is a great remedy for sore throats or at the onset of a cold.

1 inch malt whisky

2 inches boiling water, poured over a silver spoon

1 teaspoon heather honey

1 slice lemon

Other variations include a swirl of cinnamon stick, one or two cloves (*Syzygium aromaticum*), or a slice of fresh ginger root (*Zingiber officinale*).

Atholl Brose

Atholl Brose is a traditional Scottish drink based on two classic ingredients of Scottish fare: oats and whisky. According to tradition, in the year 1475 CE the Earl of Atholl went after Iain MacDonald, Lord of the Isles, who was rebelling against the king. MacDonald was known to habitually drink from a certain well, so the Earl filled it with oatmeal, whisky, and honey. When MacDonald drank from the well he became inebriated and was captured. This drink commemorates the event.

4 bottles whisky

1 pound oatmeal

1 whisky bottle full of fresh cream

1 tablespoon brandy

1 pound heather honey, slightly warmed to ease pouring

Place the whisky and oatmeal in a large container and cover with a clean linen cloth. Soak for 72 hours, then strain off the liquid and funnel it into a large jug. Gather up the remaining oatmeal in a linen cloth and squeeze out any liquid, adding it to the rest.

Mix the cream and brandy, then pour slowly into the whisky, stirring continuously. Then slowly pour in the warmed honey.

The leftover oatmeal is cooked and eaten with milk, butter, honey, or cream.

Heather Ale

*The ancient Picts are said to have made ale from heather tops (**Calluna vulgaris**) without the use of hops (**Humulus lupulus**).*

1 gallon freshly blooming heather tops

3 gallons water

2 pounds malt extract

1 pound honey

1 ounce yeast

Simmer the heather in 1 gallon of the water for about 1 hour.

Strain into the malt and honey. Stir until dissolved.

Add the rest of the water, and when the mixture has cooled to lukewarm, add the yeast.

After 24–36 hours, skim off any foam and continue to ferment. When the specific gravity of the brew reaches 1010 based on a hydrometer reading, bottle and let sit for 1–2 weeks, and then imbibe.

COOKING WITH HONEY

The darker the honey, the more nutrient dense it will be. Buckwheat honey is very dark, but some may not appreciate its strong flavor. If taste is an issue, try mixing darker honey with lighter varieties, such as clover or orange blossom.

Honey is sweeter than cane sugar per volume. In recipes use ¼ cup less honey than sugar, and if you're baking with honey add a half teaspoon of baking soda per cup of honey used and reduce the baking temperature by twenty-five degrees.

When heating honey, simmer gently (do not boil).

No-Cook Honey Syrups

Always use raw, local honey and organic fruits in your syrups. The honey will draw out the juices. For thicker syrup, use more honey and less fruit in the jar; for thinner syrup, use more fruit and less honey.

Pack a canning jar with round slices of citrus (add the zest for a stronger hit of flavor), fruits, and herbs, then fill the jar to the brim with honey. Berries can be mashed and fruit slices squeezed before putting in the honey to release their flavor.

Let the jar sit for about 4 hours, then strain and refrigerate.

The syrups will last about 2 months. Add them to sparkling water or tea, spread them on pancakes or toast, or drizzle them on yogurt or vanilla ice cream. The leftover strained-out fruit can be eaten on toast, in smoothies, on yogurt, and so on. For citrus blends, leave a few slices of citrus in the jar with the honey.

Possible combinations to try:

- lemon slices with grated ginger (*Zingiber officinale*) (1–2 lemons, 1 teaspoon grated ginger)

- clementine or tangerine with a touch of cardamom (*Elettaria cardamomum*) (1–2 sliced clementines and about 1 teaspoon ground cardamom)
- lemon slices with rosemary (1–2 lemons and 1 sprig rosemary)
- sliced limes with mint (1–2 limes, 6–8 crushed fresh mint leaves)
- orange slices with clove (½ sliced orange and 16 cloves)
- orange slices with cloves and cinnamon (½ sliced orange, 16 cloves, ½ teaspoon cinnamon)
- red rose petals (mince 1 part very fragrant, old-fashioned non-sprayed red rose petals

Other combinations to try:
- blueberries with chopped sage and lemon juice
- lemon and ginger
- strawberries with basil and lime
- peaches with lemon juice and almond extract
- chopped apple with maple syrup, cinnamon sticks, and lemon
- cherries with lemon juice and vanilla extract
- chopped pineapple with mint and lemon juice
- raspberries or cranberries with orange zest and juice

Berry-Flavored Honey

Place highly pigmented, immune-building berries such as raspberries, blackberries, strawberries, or loganberries in a non-aluminum pot. Cover with raw honey and gently bring to a simmer.

Cook for two minutes and allow to cool. Pour into jars and store in the refrigerator.

Great on waffles, pancakes, and French toast.

Herb-Infused Honey

Fill a very clean glass jar half full of fresh herbs or one-quarter full of dried herbs, such as:
- lavender blossoms (*Lavandula vera, L. angustifolia*)
- lemon balm (*Melissa officinalis*)

- chamomile flowers (*Matricaria recutita, Chamaemelum nobile*)
- basil (*Ocimum basilicum*)
- sage (*Salvia* spp.)
- mints (*Mentha* spp.)
- star anise (*Illicium verum*)
- thyme (*Thymus serpyllum*)
- vanilla beans (*Vanilla planifolia*)

Top off the jar with local raw honey, close tightly, and place in a sunny window for about a week (or longer if a stronger taste is desired). Turn the jar daily to distribute the plant matter.

Refrigerate for up to two months.

Strain and add honey to herbal or black tea, pour over vanilla ice cream, stir into oatmeal or yogurt, and mix into lemonade, sparkling water, and so on.

Ginger Ale

This is a tasty beverage that is also good for stomach flu.

Slice a large, fresh ginger root (*Zingiber officinale*), put in a pan, and cover with several cups of cold water. Simmer with a tight lid for about 20 minutes.

Remove from the heat and strain out ginger; while the liquid is still hot, add honey to make syrup.

Store in the refrigerator for up to 2 months. When you want ginger ale, place a few inches of the syrup in a glass, and then fill the glass to the top with sparkling spring water.

Cooked Honeyed Fruit

16 ounces honey
½ cup fresh fruits, such as berries, lemons, or oranges

Place your honey in a saucepan and heat gently until warmed, then slowly stir in the fruit. Please use very low heat when you do this, to preserve the flavors and nutrients.

Temper a glass jar with hot water to avoid thermal shock. Pour in the honeyed fruit, close tightly, and let stand for three days at room temperature.

Then refrigerate for up to 2 months. Use on waffles, pancakes, toast, yogurt, and so on.

AN ANCIENT BEAUTY AID

Honey protects the skin from UV rays, moisturizes, and helps lessen wrinkles, making it an ideal ingredient for beauty preparations.

Honey face mask: First lay a warm washcloth on the face to open the pores. After a few minutes, layer on some honey and leave it on the face for about fifteen minutes. Rinse off with hot and then cold water. Do this once a week for maximum effect.

To firm the skin: Mix one tablespoon of honey, one egg white, one teaspoon of vegetable glycerin, and enough flour to make a paste. Apply and leave on the face for about fifteen minutes, then rinse off.

Skin toner: Mix one-quarter cup of tomato juice with one-quarter cup of honey. Apply for about fifteen minutes and then rinse off.

Carrot face mask: Daucus carota or carrots are simmered until soft with a little honey and then applied to the face (or any area of damaged skin) as a skin conditioner.

Honey for your hair: Mix two tablespoons of olive oil, one and a half tablespoons of honey, and one egg yolk. Work into the hair and then cover with a shower cap or cloth. Leave in for half an hour and then shampoo.

12

SOME KITCHEN MEDICINES*

No herbalist should be caught without some recourse in the event of illness or injury. Sometimes the simple application of ice or cold water to an inflammation or a hot salt bath to relieve muscle pain is all it takes. And we all have herbs and spices waiting on the kitchen shelf, if we just know how to use them.

Please only buy and use organic herbs and spices. Non-organic, commercially grown herbs are sprayed with bee- and butterfly-killing pesticides such as nicotinamides, and dried non-organic herbs contain concentrated amounts of pesticide residue, which bioaccumulates in human tissue. By purchasing organic herbs and spices you will be doing your part to encourage organic farming, a practice that can ultimately preserve life on Earth.

SOME REMEDIES YOU PROBABLY HAVE ON HAND

Anise Seeds (*Pimpinella anisum*)

A tea of the seeds (you can also chew them whole) helps move gas and relieves stomachaches, coughs, phlegm in the lungs, menstrual

---

*For more on kitchen medicines, including how to use fruits, vegetables, eggs, milk, bread, and other foods to make home remedies, please see my book *The Secret Medicines of Your Kitchen* (mPowrPublishing, 2012).

cramps, and PMS. Nursing mothers can use it to increase breast milk.

To make the tea: Simmer one teaspoon of the seeds per cup of water for a minute and then remove from the heat and steep for ten minutes. Take up to one and a half cups per day in tablespoon doses.

Basil (*Ocimum basilicum*)

Use the fresh or dried leaves to soothe digestion, stomach cramps, and constipation and to ease headaches and depression. The tea will help the lungs when there is catarrh.

To make the tea: Steep one teaspoon per half cup of freshly boiled water. Take up to one and a half cups a day in tablespoon doses (adding honey will help a cough).

Every summer I collect fresh Basil leaves and steep them in vodka for at least six weeks. Then, for every two cups of vodka I add an equal amount of water into which one to two cups of organic sugar have been dissolved by heating. I let that mixture sit for six months, and it makes a lovely Basil liqueur. After experimenting with different varieties of Basil I decided I liked "Thai Basil" the best, due to its spicy flavor.

Bay Laurel (*Laurus nobilis*)

Bay leaf helps expel gas and stimulates the liver. The hot tea benefits circulation, is warming to arthritic and rheumatic conditions, and helps dispel phlegm from the head, sinuses, throat, and lungs. The tea also promotes a speedy childbirth and helps bring on suppressed menstruation. *To make the tea:* Crush three large leaves, simmer for ten minutes in one cup of water, then remove from the heat and steep for about four minutes. Add cinnamon if desired for flavor. Take one cup a day in quarter-cup doses.

Caution: Bay leaf should be avoided by pregnant women.

Laurel berries are strongly aromatic and a more powerful digestive stimulant than the leaves. The leaves and berries can be added to herbal salves for bruising and for arthritic and skin conditions. The crushed fresh fruits and leaves or a strong tea of the same can be made into a paste with honey and applied to the chest for congestion and colds.

California Bay Laurel (*Umbellularia californica*) has similar properties and is a bit stronger. When I last visited California I gathered fresh California Bay Laurel leaves and added them to a beeswax and olive oil salve. It makes a nice liniment for achy joints, bruises, and skin conditions.

Black Pepper (*Piper nigrum*)

Black pepper stimulates digestion and relieves gas. It is warming to the body and helps neutralize toxins when added to meat dishes. Add a few peppercorns to a medicinal decoction when you have a cold. You can also mix powdered black pepper with honey and eat it to help remove phlegm from your system.

Caraway (*Carum carvi*)

Caraway is another seed that helps expel phlegm, improve digestion, and move gas out of your system. Chew the whole seeds or make a tea for menstrual cramps. The tea will also help increase breast milk and, when taken by the mother, can ease colic in a baby via her breast milk.

To make the tea: Briefly simmer three teaspoons of ground or crushed seed per half cup of water or milk and then remove from the heat and allow to steep for about ten minutes. Take up to one and a half cups per day.

Cardamom (*Elettaria cardamomum*)

Cardamom is one more seed that aids digestion and strengthens the stomach; it is also mildly useful in dispelling gas. Try adding a pinch to a cup of black tea or put a few whole pods into the pot as you steep your brew.

Cayenne (*Capsicum annuum*)

My teacher, William LeSassier, taught a quick method to help a person who is having a heart attack—just pour Tabasco sauce into their mouth (be sure to also call an ambulance!). Tabasco is basically red pepper tinctured in vinegar.

Cayenne is wonderful for moving phlegm out of your system— add a pinch to any herbal tea when you are suffering a cold. It actually benefits digestion and can help ward off illness when flu and colds are making the rounds. Take a capsule a day to avoid getting a cold, but avoid overuse and never take Cayenne capsules on an empty stomach! (It won't hurt you but you will regret it; the burning can be intense.)

Mix Cayenne pepper with vinegar and rub the liniment into arthritic joints. If you cut yourself with a knife in the kitchen, reach for the powdered Cayenne. It aids in clotting and stops bleeding (just don't get any into your eyes—it stings like crazy).

Celery (*Apium graveolens*)

Many people throw away the leaves of celery, preferring to eat only the stalks, but the leaves are good medicine and can be made into tea or added to soups. The leaves help edema, rheumatism, gas, lung conditions, phlegm, and chronic skin conditions and may bring on menstruation. The leaves are diuretic so they should be avoided by those with kidney issues.

Caution: Avoid large amounts of Celery during pregnancy.

Blend Celery stalks and raw lettuce with a little water to make a drink that soothes the nerves and benefits skin eruptions that result from nervous conditions. Take it several times a day.

The seeds can be made into a tea for coughs, colds, gas, bronchitis, and nervous conditions. Regular use of the tea can help relieve rheumatic pains over time. *To make the tea:* Simmer half a teaspoon of Celery seed per half cup of water for five minutes.

Cinnamon (*Cinnamomum verum*)

Add Cinnamon to dishes such as teas, applesauce, and oatmeal to help break up a cold, break a fever, or ease rheumatic complaints. Taken over time, cinnamon capsules have been shown to help lower bad cholesterol levels, and Cinnamon tea is a great remedy for diarrhea.

To make the tea: Just break up one Cinnamon stick or put about one and a half teaspoons of powdered Cinnamon per cup into a pot of freshly boiled water and steep for ten minutes. Add milk or lemon and honey to taste.

Clove (*Syzygium aromaticum*)

Clove helps increase circulation, as it speeds up the metabolism. Simmering a few Cloves in water can make a tea to relieve nausea, gas, and hiccups and improve appetite (it's even considered an aphrodisiac!).

To make the tea: Steep one tablespoon of freshly ground cloves per cup of freshly boiled water for ten to twenty minutes. Strain and sweeten to taste. Or simply add a few Cloves to the teapot when you make black tea.

The oil of Clove is a nice stopgap measure when there is tooth pain and you have to wait to see a dentist. Pour a very small amount of clove oil on a cotton swab and apply gently to the affected area. Be careful not to swallow the oil because too much of it can damage the liver. Then call your dentist!

Cumin (*Cuminum cyminum*)

This is the herb that gives Mexican food its characteristic flavor. When added to bean dishes, it helps prevent gas, and the seeds can be chewed after a meal to relieve or prevent gas, bloating, and digestive upsets.

To make the tea: Add about one teaspoon of the seeds to a cup of freshly boiled water and steep for five minutes. Add honey to taste if desired.

Dill (*Anethum graveolens*)

Dill seeds are slightly diuretic and relaxing to the nerves of the stomach and they can help soothe menstrual pains. The seeds can be chewed for bad breath and to increase breast milk in nursing mothers (for the latter purpose try mixing the seeds with anise, coriander, fennel, or caraway).

Dill tea can help an upset stomach, gas, or insomnia and increase the appetite (add a little white wine to boost the effects). The tea has been used as an eyewash for diseases of the cornea (be sure to first filter carefully through an organic coffee filter). *To make the tea:* Steep two teaspoons of the seeds in one cup of freshly boiled water for fifteen minutes. Take in half-cup doses, up to two cups a day.

Fennel (*Foeniculum vulgare*)

Fennel seeds (and spring-gathered roots, too, if you have them) are used to dispel gas, bring on breast milk, and help digestion. Cramps and colic can be eased by Fennel tea and it is also useful to expel phlegm and catarrh. Oil of Fennel can be rubbed on painful arthritic limbs. The tea of the seeds has been used as an eyewash for eyestrain and other irritations (be sure to filter carefully with an organic coffee filter before you apply to your eyes).

To make the tea: Steep one tablespoon of seeds per cup of water for five minutes, then strain and sweeten to taste. For an eyewash, bring one cup of water and half a teaspoon of seeds to a boil and then strain carefully. Apply when cool, three times a day.

Taken with honey, Fennel is a natural cough remedy. Try mixing the slightly cooked chopped roots into raw local honey; allow the roots to steep for a few months.

Fennel leaves and flowers make a very nice herbal liqueur (see the recipe on page 33).

Garlic (*Allium sativum*)

Garlic benefits fevers and poor digestion, and it helps the liver and gall-bladder. It also helps clear plaque from the arteries and balances or lowers blood pressure. For antibiotic and antiviral effects, it is best taken raw. Please use only old-fashioned stinky Garlic. The "odorless" variety has been genetically modified and is far less effective. Soak Garlic in local raw honey, and when you need a cough or sore throat remedy, blend honey with fresh lemon juice or organic apple cider vinegar, and sip. For intestinal worms, make a strong tea of Garlic and grated fresh Ginger, strain, and use in enemas.

Everybody needs to have Garlic in the kitchen and use it liberally in their cooking. Garlic can be slipped under the skin of a chicken before roasting, added to stir-fries and soups, chopped and added to hamburgers, chopped and mixed into butter and slathered on bread, chopped into salads, or even swallowed in pill-sized pieces. Eating a sprig of fresh parsley and a teaspoon of honey after eating Garlic is supposed to prevent alliaceous breath.

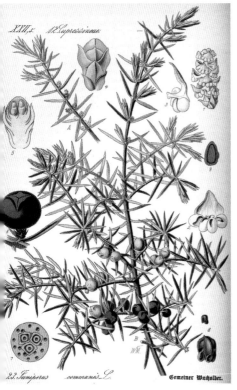

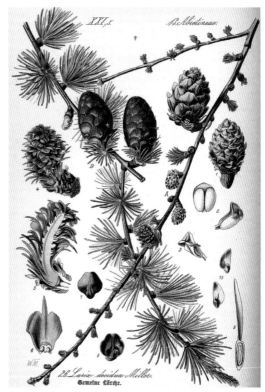

Plate 49 (left). Juniper (*Juniperus communis*)

Plate 50 (right). Larch (*Larix decidua,
L. europaea, L. laricina*)

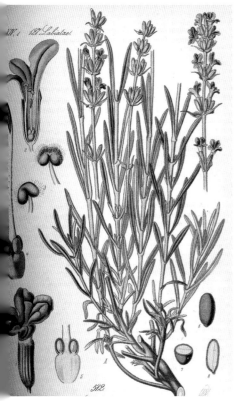

Plate 51. Lavender (*Lavandula vera,
L. angustifolia*)

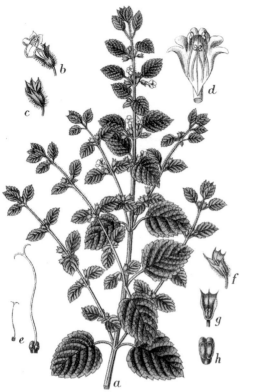

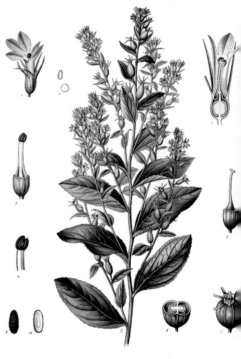

Plate 52 (left). Lemon Balm (*Melissa officinalis*)

Plate 53 (right). Lobelia (*Lobelia inflata*)

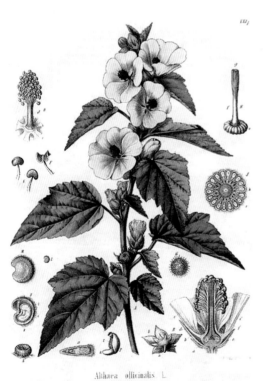

Althaea officinalis L.

Plate 54. Marshmallow (*Althaea officinalis*)

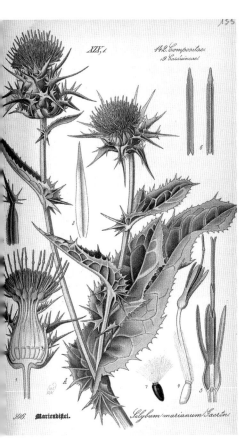

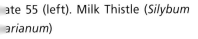

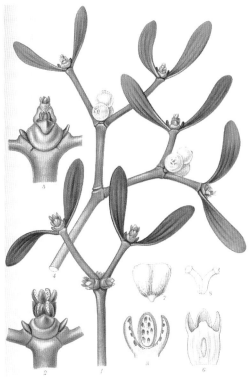

Plate 55 (left). Milk Thistle (*Silybum marianum*)

Plate 56 (right). Mistletoe (European) (*Viscum album*)

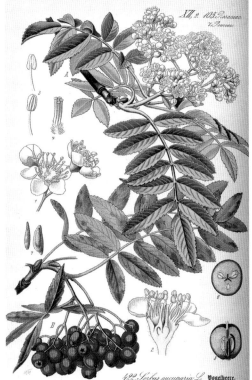

Plate 57. Mountain Ash, Rowan (*Sorbus americana, S. aucuparia*)

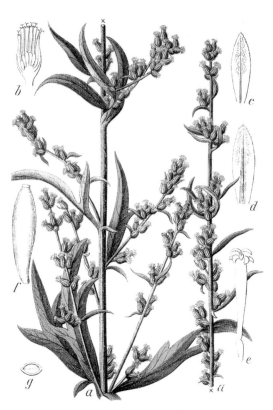
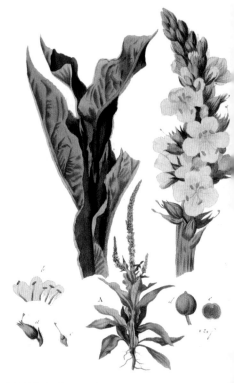

Plate 58 (left). Mugwort (*Artemisia vulgaris*)

Plate 59 (right). Mullein (*Verbascum thapsus*)

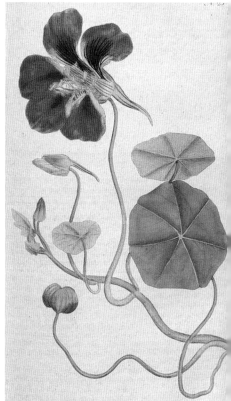

Plate 60. Nasturtium (*Tropaeolum majus*)

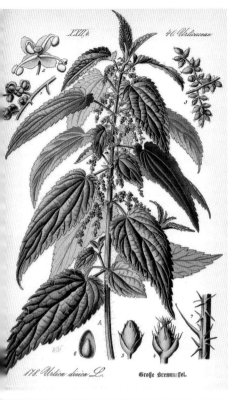

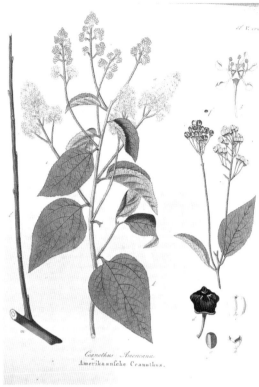

Plate 61 (left). Nettles (*Urtica dioica*)

Plate 62 (right). New Jersey Tea, Redroot (*Ceanothus americanus*)

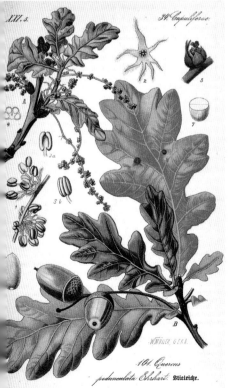

Plate 63. Northern Red Oak (*Quercus rubra*)

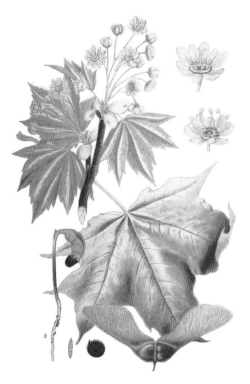

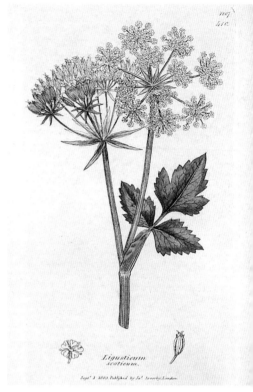

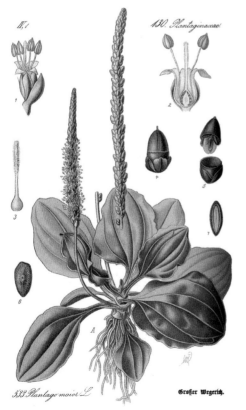

Plate 64 (left). Norway Maple (*Acer platanoides*)

Plate 65 (right). Osha, Fernleaf Licorice Root (*Ligusticum porteri, L. filicinum*)

Plate 66. Plantain (*Plantago major*)

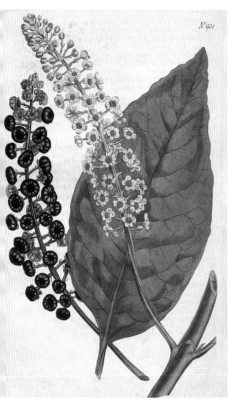

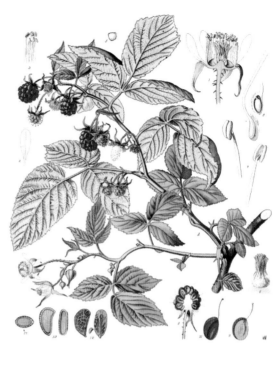

Plate 67 (left). Poke (*Phytolacca americana*)

Plate 68 (right). Raspberry (*Rubus idaeus*)

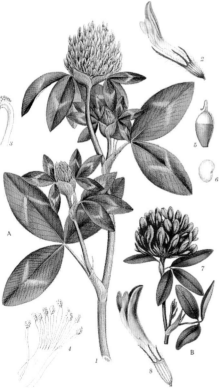

Plate 69. Red Clover (*Trifolium pratense*)

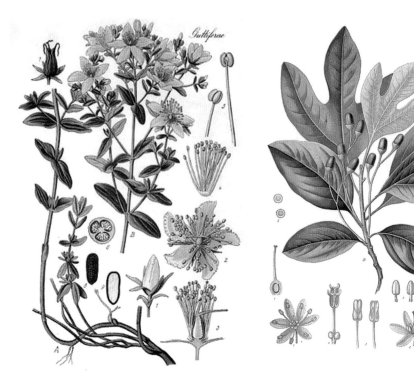

Plate 70 (left). Saint-John's-Wort (*Hypericum perforatum*)

Plate 71 (right). Sassafras (*Sassafras albidum*)

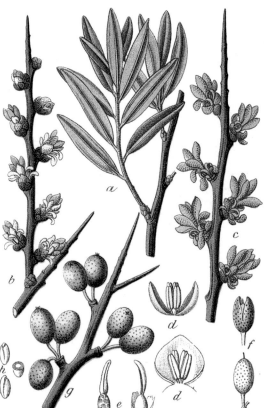

Plate 72. Sea Buckthorn, Hippophae (*Hippophae rhamnoides*)

For a sore throat remedy: Place unpeeled cloves of raw Garlic in a pan and dry-roast until they are soft to the touch. Remove from the pan and cool. Peel and eat the resulting soft Garlic paste. (It is also excellent any time when spread on toast or crackers.)

For a cold: Steep peeled cloves of garlic in brandy for two weeks, strain, and keep for up to a year. Take five to twenty-five drops in hot water every few hours.

Here is an idea for a way to use Garlic scapes:

Garlic Scapes and White Bean Dip*

⅓ cup sliced garlic scapes

1 tablespoon fresh lemon juice

½ teaspoon coarse sea salt

Ground black pepper

15 ounces cooked cannellini beans

¼ cup cold-pressed, extra virgin olive oil

Puree the scapes, lemon juice, sea salt, black pepper, and beans. Slowly stir in the olive oil, adding a little water at a time, until dip consistency is achieved. Season to taste with more lemon juice, sea salt, and black pepper as desired.

Center the dip on a plate and drizzle with olive oil on top and a little more sea salt.

Ginger (*Zingiber officinale*)

I always have fresh Ginger on hand in the kitchen. Ginger is a classic for upset digestion and in capsules it can even prevent seasickness. Sometimes if there is a very humid, long summer, the plant actually sprouts on my kitchen counter. That's when it gets potted.

In winter I often make Ginger tea, which is warming and has antibacterial properties. *To make the tea:* Use about two inches of fresh, chopped root per cup of water (simmer for fifteen minutes) or

---

*Adapted from "White Bean and Garlic Scapes Dip," www.nytimes.com/2008/06/18/dining/183arex.html.

half a teaspoon of powdered Ginger per cup of freshly boiled water (steep for fifteen minutes). Take up to two cups a day (no more or it can actually become an irritant) in quarter-cup doses. I drink the tea with honey and lemon or add it to black tea. If I have a wet cold and need to expel mucus from my system I will add a small pinch of Cayenne to the Ginger tea.

A stronger tea can be added to the bath to warm the body and help break a fever.

Horseradish (*Armoracia rusticana*)

If you are a fan of sushi you may have tried Wasabi (*Wasabia japonica, Eutrema japonica*), which is not really a horseradish but a paste that has very similar effects. You may also have noticed that it goes right up your nose to your sinuses. Horseradish does the same thing, hinting at its virtue in healing sinus infections and head colds. It is a key ingredient in Fire Cider (see page 51 for instructions) and can be mixed into tomato juice or a mixed vegetable juice (along with Lemon, Garlic, and Cayenne) to make a fabulous cold cure. You can also eat it with red meats to counteract toxins.

Juniper (*Juniperus communis*)

Traditional Dine (Navaho) birth practices included giving a newborn baby the juice of the inner bark of Juniper. A woman gathered the white inner bark and steeped it in warm water until the water gained a reddish tinge. A teaspoon of the liquid was given to the newborn to cause it to vomit mucus and any of the birth water it may have swallowed. Among the Zuni, Juniper berries and twigs were steeped and taken as tea by women during labor and afterward to cleanse the uterus.

Caution: Pregnant women should avoid the berries until the onset of labor.

Gout and rheumatic conditions will benefit from Juniper, as will colds and chills. Juniper is a gentle liver cleanser and tonic. Juniper is said to help clean and disinfect the kidneys and urinary tract (but should be avoided if you have severe kidney disease). Juniper berries can be added to red meat as it cooks to neutralize toxins. Chew Juniper berries whole (but no more than two berries a day) or make a tea to help digestion and dispel gas.

To make the tea: Steep one teaspoon of crushed berries per half cup of freshly boiled water for five minutes and strain. Take up to one cup a day in tablespoon doses.

Marjoram (*Origanum marjorana*)

According to herbal folklore, planting Marjoram around the home will help dispel melancholy. Marjoram is a digestive tonic that calms spasms, dispels gas, and helps with abdominal cramps. Taken in tea it can benefit coughs, other lung issues, and nervous complaints.

To make the tea: Steep three teaspoons of the herb per cup of water and take up to two cups a day in quarter-cup doses. A stronger Marjoram tea can be added to bathwater to calm the nerves, and the herb can be dried to make a calming sleep pillow (try adding dried Lavender, Heather, and Catnip to the pillow as well).

The flower tea helps with seasickness; women who are prone to PMS should try it starting three or four days before their period.

Mustard (*Brassica hirta, Brassica nigra*)

Warming mustard was once a stock ingredient in the medicine kit of every domestic physician. Steep three to four ounces of mustard powder in a cloth bag (or an old sock or nylon stocking) for five minutes in a basin of hot water to make a foot bath to ward off chill and lower a fever. Larger amounts (seven to nine ounces) can be steeped and then added to a bath for the whole body.

 ## Making a Mustard Plaster*

*Both white mustard (*Brassica hirta*) and black mustard (*Brassica nigra*) can be made into a plaster to pull toxins and move chest congestion.*

---

*Adapted from the Wellspring School for Healing Arts, "Mustard Plaster—For Stubborn Chest Congestion," http://thewellspring.org/mustard-plaster-for-stubborn-chest-congestion.

*White mustard is hotter and its action is more lung-centered. Black
mustard is milder and more centered on the digestive tract.*

Mix 1 part of powdered mustard seeds with 10 parts rice, buckwheat, or rye
flour (some people are allergic to white flour so it's best to avoid it). Add
enough warm water to make a paste and spread on a clean cloth.

Apply gauze to the lung area of the chest and cover the nipples with
bandages to protect them. Apply the mustard plaster over the gauze. Leave
in place for about 20 minutes (10 minutes for a child), or until the burning is
too intense. Avoid areas of sensitive skin.

Remove the plaster and thoroughly clean the area. Repeat once a day for
3 days. Any redness (this is normal) or burning will be gone in a few days.

Nutmeg (*Myristica fragrans*)

Nutmeg is the seed of a tropical tree. Small amounts of the powder
made from the seed can help digestion and improve appetite. Nutmeg
powder can be sprinkled on rich, creamy desserts to counteract mucous
formation in the body.

**Caution: eating just two of the whole Nutmeg seeds
could prove fatal.**

Oregano (*Origanum vulgare*)

Oregano leaf can be chewed or added to foods to improve digestion; it
will also help clear phlegm from the lungs and digestive tract (which
may be a reason it has been traditionally put into cheesy and pasta-rich
Mediterranean dishes). Oregano is a strong antioxidant, which may
reduce "bad" cholesterol. (Thyme does too, so why not combine them
for a stronger effect?)

Oregano is antiviral and anti-inflammatory and may even have cancer-
preventing properties. Whether eaten or taken as a tea, Oregano has been
used for urinary conditions, painful menstruation, coughing, asthma, and
arthritis. Oregano tea can also be used as a gargle for mouth irritations.

To make the tea: Steep three teaspoons of fresh herb or one teaspoon of dried herb per cup of water for five to ten minutes, then add
honey to taste.

Peppermint (*Mentha piperita*)

Peppermint tea is a nice digestive aid that also helps lower body temperature when there is a fever (drink it as hot as possible for the latter effect). Taken with honey (try adding some fresh lemon peel to enhance the flavor), it can soothe a sore throat, ease insomnia, stop nervous vomiting, lessen a headache, and even stimulate your sex life (it's a reputed aphrodisiac).

To make the tea: Steep three teaspoons of Peppermint leaf per cup of freshly boiled water. Take up to two cups a day in quarter-cup doses, for about a week. Take a break for a week and then resume if wanted.

> **Caution: Continuous use of Peppermint may result in heart issues.**

Externally, a strong Peppermint tea can be added to a cool compress for a headache and can ease heat exhaustion by being applied cold to the temples, wrists, armpits, and groin. Use it as a wash for itching skin or add it to the bath.

 ## Mint Mouthwash

This mouthwash is good for bad breath, sore gums, and canker sores.

1 teaspoon baking soda
4 drops essential peppermint oil (*Mentha piperita, M. balsamea* Willd.)
4 drops lemon or clove essential oil (*Syzygium aromaticum*)
4 drops tea tree essential oil (*Melaleuca alternifolia*)

Boil 1 cup of water for 20 minutes, allow to cool, and then pour the water into a jar that has a tight lid. Add the baking soda and peppermint, lemon/clove, and tea tree essential oils and then shake.

Do not swallow the mixture; just gargle and swish in your mouth (if more sweetness is desired add a packet of Stevia). The mixture will last about a week and does not need refrigeration—shake the jar before each use.

> **Caution: Make sure the essential oils are therapeutic grade, from an herbalist or health food store.**

Sage (*Salvia officinalis*)

Sage tea is drying to the body; it can dry up breast milk and also wet, mucusy conditions such as bronchitis. It can help dry excessive perspiration and night sweats. Nervous conditions, menstrual problems, depression, vertigo, diarrhea, and upset stomach may be eased by Sage tea.

To make the tea: Steep one teaspoon of Sage leaf per cup of freshly boiled water for thirty minutes. Take up to one cup a day in tablespoon doses for no longer than two weeks.

Sage makes a nice gargle for sore throats and the leaves or tea can be applied as a poultice or wash for insect bites and rashes.

Native American White Sage (*Salvia apiana*) has similar qualities. The wild Lyre-Leaved Sage (*Salvia lyrata*) is stronger and should only be used in mixtures. Native American herbalists used the root in healing salves and the whole plant was taken in teas for coughs and colds, nervous conditions, and asthma, as a laxative, and as a diuretic.

Sage can be taken to counter addiction to sweets and even excessive sexual cravings, but overuse of Sage could cause poisoning symptoms. My old teacher, William LeSassier, used to say that overuse of this herb will make you "boring."

Tarragon (*Artemisia dracunculus*)

Another herb that is added to bean dishes and other foods, Tarragon helps digestion, relieves colic and gas, eases insomnia, and is mildly sedative.

To make the tea: Steep half a teaspoon of herb per half a cup of water and take up to one cup a day in quarter-cup doses. Add Mint to improve the flavor of the brew.

> **Caution: Tarragon tea brings on menstruation and should be avoided by pregnant women.**

Thyme (*Thymus vulgaris*)

Another herb that improves digestion and relieves gas, aromatic Thyme is also a great herb for the lungs. Antimicrobial and expectorant, it can help with bronchitis and loss of voice, especially when gathered fresh.

To make the tea: Steep one teaspoon of dried herb or half a teaspoon of fresh herb in half a cup of water for five minutes. Take up to a cup a day in tablespoon amounts for no longer than two weeks.

Caution: Overuse of Thyme tea may irritate the thyroid gland and lead to poisoning.

A stronger tea can be added to the bath for paralysis, rheumatic pains, bruises, and swellings. Thyme can also be added to herbal salves.

Turmeric (*Curcuma longa*)

This spice is most commonly used in Indian curry. Whether eaten or made into a tea, it is beneficial to the liver, helps digestion, and can ease arthritis and rheumatism. It is an immune booster that has been recommended in anti-cancer strategies. Turmeric also benefits hypertension and can help lower blood sugar levels. Mixed into warm milk, it is a classic remedy for joint and muscle pain.

To make the tea: Simmer half a teaspoon in one cup of milk (for the joints and for tissue repair) or water (for liver detox) for few minutes.

Another method to make a nice anti-inflammatory tea is to mix powdered Turmeric with honey and powdered black pepper. When you need the tea, just put a tablespoonful of the paste in a cup, pour in hot water, and add lemon to taste if desired.

According to Tibetan medicine:

Take Turmeric before meals to benefit the lungs and throat.
Take it with a meal to enhance digestion.
Take it after meals to aid the colon and kidneys.

Turmeric powder can be combined with grated or powdered Ginger and olive oil to make a liniment for arthritic joints.

13

HEDGEROWS ARE FOOD, MEDICINE, AND MAGIC

For the ancient Celts all boundaries were liminal, magical places, whether the boundary between day and night (dawn, dusk), the boundary between the water and the land, or the portals between summer and winter (Beltaine and Samhain). The same applied to boundaries in the landscape. Offerings such as bog butter were often left for the spirits of place at the spot where two landholdings met.

In Scottish tradition it was important to *saine* (sanctify or purify) the boundaries of your land yearly by "walking the bounds" with a flaming torch, making a sun-wise circuit. The house, the barn, the herds, and the land could also be sained with salt or salt water, especially water taken from the ninth wave of the sea.

According to ancient Irish Brehon law, a boundary could be marked by a standing stone or large natural rock, a ditch, a tree, water, or a roadway. Another sturdy boundary marker was the living hedge or hedgerow.

Hedgerows have been around since the Neolithic farming revolution (four thousand to six thousand years ago), used to protect the crops and animals from predators. Bronze Age and Iron Age peoples also made walls of living plants, often using plants with thorns, as their version of modern barbed wire.

A version of this chapter originally appeared in *The Witches' Almanac* 34 (2015–2016).

Hedgerows might incorporate trees or be made of bushes or vines. Ideally the structure was half earth and half hedge. A dirt wall lay at the base, shored up with stones laid against it, to prevent erosion and stop animals like rabbits from burrowing into the sides.

MAKING A HEDGEROW

If a hedgerow is made of trees they are planted about thirty feet apart, to permit enough sun for growth, with the distances between them staggered for a more natural effect. If the hedgerow is made of bushes, these can be trimmed regularly to promote bushy growth (but it may take a few years for the hedge to produce fruit and flowers after trimming).

Interweaving or pleaching is done by making cuts at the base of stems and bending the branches between wooden stakes to form a woven wall of vegetation.

The mystical aspects of the trees and shrubs used in boundary marking should always be considered, especially if your hedgerow is designed to protect a sacred enclosure. Consider a mix of species, so that your hedge will provide flowers, fruits, and showy foliage throughout the year.

Here are samplings of useful hedge plants that will provide food and medicine for animals and people, as well as protect the sacred boundaries of the land.

Hedge Plants Suitable for Southern Areas

Camellia
(*Camellia japonica, C. reticulata, C. sasanqua,* and others)
These shrubs provide lovely, fragrant flowers and have the advantage of blooming in late fall, winter, and early spring. Camellias are an herb of the Moon.

Hibiscus or Rose Mallow
(*Hibiscus rosa-sinensis*)
The large flowers of this woody shrub come in different colors, depending upon the species and age of the plant. They attract bees, butterflies,

and hummingbirds and can be made into a delicious beverage tea that contains vitamin C and minerals, acts as a refrigerant (brings down the temperature in fevers), and lowers blood pressure.

White-flowering Hibiscus is an herb of the Moon. Pink- or red-flowering Hibiscus belongs to Venus.

New Jersey Tea, Redroot (*Ceanothus americanus*)

Deer will relish the twigs in winter and the white flowers attract butterflies. The seeds are eaten by wild turkeys and quail.

The leaves can be used as a beverage tea; the root and flowers can be used as dyes; and the bark of the root benefits colds, fevers, snakebites, stomachaches, spleen inflammation, and lung conditions such as asthma and bronchitis. The root bark tea can also help lower blood pressure.

The flowers were used by Native American women as a fragrant body wash in preparation for marriage.

Orange Jessamine, Mock Orange (*Murraya paniculata*)

An evergreen, tropical, white-flowered tree that in some species produces small orange or red fruits. In tropical areas the tree blooms year-round, attracting bees and birds. (A similar plant for more northern areas is Gardenia.) The leaf extract has been used to treat diarrhea and inflammation.

For the Javanese this herb is a symbol of wisdom and is said to protect the house from bad luck. It is used in wedding ceremonies to bring a joyful union, and in funerals to make a fragrant bed for the deceased.

North American Hedge Plants

Apothecary's Rose (*Rosa gallica* var. *officinalis*)

The advantage of this variety is that it can tolerate semi-shade. Rosehips are soothing to mucous linings in the throat and intestinal tract and contain vitamin C to boost the immune system and ward off colds. The flowers are very fragrant and the scent of rose is a natural antidepressant. The petals can be used as a beverage tea, in jellies, as a douche, and to wash sore eyes.

Rose is an herb of the Moon and belongs to Venus. Roses symbolize love, beauty, and joy and bring passion to a wedding or handfasting.

Barberry (*Berberis vulgaris*)

This thorny bush produces yellow flowers in the spring and showy berries that turn from green to yellow to red in the fall. The berries are edible and rich in vitamin C. They contain a good amount of pectin and are used to help jams gel. They are added to rice pilaf in Iran.

The ripe berries are used in teas and syrups to treat colds, flu, fever, and infections, and they may be rubbed on sore gums. The fall-gathered bark of the root is a liver medicine. The berries, root, or leaves can be sewn into an amulet for protection from evil. Barberry is an herb of Mars.

Blackberry (*Rubus villosus*)

Walking along country roads in Ireland, you may come upon large hedges of blackberry. The thorny bush provides protection for the farm and luscious fruits for jams, jellies, and ice cream. The berries are slightly astringent and help with diarrhea; the bark of the root is a much stronger antidiarrheal. The leaves are applied to burns to relieve pain and chewed to help bleeding gums. Blackberries are sacred to Brighid, a triple fire goddess. This is an old healing charm used when applying the leaves to a burn:

> *Three ladies come from the east,*
> *One with fire and two with frost.*
> *Out with fire and in with frost.*

Blackberry is an herb of Venus.

English Holly (*Ilex aquifolium*)

This hedge plant makes a dense evergreen wall with lovely white flowers and, later, the classic red berries. It has leaves that can be used as tea for coughs, colds, flu, and bronchitis. Holly tea also benefits gout, bladder conditions, and arthritic complaints.

Prickly Holly is a warrior herb that sharpens the wits and bestows courage. Make Holly water by steeping the herb in water under the full moon, and sprinkle the water on any person, place, or thing in need of protection; use it to bless a newborn; and so on. Holly is placed on the door at winter solstice as a symbol that the nature spirits are welcome into your home. Holly is an herb of Mars.

Hawthorn (*Crataegus* spp.)

This tree was an important one for the Druids, who would watch for the blooming of the Hawthorn to announce the festival of Beltaine (May Day). The young leaves and flowers are tinctured in alcohol in the spring and the red fruits are tinctured in the fall to make a cardiac tonic (see page 172 for instructions). Hawthorn is an herb of Mars.

Lavender (*Lavandula vera, L. angustifolia*)

Single hardy flower species such as Lavender have been used to mark boundaries in some areas. Plant a thick row of winter-hardy Lavender on a raised earthen bank, shored up with flat stones along the base. Bring Lavender into your home to foster peace, love, and healing. Lavender tea is a natural antidepressive and the scent is calming to those in pain. The flowers have antiseptic qualities and can be added to herbal salves. The leaf tea helps with nausea and vomiting.

To make the tea: Steep two teaspoons of the flowers per cup of water for twenty minutes. Drink a quarter cup four times a day.

Lavender flowers and rose petals can be soaked in vinegar for a few weeks and then strained. The vinegar is applied to the temples and forehead, using a compress, to soothe headaches. An ingredient of love spells, the scent of Lavender is said to attract men. Offer the flowers to the Midsummer fire to honor the gods and goddesses. Lavender is an herb of Mercury, especially sacred to Hecate and Saturn.

Mountain Ash, Rowan (*Sorbus americana, S. aucuparia*)

This is the ultimate tree for magical protection, according to Scottish lore, with lovely white flowers in the spring and bright red or orange berries in the fall. Rowan branches were once placed in the cradle, hung over the door, and hung over the entrance to the barn to protect against sorcery. Highland ladies once wore necklaces of red Rowan berries as a form of magical protection. Planted near the home, Rowan is said to be protective against fire; planted near graveyards, it keeps the dead from rising. Walk with a Rowan stick to safely enter fairy forts and to avoid being "taken" by the fairies.

The berries are rich in vitamin C and were once made into syrup, with apples and honey, for fevers, bronchitis, and other lung ailments. The berries are made into jam, which helps treat diarrhea in adults and children. The jam is also used as a condiment for meats such as wild game and lamb. The berries should be picked just after the first frost, when they have a deep, bright color.

Rowan is an herb of the Moon.

> **Caution: Children should not eat raw Rowan berries but they may safely eat the jam.**

Rowan Berry Jam

Place equal parts ripe rowan berries and finely chopped apples, including the cores, into a pan. Bring to a simmer and cook until the fruit is soft (the berries will lose their color).

When the fruit is soft enough, press through a sieve and then discard the seeds and skins.

Place 1 part organic sugar (or ½ part honey) into a separate pan with a little water and simmer until the sugar dissolves.

Bring the sugar water to a boil, add the pulp, and bring back to a boil. Boil for 5 minutes. Test by dropping the jam onto a plate and see if, when cooled, it forms sticky ridges.

Sea Buckthorn, Hippophae (*Hippophae rhamnoides*)

This is another plant that makes a great barrier hedge or windbreak with colorful, edible berries and strong roots that will hold back soil. Common along sandy seacoasts in Europe, the plant also thrives in desert areas of Asia. It needs full sun to thrive. It is important to plant both male and female plants; the female plant produces the orange berries that are an important winter food for birds and also useful for us humans.

The fruits are anti-inflammatory and benefit the lungs, digestive tract, heart, liver, skin, reproductive organs, and metabolism. The leaves and bark are astringent and used externally to treat wounds, suppuration, and bleeding, and internally for diarrhea. The berries are bitter and taste best after they have been frozen. They are rich in vitamins C and A and their juice can be added to other sweeter juices, such as apple, to improve flavor. The fruits can also be used to make jams, pies, fruit liqueurs, mead, and wine.

The branches have thorns, which makes harvesting a challenge. An old technique was to break off an entire branch, freeze it, and then shake off the berries. The berries were then kept frozen for later use. A less destructive method is to shake the branches to allow the berries to drop onto a cloth.

Sea Buckthorn is an herb of Saturn that is said to foster communication with animals, especially between a horse and rider.

> **Caution: Sea Buckthorn leaves and bark are not for long-term use internally due to their high tannin content.**

Shadbush, Serviceberry, Juneberry, Saskatoon (*Amelanchier* spp.)

A native plant that goes by many names and is found across the USA and in Canada, *Amelanchier* has a cherry-like berry with a soft inner seed. Moths and butterflies appreciate the leaves, and deer and rabbits will browse the branches. Juneberry species have differing qualities: some are bushes and some are small trees. They produce white, pink, yellow, or red-streaked flowers in early spring, at the time of the shad run. The flowering of these trees was once a signal to Native American tribes in New England that it was time to go fishing. In Appalachia their blooming meant that roads were again passable and that the ground was thawed enough to bury those who had died over the winter. In the plains, the blue berries heralded the return of the bluebirds from their winter nesting grounds.

As the name implies, the bushes produce iron-rich blueberry-sized fruits in June that can be eaten raw or made into pie or jam. They can also be added to breads, muffins, salads, granola, and pancakes. They can be frozen on a cookie sheet and then kept frozen in a container for later use.

Native Americans used the berries to make pemmican, a mixture of fruits, chopped dry meat, and fat. The wood was once used to make arrow shafts, tool handles, and fishing rods.

 Juneberry Sauce
(for pancakes, cheese cake, ice cream, etc.)

1 cup Juneberries

½ cup water

½ cup sugar

1 tablespoon lemon juice

2 tablespoons cornstarch

Place all the ingredients in a small saucepan and stir continuously while heating until a thick sauce results.

Trifoliate Orange, Chinese Bitter Orange
(*Poncirus trifoliata*)

This citrusy plant is hardy to zone 5 and tolerates frost and snow. It is thorny and deciduous (drops its leaves in winter), bears fragrant leaves and flowers, and has small, bitter orange fruits that can be used for marmalade. "Flying Dragon" is a variety with interesting twisted stems.

The fruits are used to relieve allergic inflammation in Chinese medicine and show antitumor and antiviral properties. They contain vitamin C and can be juiced to help with colds.

Oranges symbolize the Sun, luck, and good fortune and are said to attract good business. The flowers are used in weddings to bring good fortune and happiness and added to the bath to make one more alluring. Oranges may be used to invoke Apollo, Hera, and Gaia.

14

DECIDUOUS TREES FOR HEALING

When I first moved to the hills of western Massachusetts I was struck by the shortness of the growing season. I had migrated north from Philadelphia, where we had roses blooming until December and you could start planting flowers in early March. In our neck of the woods it is only safe to plant after Memorial Day (the end of May) and the first frosts can appear by mid-September. That means there are only three months or so to harvest food and medicine from the wild. (At least that was the rule of thumb when I got here in the mid-1980s. These days we seem to have moved into a completely different planting schedule.) I had a very hard time imagining how the native peoples and white settlers survived in this climate, with such a short gardening and wild-crafting window.

One day I looked out the window and it dawned on me that part of the secret to survival in this climate must have been the trees. Surrounding the house were Pines, Cedars, Oaks, Birches, and Sassafras. There were Willows nearby in boggy areas, and also Alder, Maples, Poplars, Ash, Witch Hazel, and American Hawthorn. I reasoned that the native peoples must have been using these trees for food and medicine.

I started looking for a tree herbal that would teach me how to gather these things; there was no Internet at the time, so I went to local bookstores and libraries. I searched and searched but could not find a book that would tell me the herbal uses of trees. Then I made a profound leap of illogic and decided to write such a book. That was how my first herbal, *Tree Medicine, Tree Magic* (now out of print) came to be.

In the years since I have made a DVD on the herbal uses of trees and wild weeds, called *Gifts from the Healing Earth* (from local producers Sawmill River Productions), and I have a tree herbal out called *A Druid's Herbal of Sacred Tree Medicine* (Destiny Books) that covers the herbal and spiritual aspects of twenty trees.

A LITTLE TREE LORE

"Where Oak and Ash and Thorn grow together one is likely to see fairies." So goes the old adage, passed down through the generations to impress upon us the value and sanctity of trees. For our ancestors, these three trees and many others were the basic tools of survival. Through the ages trees have given us shelter, medicine, tools, and household items such as cups, bowls, and dishes. They gave us paper, building materials, and cloth. They cooled us in summer and warmed us in winter. For these reasons alone they deserve reverence. We are also the inheritors of a rich compendium of knowledge and spiritual tradition involving trees. Here are just three of the many important trees that surround our homes and offer their medicine, if we are wise enough to pay heed. Understanding the value and sanctity of trees is the birthright of every human being, and we must all strive to pass on the trees' wisdom to future generations.

The Mighty Oak, Tree of Balance

The Indo-European cultures of Europe and Asia were cradled in a vast Oak forest that once stretched from the west coast of France to the Caucasus. Most homes and shelters in this area were made of Oak. Oak is a dense and hot firewood and was used to make bows, spears, oars, and boats. The bark, leaf, and galls were used to tan hides and fishing nets and to make a wound wash that would help healing by pulling the edges of a wound together. The bark and leaves of White Oak were especially valuable as a medicinal tea for coughs, colds, and mucous congestion. The acorns provided a carbohydrate-rich food for humans, pigs, and wild game.

Oaks were known to attract lightning and became associated with the sky gods such as Taranis, Indra, Jupiter, Yahweh, Ukho, Rhea, Kybele, Thor, Artemis, Brighid, Balder, the Erinyes, the Kikonian Maenads, Perun, and Perkunas. The roots of an Oak go as deep as the tree is high, making its spirit a powerful ally in shamanic travel between the worlds. There is a spirit in each Oak that can take you down to the underworld through its roots and up to the sky world via its branches.

Druids of the past and of today revere the Oak as the symbol of a balanced life: feeding and sheltering the people, with its feet firmly on the ground, and its head in the highest heavens. The Druid orders to which I belong (Ord Na Darach Gile—Order of the White Oak—and Fine na Darach—Tribe of the Oak) honor this tree above all others.

According to tradition, carrying an acorn on your person will bring luck and fertility to all your projects. Druids carried acorns and Hazel nuts for luck. Hazel nuts and acorns were also a symbol of the compact wisdom that a Druid carried in her head.

An ancient Welsh belief is that good health is maintained by rubbing your hands on a piece of Oak on Midsummer's Day, while keeping silence. The dew under Oak trees is said to be a magical beauty aid.

The Sacred Ash

Another sacred tree for our ancestors was Ash. Ash has a denser wood than Oak and can even be burned green. It is a tree that was especially sacred in Scandinavia. The ancestors used it to make spear shafts, household crafts, and bows. Neolithic farmers relied on the leaves as winter fodder for their animals. The ancient Greeks said that Zeus created humanity from Ash trees, and the Scandinavians said that after Ragnarok, the destruction of the world, a male and a female will emerge from Yggdrasil, the cosmic Ash, to begin life on Earth all over again. It was Yggdrasil upon which Odin hung for nine days, until he discovered the runes.

On-Niona was the Gaulish goddess of Ash groves. The Irish word for Ash, *nion,* was also the word for heaven, *nionon.* Ash is considered a solar tree, and its wood is used to make the Yule log. A Druidical Ash wand from the first century CE, decorated with spirals, was found on the island of Anglesey, Wales. Ash divining rods are cut on summer solstice. Witches' brooms, used for flying and sacred ceremony, are traditionally made of an Ash pole, with Birch twigs and Willow bindings. Eating red Ash buds at Midsummer is said to protect one from sorcery.

The Fairies' Favorite: Hawthorn

Another sacred tree by tradition is Hawthorn, which must never be felled because to do so will anger the fairies. A solitary Hawthorn on a hill, and especially if there is a well or a spring nearby, is said to mark an entrance to the Land of Fairy.

I have been a Druid initiate and priestess since 1985. One of the duties of a Druid is to keep an eye on the local Hawthorn tree because the day it first blooms is the official start of summer. When the Hawthorn blooms it is a signal that the weather is warm enough to move the cows to their summer pasture, high in the hills. It was once the job of the local Druid to set the date for the all-important purification ceremonies that were done to bless the herds on their way. I keep several Hawthorns around the house for this purpose, including one grown from seed brought back from Uisneach in Ireland, the seat of the arch Druid in ancient times. I like to know the exact date of the start of summer, even if I don't presently have any cows!

Hawthorn flowers may be used to decorate the tops of Maypoles (or Maybushes in Celtic areas) but must never be carried into the house or mischievous fairies might come in with them.

TREES FOR OUR FUTURE

Our future survival may hinge on trees. As carbon dioxide emissions heat the planet by encasing it in a warm blanket of smog, the oceans are warming, storms are becoming stronger and more destructive, and tropical diseases are moving ever northward. The threat of coastal flooding threatens massive population displacements and eventual conflicts over resources.

One way to mitigate global catastrophe is to plant trees. A single tree can absorb a ton of carbon dioxide over its lifetime. But where the tree gets planted matters. Forests are darker than fields and pastures and as a result they actually absorb heat in northern latitudes. (Snow on an empty field reflects more sunlight back into space than does a snow-covered forest.)

It is in the tropics that trees are most valuable for global cooling. The trees that grow in these areas are deep rooted, bringing up water from the earth, which they evaporate through their leaves, forming clouds that reflect sunlight back into space. The massive clear-cutting and deforestation that is now occurring in tropical forests is a tragedy for the animals and humans who live there, and for our entire planet's ecosystem.

Of course, the best solution of all is to cut our dependence on greenhouse-gas-producing fossil fuels. We have many positive options before us: wind and solar energy, biomass, geothermal energy, conservation, and hydrogen- and solar-powered cars, just to name a few. (Nuclear energy is not a positive option, because we still have no idea what to do with the lethal, cancer-causing waste other than produce more nuclear weapons.)

USING DECIDUOUS TREES FOR MEDICINE

In celebration of the trees, here is a sampler of the medicinal and edible properties of some of them. A reminder: when a suggestion is made to use "the bark" I mean the inner living green layer of bark, taken from a branch (not the trunk) or from a root.

> **Caution: Deciduous tree leaves should only be gathered for medicinal purposes before summer solstice, June 21; after that they will contain too many plant alkaloids.**

Alder (*Alnus* spp.)

The inner bark of Black Alder (*Alnus glutinosa*) is simmered to make a wound wash and a wash for sprains, bruises, headache, and back pain. Being highly astringent, Alder helps pull the edges of a wound together (be sure the injury is very clean before you attempt this). It is also a good wash for skin problems such as eczema and swellings. The inner bark can also be tinctured in vinegar to make a wash for lice and scabies. *To make the tincture:* Soak the bark for about two weeks in apple cider vinegar, strain, and apply.

To use the bark tea internally you must first dry the bark (the fresh bark is emetic). A dried bark tea can be taken to stop internal bleeding and for cramps, vomiting, diphtheria, and rheumatic pains. The bark tea is also used as a gargle for sore throats and gums.

To make the tea: Simmer one teaspoon of the dried inner bark per cup of water for about twenty minutes, and take up to two cups a day in very small doses. Alternatively, the tea can be made from a combination of spring-gathered leaves and the inner bark; this tea can be taken for fevers, internal hemorrhage, and bleeding from the lungs.

Red Alder (*Alnus rubra*) and Smooth Alder or Hazel Alder (*Alnus serrulata*) can be used in the same way.

Apple (*Malus* spp.)

Apple is the tree of love sacred to the Greek goddess Aphrodite. In European folklore apples are associated with love magic. You will know that you have been visited by a woman from the fairy realm if she appears bearing an apple branch with fruits, leaves, and flowers upon it.

And what would New England be without apples? They are our classic fruit. The best variety of apple to eat is the sour green variety called "Granny Smith," which has the least hypoglycemic effect on the pancreas. Other sweeter varieties like yellow and red are loaded with carbs and sugar. Eating peeled, grated raw apples will help diarrhea. Add cinnamon for an even more effective remedy. Apples eaten whole (with the peel on) or baked have the opposite laxative effect. Apply warm baked apples as a poultice for inflammations and sore throats.

After a course of antibiotics (including natural ones like Goldenseal), drink or eat raw, unpasteurized apple cider or applesauce that has been left out for a day or two, well covered and at room temperature, to promote the growth of bacteria. These are the exact bacteria needed by the human gut, important after any dose of antibiotics to replenish the intestinal flora and prevent candidiasis (an overgrowth of yeast in the system).

The tea of the inner bark of apple trees and the bark of the root is used to treat fevers and in Appalachian folk medicine to soothe a "sour or burning stomach." *To make the tea:* Simmer two teaspoons of inner bark or root bark per cup of water for twenty minutes. Take quarter-cup doses throughout the day.

Apple cider vinegar can be taken with water to improve digestion and in Appalachian folk medicine is applied externally to diaper rash, prickly heat, and poison ivy rash. Use it with White Oak to poultice varicose veins.

Ash (*Fraxinus* spp.)

An old saying, "Beware the Ash, it courts the flash," reveals Ash's association with lightning, the sun, and the high gods. In Scandinavian and Celtic tradition Ash was chosen for thrones, spears, shields, and other royal accoutrements.

A tea of the young leaves and bark of the root is diuretic and laxative. Harvest the young leaves in spring and use them fresh, or dry them for later use as a gentle laxative. *To make the tea:* Steep one or two teaspoons of leaf or mixed leaf and bark per half cup of freshly boiled water for about five minutes. Take up to one and a half cups per day in teaspoon doses.

In winter you can gather the inner bark of a branch or the bark of the root to make a tea for fevers. *To make the tea:* Simmer one teaspoon of bark per half cup of water for about ten minutes. Adults can take up to a cup a day in teaspoon doses.

Beech, American Beech (*Fagus grandifolia*)

A tea of the inner bark is used for lung conditions and the leaf tea makes a nice wash for burns, rheumatic swellings, and acne. The tea can be used as a gargle and mouthwash for mouth sores.

Birch (*Betula* spp.)

In European folklore Birch is called "the tree of new beginnings." Birch is the first letter of the ancient Irish tree alphabet called Ogham, and its twigs were once used to make brooms to clean the house and barn. Fragrant Birch tea can also be used to clean grease from dishes and kitchen surfaces. All the Birches make excellent syrup when tapped in the spring. Betulinic acid from the sap benefits cancers.

All Birches (such as Black Birch, River Birch, and so on) except the

White Birch make an excellent beverage tea from spring through fall. White Birch is not good for tea because it is tasteless. Snap a bit of twig and give it a sniff. If it smells like wintergreen you have the right one. The tea also has sedative qualities to help you sleep and to ease muscle pains. The tea can be made from the twigs, inner bark, root bark, or a combination.

To make the twig tea: After removing the leaves, break the twigs into two-inch pieces. Barely cover them with water and then simmer (do not boil) for about twenty minutes, in a pot with a tight lid (please don't use aluminum pots; any other pot will do). *To make the bark tea:* Use one teaspoon of bark per cup of water, and simmer for twenty minutes. Take up to two cups a day in quarter-cup doses.

Add the tea to a bath or use it as a wash for eczema, psoriasis, sores, and other moist, oozing skin conditions.

Cucumber Tree (*Magnolia acuminata*)

The inner bark tea is taken for fevers and as a laxative, and also for stomachaches, rheumatic complaints, and cramps. It can be snuffed for sinus problems.

Elder (*Sambucus canadensis*, *S. nigra*)

A female spirit of the forest called the Elder Mother lives in this tree, so it is very disrespectful to cut one down. The berry is edible when processed; taken as tea or tincture, it cleans the bone marrow, eases rheumatic pains and neuralgia, and benefits coughs, colds, bronchitis, flu, and asthma (see page 54 for the tincture recipe). The berries are also used in wines, pies, and preserves.

To make the tea: Simmer one teaspoon of berries per cup of water for twenty minutes, and take in quarter-cup doses throughout the day.

Caution: Do not eat Elder berries raw; they must be cooked, dried, or tinctured.

The flowers of Black Elder (*S. nigra*) are particularly fragrant, make a nice addition to drinks, and are soothing to the nerves. They can be dried or tinctured in vodka as a remedy for pneumonia, bronchitis, fevers, and measles. Use a few drops (three to five) of tincture in water, three times a day. The older leaves are made into a tea with tobacco to repel insects, while the young leaf (gathered before summer solstice) is used in healing salves.

The bark of the fresh root of American Elder (*Sambucus canadensis*) makes a tea for headaches and mucous conditions, to promote labor, and to poultice mastitis. The green and fresh inner bark is used in healing salves. *To make the tea:* Simmer about one teaspoon of inner bark per cup of water for about twenty minutes. Take no more than one cup a day in tablespoon doses.

> **Caution: Use sparingly, as large doses of Elder bark are emetic and purgative.**

Elm (*Ulmus* spp.)

This tree was called "Elven" in ancient Britain because it's a tree that is popular with the wood elves. The leaves (picked in the spring before summer solstice) and inner bark of the European or English Elm (*Ulmus procera = Ulmus campestris*) can be tinctured in apple cider vinegar for a few weeks to make a wash for skin eruptions and diseases. The leaves, bark, and roots can also be made into a strong tea and added to bathwater to help heal broken bones.

Slippery Elm (*Ulmus fulva = Ulmus rubra*) is a smaller variety that has a fragrant, glue-like inner bark. In Appalachian folk medicine the bark is chewed for coughs and colds and to benefit the stomach. Powdered Slippery Elm bark can be mixed with water and fed to babies who cannot tolerate cow's milk. As a tea the inner bark is mucilaginous and soothing to the throat, stomach, and bowels. It can help heal gastritis, colitis, enteritis, bronchitis, coughs, and bleeding from the lungs. It is also calcium rich and eases insomnia.

To make the tea: Add one teaspoon of the bark to a pint of freshly boiled water. Steep for an hour, then bring to the boil again. Let stand for another hour, then bring to a boil one more time. Take one-quarter cup three times a day.

I always add Slippery Elm to my poultices, along with other skin- and bone-healing plants such as Comfrey (*Symphytum* spp.) and

Plantain (*Plantago* spp.). These poultices are great for burns, ulcers, and wounds, to heal surgery incisions, and for sprains, fractures, poison ivy rashes, and skin inflammations.

To make the poultice: Blend your herbs with enough water to liquefy them. Pour the liquefied herbs into a bowl and add enough powdered Slippery Elm bark to achieve a "pie dough" consistency, then roll out with a rolling pin on a clean cloth. Apply for one hour, then discard.

Slippery Elm is a plant that can also be added to healing salves.

Eucalyptus (*Eucalyptus* spp.)

Eucalyptus leaves are a natural disinfectant and fever reducer. If you are lucky enough to live near these trees, you can make your own tincture. *To make the tincture:* Pack young leaves into a jar and just barely cover them with vodka. Allow the leaves to steep for about two weeks (be sure to shake the jar every few days), strain, and store in a cool, dark place or put into brown or blue glass bottles.

For colds, bronchitis, and sinusitis, three drops of the organic essential oil (no more!) can be added to three drops (no more!) of organic Peppermint oil (*Mentha piperita, M. balsamea* Willd.) and the juice of half a lemon, in a cup of freshly boiled water. Start by inhaling the brew and, when cooled enough, drink the tea.

> **Caution: More than three drops per day can damage the kidneys, and large doses can be fatal. Avoid this remedy if you have any kidney or liver issues.**

Place a few drops of Eucalyptus essential oil in a vaporizer to ease asthma and bronchitis attacks. Take a few drops of the oil in hot water as a tea to ward off flu and pneumonia, when gonorrhea is suspected, and for malaria and recurrent chills, leukemia, internal hemorrhage, typhoid, exhaustion, and gastrointestinal and genitourinary infection and pain. One drop (no more!) taken in water three times a day stimulates the heart. Two drops of the oil in warm water may be used as a gargle for sore throat and a rinse for gum diseases such as pyorrhea, and it may be used externally as a wash for burns.

> **Caution: Do not take the oil for more than a few days.
> Not for long-term use.**

Externally, the oil is antiseptic for wounds and ulcers; try soaking infected parts in very hot water with about an ounce of Eucalyptus oil per pint of water (add sea salt if desired) for speedy healing.

Eucalyptus has been added to water for animals (just a few drops given one time only) when distemper was moving through the neighborhood, as a preventive measure.

Eucalyptus is an herb of healing and protection when hung in the room.

Fringe Tree, Old Man's Beard, Snowdrop Tree (*Chionanthus virginicus*)

A tea of the dried inner bark can be used to benefit liver complaints (do not use if there is an active gallbladder attack going on). The tea is a spring tonic and good for colds, eczema, and acne. Externally, it is used as a wash for burns and sores.

Hawthorn (*Crataegus* spp.)

Hawthorn is a great favorite of the bees. The young leaves and flowers and the red, ripe berries are cardiac tonics. Tincture the leaves and flowers in spring and the berries in the fall, combine the two, and take a few drops daily for angina, myocarditis, high blood pressure, atherosclerosis, stress, insomnia, and nervous tension. Hawthorn can also be taken as a general tonic for those who feel "run down."

To make the tincture: In the spring, put the fresh young leaves and flowers in a jar and barely cover with vodka. Cap tightly and steep until the plant matter begins to break down. Strain and store in a brown or blue glass container (or in a dark cupboard). You can use the flower and leaf tincture by itself or combine with the berry tincture. In the fall, pick the berries just after the first frost when they are bright red and put them in a jar. Barely cover with vodka and steep, tightly capped, for about a week. Strain and add the berry tincture to the leaf and flower tincture.

> Caution: Do not take this herb with blood-pressure-lowering drugs, as it can cause a precipitous drop in blood pressure over time (I have seen this). Be sure to monitor blood pressure carefully when using this herb, and use only with medical supervision.

Holly (*Ilex* spp.)

The leaf tea of English Holly (*Ilex aquifolium*) can be taken for fevers, flu, coughs, colds, pleurisy, smallpox, intermittent fever, and rheumatic conditions. The leaf tea is a mild diuretic that produces sweating. *To make the tea:* Simmer two tablespoons of leaf per cup of water for twenty minutes in a non-aluminum pot with a tight lid. A 150-pound adult may take a quarter cup four times a day.

> Caution: Make sure you are using English Holly and not another Holly species because some species are emetic (they will cause vomiting).

The leaf tea of American Holly (*Ilex opaca*) also benefits colds, flu, measles, and lung conditions and is used as an external wash for itching and sores. Use the leaves fresh or dried and please collect them before the summer solstice. *To make the leaf tea:* Steep two teaspoons of the chopped leaves per pint of freshly boiled water for about twenty minutes. Take up to two cups a day in quarter-cup doses.

The dried and powdered berries can be applied externally to stop bleeding.

> Caution: Do not eat Holly berries, as they are emetic and purgative.

The root bark of American Holly can be used as a tonic for coughs and pleurisy, and the tea of the inner bark was once used for epilepsy and malaria.

Horse Chestnut (*Aesculus hippocastanum*)

A little folk magic: as an herb of Jupiter, Horse Chestnuts attract financial success when placed into a bag of oats, sewn with green thread.

A tea of the inner bark was once taken for malaria and dysentery and used as a wash externally for lupus and ulcers on the skin. The leaves are antitussive and can be added to cough mixtures; the leaf tea (gather the leaves before the summer solstice) can be taken for fevers. According to Appalachian folk medicine the leaves will help with dropsy or "fluid retention."

The peeled roasted nuts are simmered to make a tea for diarrhea and prostate problems. The nuts are used in salves because they are anti-inflammatory and kill pain, providing a classic remedy for piles, sunburn, diaper rash, minor kitchen burns, scrapes, and dry flaky skin conditions (do not apply to deep wounds or serious burns where the skin is broken).

> **Caution: The spiny outer husk of the Horse Chestnut nut should not be used and can be toxic.**

Healing Horse Chestnut Salve

Remove the spiny outer hulls and put the smashed nuts (the brown shiny hulls and the meat of the nuts) into a pot with other skin-healing herbs. Add equal parts of three or more of the following:

- plantain leaves (*Plantago* spp.)
- pine needles (*Pinus* spp.)
- comfrey leaves (*Symphytum officinale*)
- elecampane roots (*Inula helenium*)
- baby oak leaves (*Quercus* spp.)
- chopped white sarsaparilla root (*Aralia nudicaulis*)
- English ivy (*Hedera helix*)
- bee balm leaves (*Monarda* spp.)
- fresh, chopped green outer hulls of walnut (*Juglans* spp.) (not the nuts)

Add fresh or dried Calendula (*Calendula officinalis*) blossoms, which stop bleeding, and fresh or dried Lavender (*Lavandula angustifolia, L. vera*) flowers, which have antiseptic properties.

Just barely cover with a good-quality olive oil (carefully record how many cups of oil you use) and bring to a simmer (do not boil!). Cover tightly and simmer for about 20 minutes.

At the same time, in a separate pot or double boiler (bain-marie), melt beeswax and bring it to a simmer.

When both pots are of equal temperature, remove them from the heat. For every cup of oil you used, add 3–4 tablespoons of melted beeswax. Stir, strain, and pour into very clean glass jars. Cap tightly. The salve will keep nicely for years in a dark, cool place.

> **Caution: Do not apply the salve to broken skin, deep wounds, or serious burns.**

For primitive-skills fans and hunters, try using deer tallow, beef tallow, or bear fat as the basis of your medicinal salve. That is what our ancient ancestors would have done.

Ohio Buckeye (*Aesculus glabra*) can also be used to make the salve. A very tiny pinch of the dried, powdered nut was once taken for asthma with a tight chest and coughs.

Larch (*Larix decidua, L. europaea, L. laricina*)

Larch is the sacred tree of the Turanian people of Siberia. The inner bark is styptic. Dried and powdered, it can be applied to bleeding wounds. Taken internally as a tea, it can stop internal bleeding. Native Americans used *L. laricina* (Tamarack) as a cough remedy by making a tea of the inner bark and needles. A poultice of the needles and inner bark was applied to infected wounds. Western tribes used *L. occidentalis* (Western Larch) similarly. Make a tea of the fresh needles and twigs and add it to the bath.

Sap (tree resin) will emerge if a hole is bored in the tree. This resin is made into "Venice turpentine," which provides a good remedy for humans with wounds and also for horses with sore feet (and it helps harden their hoofs). Venice turpentine can be bought from veterinary supply houses. For external use, add a few drops to a hot cloth and apply for thirty minutes. Do this only once a day.

> **Caution: Wear rubber or plastic gloves when handling Larch sap or Venus turpentine to avoid skin irritation.**

> **Caution: Pregnant women should avoid Larch.**

Linden Tree, American Basswood (*Tilia americana*)

A tea of the inner bark can be used for lung conditions and heartburn, and a tea of the bark or flowers is good for coughs and colds. A tea or tincture of the leaves, flowers, and buds has been used for painful digestion.

> **Caution: Linden is for short-term use only;
> long-term use could cause heart damage.**

Maple (*Acer* spp.)

The Seneca say Maple is the most creative tree, as one can see from the bright colors it shows in the fall. For this reason, it is the wood of choice for musical instruments.

Maple leaf oil is massaged into nerves and muscles to heal them. *To make the oil:* Gather the young leaves before summer solstice and layer them in a pan with a nice massage oil such as almond. Bake in a very slow oven (about 110 degrees) for six hours, strain, and use.

The powdered leaf is applied to skin cancers.

The inner bark of Striped Maple (*Acer pensylvanicum*) was made into a tea by Native American healers, then used for coughs and colds, bronchitis, kidney affections, gonorrhea, and spitting up of blood. The tea was applied externally for swollen limbs, paralysis, and skin eruptions. A large dose of the leaf and twig tea is emetic. A small, dilute dose can ease nausea. In Appalachian folk medicine Maple tea is said to help both men and women through the change of life.

Sugar Maple (*Acer saccharum*) is familiar to most of us as the source of maple syrup. Native American healers used the inner bark tea for coughs and diarrhea, as an expectorant, and as a blood purifier. They considered maple syrup to be a liver and kidney cleanser and added it to cough syrups.

Oak (*Quercus* spp.)

Like the Ash, Oak "courts the flash" and lives, all the while providing food (acorns), medicine, shelter, and warmth for animals and people. The bark of Oak is loaded with tannins and a strong tea of the inner bark can be used as a wound wash, to shrink goiters, varicose veins, and glandular inflammations, and to shrink fistulas and swellings. Just soak a cloth in a strong tea made with Oak bark or bark and leaf and apply.

For internal use, choose the inner bark of White Oak. The tea removes mucus and tones the stomach. Collect the bark from twigs in the early spring. *To make the tea:* Simmer one tablespoon of inner bark per pint of water for ten minutes. Adults can drink up to three cups a day.

To make an enema or douche: Simmer one tablespoon of inner bark per quart of water for about twenty minutes. *To make a wound wash or other external application:* Use about a pound of bark or leaves or both per quart of water; simmer for twenty minutes.

Peach (*Prunus persica*)

The leaves are used for morning sickness and to soothe the nerves. The tea is slightly sedative and also expectorant for bronchitis and other chest problems with phlegm. The powdered leaf can be applied externally to wounds and sores. *To make the tea:* Steep one teaspoon of leaf per cup of water. Take up to three cups a day, the first being before breakfast.

Caution: Use too much Peach leaf and it becomes a laxative.

Poplar (*Populus* spp.)

The fluttering leaves of Aspen can be used to send out a wish to the winds.

The inner bark of Quaking Aspen (*Populus tremuloides*) is used as a tea for fevers and to improve digestion. *To make the tea:* Simmer two teaspoons per cup of water for twenty minutes, and take one-quarter cup four times a day.

The inner bark of White Poplar (*Populus alba*) makes a tea for colds. *To make the tea:* Simmer two teaspoons per cup of water for twenty minutes, and take one-quarter cup four times a day.

Collect the resinous winter buds of Quaking Aspen and add

them to healing salves, or use them as a tea for colds and sore throats, and as a gargle. *To make the tea:* Simmer two teaspoons per cup of water for twenty minutes, and take one-quarter cup four times a day. Make a stronger bud tea for external use; it makes a nice wash for burns, inflammations, and wounds. The buds of Balm of Gilead/ Tachamahac (*Populus candicans, Populus balsamifera*) are used the same way.

Rowan, Mountain Ash (*Sorbus* spp.)

The inner bark tea has been used for pleurisy, to purify the blood, and to increase appetite. The root tea has been used to treat colic. Rowan leaves can be added to formulas for pneumonia, diphtheria, and croup.

> **Caution: Too much of Rowan leaf tea is emetic, so use it very sparingly. Gather the leaves before summer solstice, and use them fresh or dry them for later use.**

The berries are full of bioflavonoids and vitamins A and C. Gather them just after the first frost when they are a deep red or orange, depending on the species. The fresh berry juice is laxative and a teaspoon can be added to warm water to make a gargle for sore throat or mouth sores. *To make the juice:* Simmer one teaspoon of berries per cup of water for twenty minutes. Another method is to soak one teaspoon of dried berries per cup of water for ten hours. Take one cup a day in quarter-cup doses.

Sassafras (*Sassafras albidum, S. variifolium*)

Sassafras is a tree of faith, organization, and efficiency. The bark of the root can be added to Birch bark as a spring tonic. It also cleans the blood and lowers fever by producing perspiration.

> **Caution: Do not overuse Sassafras; long-term use carries a risk of cancer.**

Each spring I like to dig up a Sassafras root and use it to make non-alcoholic birch beer.

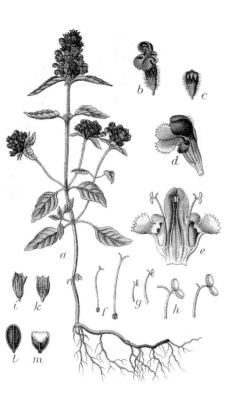

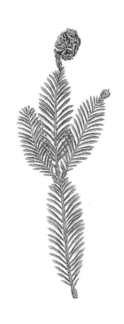

Plate 73 (left). Self-heal (*Prunella vulgaris*)

Plate 74 (right). Sequoia, Redwood
(*Sequoia sempervirens*)

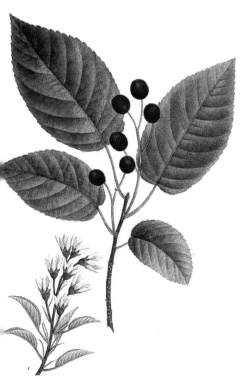

Plate 75. Shadbush, Serviceberry,
Juneberry, Saskatoon, or Chuckley Pear
(*Amelanchier arborea*)

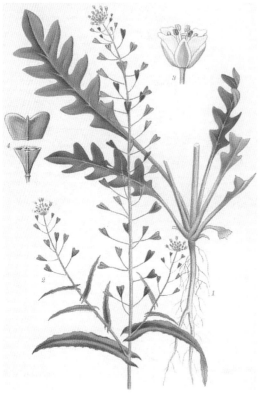

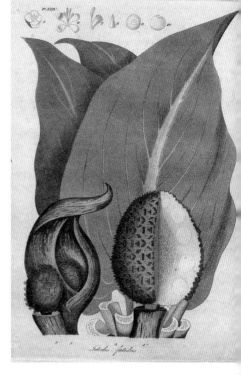

Plate 76 (left). Shepherd's Purse (*Capsella bursa-pastoris*)

Plate 77 (right). Skunk Cabbage (*Symplocarpus foetidus*)

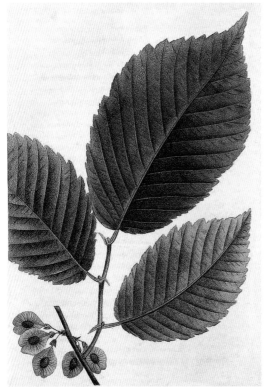

Plate 78. Slippery Elm (*Ulmus fulva, U. rubra*)

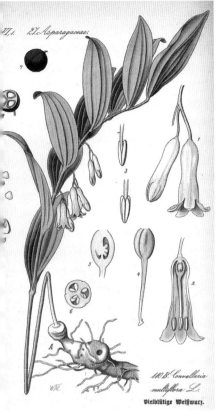

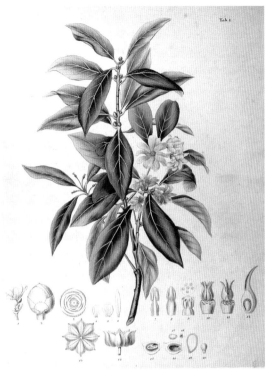

Plate 79 (left). Solomon's Seal
(*Polygonatum multiflorum*)

Plate 80. (right) Star Anise
(*Illicium verum, I. anisatum*)

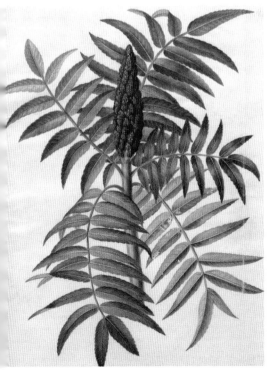

Plate 81. Sumac
(*Rhus typhina*)

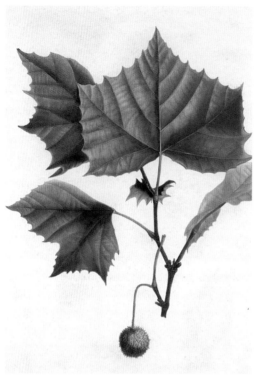

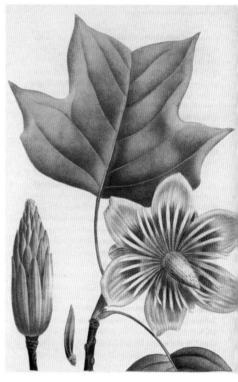

Plate 82 (left). Sycamore (*Platanus occidentalis*)

Plate 83 (right). Tulip Poplar, Tuliptree (*Liriodendron tulipifera*)

Plate 84. Uva Ursi, Bearberry (*Arctostaphylos uva-ursi*)

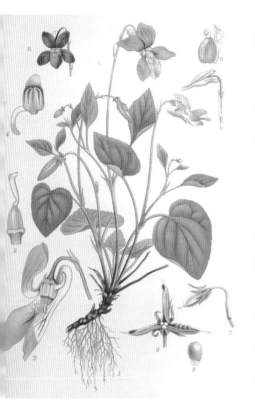

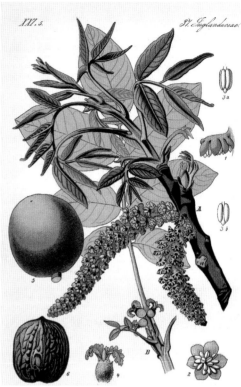

Plate 85 (left). Violet (*Viola riviniana* and *V. canina*)

Plate 86 (right). Walnut (*Juglans regia*)

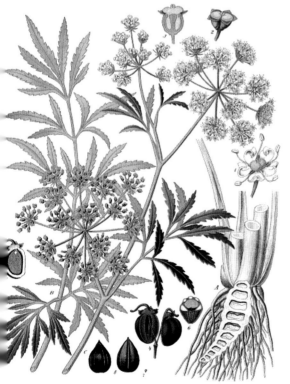

Plate 87. Water Hemlock (*Cicuta virosa*)

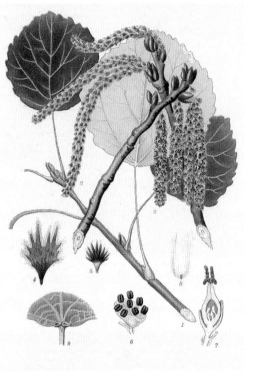

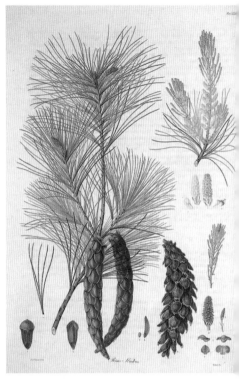

Plate 88 (left). White Aspen (*Populus tremula*)

Plate 89 (right). White Pine (*Pinus strobus*)

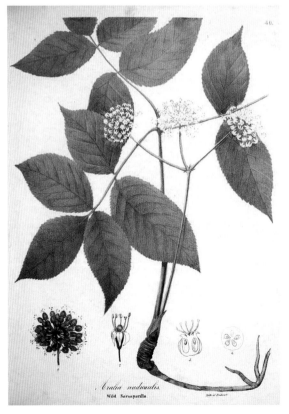

Plate 90. White Sarsaparilla, Spikenard (*Aralia nudicaulis*)

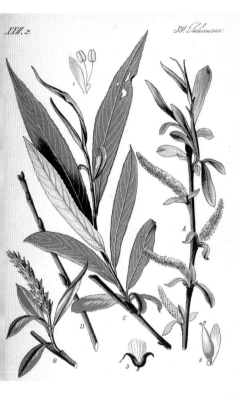

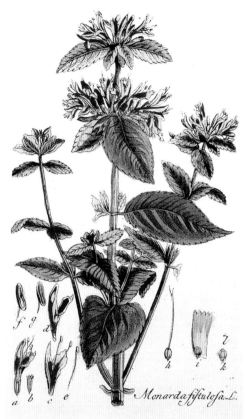

Plate 91 (left). White Willow (*Salix alba*)

Plate 92 (right). Wild Bergamot, Bee Balm (*Monarda fistulosa*)

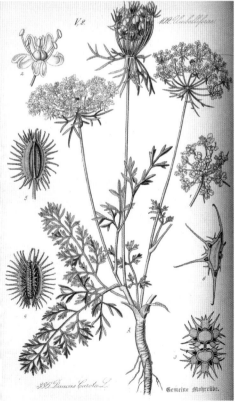

Plate 93. Wild Carrot, Queen Anne's Lace (*Daucus carota*)

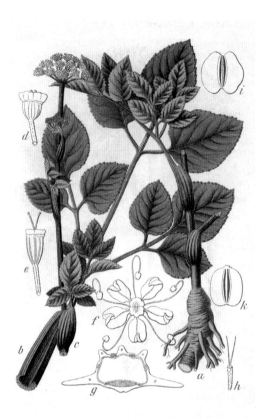

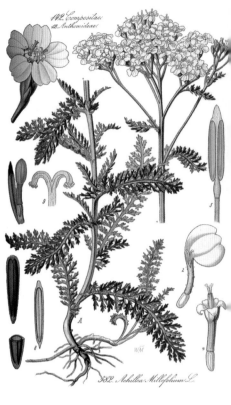

Plate 94 (left). Woodland Angelica (*Angelica sylvestris*)

Plate 95 (right). Yarrow (*Achillea millefolium*)

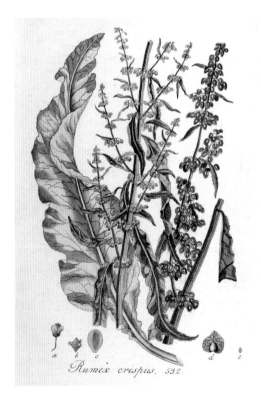

Plate 96. Yellow Dock, Curly Dock (*Rumex crispus*)

◊ Making Nonalcoholic Birch Beer

Find a sassafras grove and dig up one small tree. The part you will need is the bark of the root. Clean off any dirt from the root and then soak it for 20 minutes in cold water with a few tablespoons of vinegar or salt added, to remove parasites. Rinse well.

Peel off the root bark and put it in a pot with birch twigs broken up into 2-inch pieces and a few slices of fresh ginger root. Put everything into a non-aluminum pot with a tight lid and barely cover with cold water. Bring to a simmer and then simmer for 20 minutes (do not boil).

Add a natural sweetener, such as Sucanat, maple syrup, sorghum, or honey, to make a syrup. When you want birch beer, just add sparkling spring water to taste and voilà!

Caution: Use Sassafras sparingly; I only make the brew about once a year.

Tulip Poplar, Tuliptree (*Liriodendron tulipifera*)

The root bark tea improves digestion, benefits fevers and rheumatism, and can be added to cough mixtures. Externally, the root bark tea makes a wash for wounds, boils, and snakebites. The buds are added to salves and ointments for burns and inflammations.

Walnut (*Juglans* spp.)

Walnut is sacred to the Greek god Adonis, the young god of love and spring. The green outer hull of the nut is antifungal and has manganese, a skin-healing agent. It is a good addition to salves for dry skin and wound healing. The green outer hull of the nut of Black Walnut (*Juglans nigra*) can be applied as a poultice to ringworm.

The inner bark of Black Walnut can be made into a tea used for diarrhea, to dry up breast milk, as a douche for vaginal infections, and as a mouthwash for sore throat, tonsils, and gums. Native Americans used the tea as a wash for sores.

Juglans cinerea (Butternut, White Walnut) is used as a tonic laxative (it strengthens the bowels as it works); the inner bark tea is also taken for colds and flu and can help expel worms. *To make the tea:* Simmer one teaspoon of inner bark per cup of water. Take up to one cup a day in tablespoon doses.

The inner bark can also be used in syrups; simmer it in water until half the liquid is removed, add a sweetener, and simmer again until a syrup consistency is reached. If the inner bark is tinctured in alcohol the dose is fifteen drops, three times a day.

Willow (*Salix* spp.)

In Celtic tradition Willow was the "tree sacred to poets." Harps were once made of Willow wood. About forty varieties of Willow grow in the United States and all of them have medicinal bark. Find a Willow twig and scrape off the bark (never take bark from the trunk of a tree or you will kill the tree!). The inner bark contains salicylic acid, which is the "active ingredient" in aspirin, which is basically synthetic Willow bark.

Willow bark tea is helpful for fevers, muscle aches, toothaches, arthritic conditions, and any condition where you would normally think of aspirin. *To make the tea:* Steep about three teaspoons of the inner bark per cup of cold water for five hours, and then bring to a simmer briefly. Adults can take up to one cup a day, in tablespoon doses. It is a good herb to add to cough and cold mixtures.

> **Caution: Persons with sensitivity to aspirin will also be sensitive to Willow bark. Teenagers and children should avoid it, to prevent Reye's syndrome.**

15

CONIFERS FOR HEALING

Everyone needs to learn how to use evergreen conifers, herbal remedies that are available all year round. Here is a closer look at three conifers that offer us significant gifts.

JUNIPERS

This tree (*Juniperus* spp.) is an important healing and magical plant in Scottish lore. At Hogmanay (New Year's), Juniper was burned in the house with the object of fumigating every room. Like Native American smudging (usually done with Sage or Cedar), the smoke was seen as a kind of purification to drive out evil and start the year afresh.

The tree branches were ritually gathered by men at dusk and brought home and placed before the fire to dry out. Someone else went to the "dead and living ford" (a place where the dead and the living crossed over, such as a bridge over a stream where coffins were carried to the graveyard) to collect water.

The next morning everyone living in the house gathered to drink the water, and then the head of the clan went from room to room, ritually sprinkling water on beds and on the servants and other household members.

All window openings and even the keyholes were stuffed with rags, then branches of flaming Juniper were carried from room to room. When the house was deemed completely *sained* (cleansed) by smoke, the doors and windows were opened once more and a whisky bottle was passed around. The same ritual was done in the barn. Only then could everyone sit down to eat New Year's breakfast.

Using Junipers

The berries and branches are burned as incense and in the sweat lodge to purify the area and drive out negative forces. Branch tips can be gathered, bundled together, and hung to dry inside a brown paper bag on a clothesline. That way the needles will collect in the bag as they fall off the branch. When eating the berries, consume no more than two a day. Juniper berries should be picked when they are fully ripe and then placed in doubled-over cheesecloth to dry (always in the shade, never the sun). The berries can be used for flavorful cooking, such as in the following recipe.

 ## Juniper Cookies*

8 ounces butter, softened

1½ cups plus 2 tablespoons organic sugar

2 eggs

1 teaspoon gin (remember that gin is flavored with juniper berries and cooking will drive off the alcohol—but this is optional)

2¾ cups flour or gluten-free substitute

2 teaspoons baking powder

½ teaspoon sea salt

15–20 juniper berries

Cream the butter, 1½ cups sugar, eggs, and gin until fluffy.

In a separate bowl, sift together the flour, baking powder, and salt.

Combine the two mixtures, the wet and the dry, into a soft dough.

Use a food processor or a mortar and pestle to grind the berries with 1 tablespoon of sugar. When finely ground, add the remaining tablespoon of sugar.

Roll 1-inch balls of the dough in the juniper sugar and space evenly on

---

*Adapted from Hunger and Thirst, "Juniper Snickerdoodles," http://hungerandthirstforlife .blogspot.com/2012/10/juniper-snickerdoodles.html.

a baking sheet (the cookies will spread a bit, so leave room for that). Press a glass gently on top of each cookie to flatten it slightly.

Bake at 350 degrees for 10–12 minutes, or until the edges start to turn golden.

Cool on a rack and allow to sit for a few days in a covered tin (the longer you wait, the more intense the flavor will be).

> **Caution: Juniper should be avoided by pregnant women until the onset of labor.**

Think of Juniper tea for urinary tract infections. *To make the tea:* Use about one teaspoon of crushed berry or one teaspoon of needles per cup of water. Steep for about fifteen minutes, and take up to three cups a day in quarter-cup doses.

> **Caution: If the kidneys are infected or weak, Juniper should be avoided, as the oils could be irritating.**

Alligator Juniper, Checkerboard Juniper
(*Juniperus deppeana*)

The berries of *Juniperus deppeana* can be eaten raw or cooked. The berries were used by indigenous healers for diabetes and stomach ailments and were taken as tea before and after childbirth. The Yavapai pulverized the berries of *J. deppeana* and, after soaking them in water, put them into the mouth, sucked all the juice out, and then spat out the solid matter. Zuni children use the pitch as chewing gum.

Blueberry Juniper, Mountain Cedar, Ashe's Juniper
(*Juniperus ashei*)

Juniperus ashei is found in the southern United States, from Missouri to Texas and south to Mexico. Its fruits can be eaten cooked or raw.

California Juniper, Desert White Cedar
(*Juniperus californica*)

This Juniper is found in the southwest of the United States. The fruits of *Juniperus californica* are eaten raw or cooked, and they are dried and ground into a powder used to flavor foods. The leaf tea has been used for high blood pressure, coughs, and colds and as a hangover remedy. The tea can be safely used by pregnant women to help relax the muscles just before the onset of labor.

Common Juniper (*Juniperus communis*)

This is a small tree in New England and in other areas of the north-eastern United States. In the West it does not usually grow larger than a shrub. *Juniperus communis* berries are used to flavor dishes such as sauerkraut, stuffings, and meat dishes and can be dried and ground as a pepper substitute. They are the berries that give gin its distinctive taste.

A tea made from the berries can help digestive problems such as lack of appetite, cramps, and gas as well as mild kidney and bladder ailments, but it should be used sparingly. Cystitis and other infections can benefit from the tea because of its cleansing and antiseptic properties.

Caution: When overused, *Juniperus communis* can lead to kidney damage, irritation of the urinary passages, and possibly diarrhea. Do not use for more than a month without taking a break of a few weeks.

Arthritis, gout, and rheumatism also have been helped by the berries, which are warming to the system. The oil of the berries can be applied externally to arthritic inflammations and the berries can be used in healing salves. The oil or a strong tea can be inhaled in steam or added to the vaporizer and inhaled to relieve bronchitis and other lung infections.

Caution: Pregnant women should avoid *J. communis* as it can be abortive. It should also be avoided by those with kidney disease and by women who typically experience heavy bleeding during the menses, as that could be exacerbated.

Creeping Juniper (*Juniperus horizontalis*)

Juniperus horizontalis is another edible variety. A northern species, it is found from Newfoundland to British Columbia and south to Washington and Maine. Make a tea from the new growth of the branches or roast and grind the berries to make a coffee-like beverage. The branch tea is used or the cones chewed for coughs, colds, tonsillitis, and fever. The berry tea, which is slightly sedative, has been used for kidney conditions (however, see Caution below).

Caution: *J. horizontalis* **berries are strongly diuretic.**

Native Americans used a tea of the roots as a bath to give their horses shiny hair. The leaves were burned as a smudge to prepare for childbirth.

Oneseed Juniper, Cherrystone Juniper (*Juniperus monosperma*)

Juniperus monosperma berries and inner bark were once eaten by Native Americans of the southwest from Wyoming to Mexico as an emergency food, raw or cooked. The gum was chewed and used as a temporary filling in decayed teeth.

Caution: *J. monosperma* **berries are strongly diuretic.**

The leaves were taken as tea for fever, as a laxative, for lung complaints, and by women as a muscle relaxant before childbirth and after childbirth to stop blood flow. The chewed bark was used to poultice insect bites and as a burn dressing. The leaves were burned as a smudge to bless mothers and their new infants.

Rocky Mountain Juniper, Rocky Mountain Red Cedar (*Juniperus scopulorum*)

Juniperus scopulorum grows from British Columbia to California and Mexico. The berries can be eaten cooked or raw. Dried and roasted, they can be added to coffee or used as a coffee substitute. Dried and powdered, they make a flavoring.

Native American healers made a tea of the shoots for venereal diseases. A tea of the twigs was taken for pneumonia, fever, coughs, and colds. The leaf tea was taken for internal hemorrhage, constipation, and chronic coughs. The berry tea was taken for stomach issues and kidney and bladder problems. A poultice of the branches was used on sores and the leaves were rubbed into the scalp to treat dandruff.

Savin Juniper or Savin (*Juniperus sabina*)

This Juniper is a native to Europe and western and central Asia. It should be used only as an ornamental.

Caution: *J. sabina* is toxic and abortive.

Utah Juniper, Desert Juniper (*Juniperus osteosperma*)

Called *sammapo* by the Shoshone, *wapi* by the Paiute, *paal* by the Washoe, and *bat-they-naw* by the Arapaho, *Juniperus osteosperma* grows in the southwestern United States from California to New Mexico and Wyoming. The leaf tea was used by Native American healers as an antiseptic blood tonic and as a laxative. The leaf poultice was held to the jaw for toothache and sore gums.

A tea of the young twigs was taken for kidney and stomach problems, coughs, colds, and hemorrhage. A strong tea made from the branches was used as a wound wash and the mashed twigs were used to dress burns and inflammations. The smoke of the burning branches was inhaled for headache and for colds.

The berries can be eaten raw or cooked. A tea of the berries was taken for menstrual cramps, bladder problems, kidney complaints (it is diuretic), coughs, colds, and fevers and was applied externally to rheumatic joints. Bladder problems were also addressed by eating the berries. Arthritis and rheumatism were relieved by drinking the berry tea while lying down and inhaling the smoke of the burning fresh branches. Drinking a cup of the berry tea for three days was a form of birth control.

Caution: Pregnant women should avoid *J. osteosperma* berries.

Virginia Juniper, Eastern Red Cedar, Southern Red Cedar (*Juniperus virginiana, J. silicicola*)

Found in central, southern, and eastern North America from Canada to

Georgia and Texas, *Juniperus virginiana* fruits are eaten cooked and raw and used to flavor stews and soups.

Native American healers use a tea of the leaves for lung conditions, venereal warts, and skin problems. The leaf tea is also a deworming agent. It is used for coughs and colds and as a strengthening tea for invalids. The twig tea is diuretic and is used in the sweat lodge as a tea and also as a steam bath for rheumatism (by pouring it onto the hot rocks in the lodge).

The berry tea and the berries are anthelmintic (drive out worms). The berries are chewed for mouth sores or taken as tea for colds, rheumatism, worms, and menstral difficulties.

Caution: Pregnant women should avoid *J. virginiana* berries, as they are emmenagogic (they bring on menstruation).

Western Juniper (*Juniperus occidentalis*)

Juniperus occidentalis occurs from British Columbia to the Sierra Nevada. Its berries can be eaten raw or cooked. Its leaves were used by Native American herbalists as a laxative, as a blood tonic, and for colds and coughs. The leaf tea was also taken by women just before labor as a muscle relaxant. A poultice of the leaves was applied to the jaw for toothache and sore gums.

The young twigs were simmered to make a tea for kidney problems, fevers, upset stomach, flu, hemorrhage, and even smallpox, and it was used externally as a wound wash. A poultice of the twigs was used to dress burns and to pull boils and splinters. The smoke of the burning twigs was inhaled for headaches and colds.

A tea of the berries was taken as a blood tonic, to relieve menstrual cramps, and as a diuretic. A berry poultice was used on rheumatic parts.

REDWOODS

Sequoia, Redwood (*Sequoia sempervirens*)

This tree was named for Cherokee chief Sequoyah, inventor of the Cherokee alphabet. The inner bark tea was used by Native American healers to clean the liver and the blood. A hot leaf poultice was applied to sore ears and an infusion of the gummy sap was used as a tonic for those who were weak and run down.

As with most conifers, the new spring growth is tasty and edible, right off the tree. Try using the new growth as a tea for coughs and colds. *To make the tea:* Bring water to a boil, remove from the heat, and place the new branch tips into the pot. Steep for about twenty minutes, with a tight lid on the pot. Take a cup a day in quarter-cup doses.

The young leaves and twigs can be added to healing salves.

PINES

All Pines are antiseptic and Pine pitch or resin is a great skin healer. Gather loose or dripping resin from the outside of the tree. The resin can help draw dirt and infection from a wound. (Bear in mind that the tree is likely dripping resin because it has been wounded in some way. The resin is a "tree scab," so be mindful how much you take.)

Add the resin to salves by freezing the pitch, folding it into a cloth, and then shattering it into small bits with a hammer. Put the resin pieces in a glass jar and barely cover with cold-pressed, organic olive oil. Depending on your local climate, leave the jar on a woodstove, heat in a double boiler, or place it in the hot sun or in a sandbank for a few weeks until the chunks are dissolved into the oil. Strain out any debris and use the oil with beeswax to make a healing salve.

A resinous tea can also be used for sore legs in humans and horses. Make a strong tea of the twigs and needles and soak sore or tired feet in the hot brew, or add it to bathwater for the whole body. The scent of Pine is calming to the senses and makes a good bath for nervous debility.

For tinctures, the spring-gathered shoots of new growth and needles are best (though you can gather them year-round). *To make the tincture:* Place the shoots and needles in a jar and barely cover with vodka. Allow the needles to steep for about eight days, shaking from time to time (be sure the jar is tightly capped). Strain and store the tincture in a brown or blue glass container. Add the tincture to herbal teas or take in water for colds, bronchitis, flu, fever, coughs, tonsillitis, and laryngitis. Pine has even been used as a remedy for tuberculosis. A suggested dose is twenty drops three or four times a day.

White Pine, Symbol of Peace

For the Haudenosaunee (Iroquois) Confederacy, White Pine's bundles of five needles represent the family. Each family is attached to a twig, which symbolizes the clan, and each twig is attached to a branch, which symbolizes the nation. All the nations are joined to one trunk, which symbolizes unity. White Pine is soft and bends easily, indicating its willingness to be humble and reach compromise. All this makes White Pine the sacred tree of peace. In a time of strife between the nations, a peacemaker was born who created a ritual involving the planting of a White Pine. That ceremony is still done to this day.

In Germany, Martin Luther chose Pine to symbolize the Christmas season when, according to tradition, the biblical "King of Peace" was born.

White Pine (*Pinus strobus*)

The best conifer for internal use is probably White Pine; the way you know you have it is to look for the bundles of five needles. The Kanienkeha (Mohawk) ate the inner bark of White Pine as an emergency food, earning them the derogatory nickname of "bark eaters" (given as a taunt by the Abenaki). Among the Mohawk, pregnant women would take a tea of White Pine, Cranberries, and the inner bark of Sumac (*Rhus typhina, R. hirta*) to prevent urinary tract infections.*

White Pine has more vitamin C than lemons and is available even in the dead of winter. It is antiseptic and anti-inflammatory and promotes tissue repair while easing pain in sinusitis, bronchitis, and flu. It can also help relieve asthma. It is especially powerful for lung conditions with green phlegm. White Pine is stimulating and increases circulation,

---

*Please note: to be effective in preventing urinary tract infections and to prevent the growth of bacteria, Cranberry juice should be taken without added sweeteners.

which means more oxygen is carried to lung tissues and cleansing and expectoration are enhanced.

To make the tea: Gather the fresh twigs and needles and place them in a non-aluminum pot with a tight lid. Just barely cover with fresh cold water and simmer for twenty minutes. The lemony tea will help with coughs, colds, sore throats, and chest conditions.

Cooking with Pines

As this sampling of recipes will show, Pine is very versatile in the kitchen!

 ## White Pine Cookies

Gather fresh White Pine needles and then dry them in a food dehydrator or in a very slow oven (I like to dry herbs at about 110 degrees for several hours). The needles are ready when you can crumble them into a powder.

1 cup butter, softened

½ cup organic sugar

¼ cup raw honey

1 egg

2½ cups whole-wheat flour

1 teaspoon ground pine needles

1 teaspoon baking soda

1 teaspoon sea salt

Cream together the butter, sugar, honey, and egg. In a separate bowl, mix together the flour, pine needles, baking soda, and salt. Add to the butter mixture and mix well.

Place the dough in the refrigerator in a covered container for 2 hours.

Roll out the dough on a floured board to ¼ inch thickness. Cut with a cookie cutter (for simple round shapes you can use an upside-down glass).

Bake at 350 degrees for about 7 minutes.

Icing

1¼ cups coconut oil

¾ cup softened raw honey

2 tablespoons lemon juice (or juice of 1 lemon)

¼ cup tapioca starch

Cream the oil and honey, then whip. Add the lemon juice and tapioca and continue whipping until all are well combined. Ice the cookies when they are completely cooled.

Pine Gingerbread*

5 tablespoons butter, softened

9 tablespoons brown sugar

4 teaspoons grated ginger

¾ teaspoon vanilla extract

¾ cup plus 2 tablespoons wheat flour or gluten-free flour

½ teaspoon baking powder

¼ teaspoon sea salt

1 teaspoon ground black pepper

2 teaspoons ground pine needles

¼ cup milk

Cream the butter and sugar until fluffy, then mix in the grated ginger and vanilla.

In a separate bowl, combine the flour, baking powder, salt, pepper, and ground pine needles.

Add half of the milk to the creamed butter and mix well, then add half of the dry ingredients and mix again. When the batter is smooth, mix in the rest of the milk and then the rest of the dry ingredients.

Spread half of the batter onto a parchment-lined half-sheet pan. Spread the rest onto a second parchment-lined half-sheet pan.

Bake at 325 degrees for 15–18 minutes. The batter will be thinly spread, so watch carefully to see that it doesn't burn (rotate the sheets once during baking). Remove from the oven when the cookies are a medium brown.

---

*Adapted from Hunger and Thirst, "Fairy Gingerbread with Black Pepper and Pine," http://hungerandthirstforlife.blogspot.com/2012/12/fairy-gingerbread-with-black -pepper-and.html.

Cut the cookies into rectangles the moment they emerge from the oven (use a paring knife or, even better, a greased pizza wheel if you happen to have one).

When cooled, go over the cuts a second time, then peel off the parchment paper.

Pine Syrup

Gather about a quart of fresh white pine needles. Pour into a pot and just barely cover with a mixture of half water and half organic sugar. Simmer for about 20 minutes, tightly covered. Loosen the lid so steam can escape and simmer for another 20 minutes. Strain, allow to cool, and refrigerate.

Pine Elixir*

Pack fresh pine, spruce, or fir needles into a glass jar. Small twigs too. If you have a few small pieces of pine resin, add those to the mix (resin is found on the outer bark of the tree and on pine cones). Fill the jar three-quarters full of vodka and top off with raw local honey. Cap tightly and shake every few days. After a month strain out the liquid and store in a brown or blue glass bottle or in a dark cupboard.

Clarified Pine Butter

Pine butter is especially well suited for cooking meats and fish. Pansear the meat in pine butter oil or dot a fish with it as it bakes.

Gently heat organic butter until it is liquid. Pour off the ghee (the yellow liquid) and reserve. Discard the white fat globules that remain in the bottom of the pan.

Return the yellow clarified butter to the pan and stir in slightly dry pine needles. Heat the mixture until warm, then remove from the flame and cover with a lid.

Let it sit for 8 hours or so (leave a small crack on the side of the lid where

---

*You can also do this with fresh mint leaves, lemon balm, basil, fennel, or freshly sliced ginger.

steam can escape). Strain out the needles and store the ghee in a tightly capped jar.

Pine Oxymel

A variant of Fire Cider (see page 51), this is a remedy for coughs, colds, and flu.

1 part pine needles
1 part organic orange peels
1 part elderberries
1 part rosehips
Raw honey
Organic apple cider vinegar

Place the herbs in a glass jar and cover with honey (no more than one-third of the jar). Fill the rest of the jar with apple cider vinegar. Steep for about a month and then strain.

Pine Vinegar

Vinegar is used to tincture herbs such as cayenne and is a good agent to leach minerals out of plants (see goldenrod, for example, on page 33). Vinegar benefits bone health, digestion, and circulation.

Pack a jar about one-quarter full of pine needles and then fill the rest of the way with raw apple cider vinegar. Allow to steep for about a month and then strain.

Other Uses for Pine

The fresh scent of Pine makes it a good ingredient in preparations for the home and body.

Forest Incense

Combine pine needles and small twigs and those of other conifers with dried roses, sage, cedar, sweet grass, lavender, rosemary, copal, frankincense, myrrh, mugwort, or holy wood (*palo santo, Bursera graveolens*). Experiment with different combinations, using just two or three at a time, burning the mixtures in a ceramic dish or in an abalone shell that has been filled with sand.

Pine Bath Sachets

Fill a small cloth bag (or even an old cotton sock) with pine needles (or other conifer needles such as spruce), dried rose petals, and dried peppermint. For itchy skin, add oatmeal, and for sleep, add chamomile, lavender, hops, or jasmine instead of mint. Soak the bag in the tub for a while before you get in.

Pine, Peppermint, and Orange Bath Scrub

Mix together in a large bowl equal parts coarse kosher salt and fine sea salt. Add a large drizzle of cold-pressed olive oil and then essential oils of peppermint, sweet orange, and pine. Mix well with a wooden spoon and store in plastic containers (salt corrodes metal so avoid metal containers or metal lids). This one really wakes you up!

OTHER CONIFERS FOR HEALING

Cedar, Arborvitae, Thuja (*Thuja occidentalis*)

Cedar is the sacred tree of the Algonquin Nation and the sacred World Tree of the ancient Assyrians, and it was used in Babylonian and Chaldean healing rituals. The Algonquin say that the scent and taste of Cedar harmonize the emotions and "put one in the proper state of mind for prayer." The smoke of burning Cedar is used to consecrate and purify an area. The leaves are used as a "smudge" or incense for sacred ceremonies, burned fresh in the fire during rituals, and placed on the floor of the sweat lodge.

For the Algonquin, Arborvitae (tree of life) is the universal remedy that is taken for any illness. Centuries ago they gave Cedar tea to the first English settlers who arrived sick with scurvy on the shores of New England. It has more vitamin C than lemons and you can gather Cedar leaves and twigs year-round.

To make the tea: Gather the fresh twigs and "bracts" (the green leafy portions) and place in a pot. Barely cover with cold water; cover and simmer until the water starts to turn brown (do not boil). Lemony Cedar tea is delicious in any season and benefits the kidneys, rheumatism, coughs, and colds, and it can be taken as a general tonic.

Hemlock (*Tsuga canadensis, Abies canadensis, Pinus canadensis*)

I once heard the fairies singing in an old-growth Hemlock forest in western Massachusetts. I learned to eat the new growth on these trees from Chippewa-Cree elder Ron Evans. He said his people learned about it from the deer that graze on the branch tips in spring. The new growth is soft, lemony, and delicious and can be used in teas, salads, and healing salves. The pale green new branch tips are very well suited for sore throats and colds: try freezing them in ice cubes for use as tea throughout the year. They are also used as a tea for kidney problems and in the sweat lodge for rheumatic conditions, coughs, and colds.

To make the branch-tip tea: Bring water to a boil, remove from the heat, and place the new branch tips in the pot. Steep for about twenty minutes, with a tight lid on the pot. Take a cup a day in quarter-cup doses.

The inner bark is made into a tea for colds, diarrhea, fever, and scurvy and can be used externally to poultice bleeding injuries. *To make the bark tea:* Place the inner bark in a pot, just barely cover with cold water, and simmer for twenty minutes, with a tight lid on the pot (do not boil).

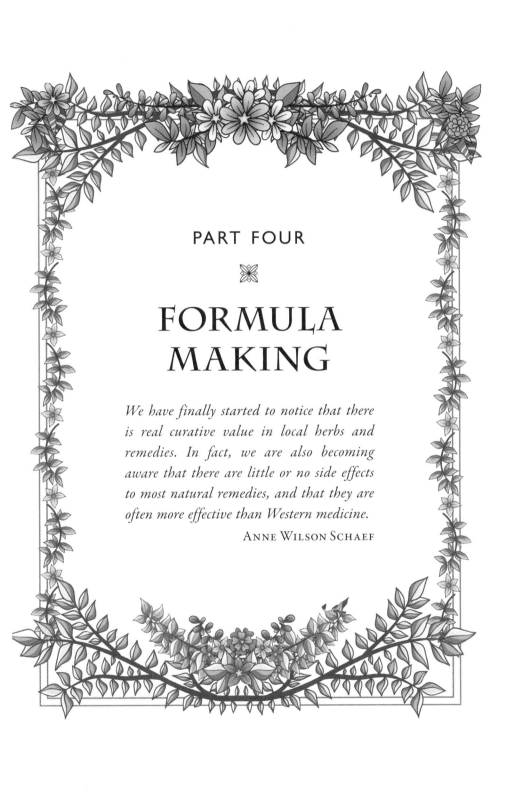

PART FOUR

FORMULA
MAKING

We have finally started to notice that there is real curative value in local herbs and remedies. In fact, we are also becoming aware that there are little or no side effects to most natural remedies, and that they are often more effective than Western medicine.

ANNE WILSON SCHAEF

16

GENERAL FORMULAS

From Tinctures to Poultices

Now that you have become familiar with herbs in your garden and kitchen, you will want to explore a few ways of creating formulas for "acute" (short term) and "chronic" (longer duration) conditions. Single plants can be used for short periods of time (no more than a few weeks) to address acute conditions. If a single plant is used month after month, it eventually irritates tissue and may actually harm an organ (unless it is an *alterative*, that is, an herb that is very gentle in action and suitable for long-term use).

For longer-term herbal therapy, it is wise to use at least three plants. This chapter includes a system of formula making, used by herbalist Michael Tierra and others, that uses several herbs, along with a system of constitutional prescribing that builds on a basic triangle of plants (a builder, a cleanser, and a tonic). *Builders* are plants that will nourish an organ or a body system, *cleansers* will clean the organ or body system, and *tonics* help balance both functions.

DELIVERY METHODS FOR HERBAL FORMULAS

Whichever system you use, your formula can take a number of different forms, some for internal use, and some for external application.

Preparations for Internal Use

Herbal formulas are usually taken between meals (one hour before or after). If taken *with* food, a formula becomes a tonic for a weak person. Formulas taken immediately *after* a meal can help address gas and digestive problems and urinary tract issues. Taken *before* a meal, a formula can benefit nervous conditions, tone the intestines, or aid in weight loss.

Capsules

The formula you create can be milled and put into "00"-size gelatin capsules. Capsules are taken two at a time, four times a day, between meals.

Tinctures

Another method is to combine the alcohol tinctures of all the plants you want into one bottle and take about twenty drops in water, four times a day. This is a good method for those who are travelling, since a single bottle of tincture is easy to carry. However, some herbs should only be tinctured in vinegar, not alcohol. Lobelia (*Lobelia inflata*) and Cayenne (*Capsicum annuum*) fit this category.

Herbal Glycerites

Glycerites are sweet vegetable glycerin extractions that make herbs palatable to children. Cold and flu herbs such as Elderberries (*Sambucus nigra*) and Echinacea (*Echinacea angustifolia, E. purpurea, E. pallida*) can be painlessly delivered to a small child using this method.

To Make an Herbal Glycerite

Fill a jar to the top with fresh chopped herbs or half full with dried herbs.

Cover fresh herbs with glycerin to within 1 inch of the top of the jar. For dried herbs use 1 part glycerin to 3 parts water and fill the jar to within 1 inch of the top.

Stir and poke with a spoon to remove air bubbles from the jar, then cap the jar and let it steep for 6 weeks. Shake every few days, and add more glycerin or glycerin and water if the plants absorb the liquid.

Strain the liquid through cheesecloth into dark glass bottles (or clear glass bottles that can be stored in a cool, dark cupboard). Be sure to label the mixture with the herbs used and the date!

To improve the taste of herbs for children, try adding licorice, fennel, peppermint, or spearmint. Give 10–60 drops, one to four times a day.

Herbs for Babies

The safest way for a baby to get an herbal formula is through his or her mother's breast milk. Mom drinks the tea and the child gets the milk. Herbs that are safe for babies can also be given with a dropper bottle; examples are Catnip (*Nepeta cataria*) for colic or Slippery Elm (*Ulmus fulva*) for gas.

Herbal Tea

Roots, barks, and berries are simmered. Leaves and flowers are steeped. Store teas in a large container in the refrigerator; they'll keep for up to a week. The usual adult dose is a quarter cup four times a day, not with meals.

Powdered Herbs

Powdered herbs can be infused overnight in cold water. Powdered herbs can also be added to soups, butter or ghee, warm milk, oil, or honey, or mixed with raw organic sugar. In medieval times the herbalist and abbess Hildegard of Bingen advised sprinkling powdered herbs on bread spread with lard or butter. (But do bear in mind that powdering herbs exposes more of their surface to oxygen and their maximum effectiveness lasts for only about three months.)

Some herbs have active principles that are actually harmed by heat and have to be cold-infused; examples are Apricot seeds (*Prunus armeniaca, Amygdalus armeniaca*) and Cherry bark (*Prunus serotina, P. virginiana*).

Salt and Vinegar

Add a pinch of salt to a formula for urinary tract toning, or to help carry herbs to the kidneys (to clean those organs adopt a salt-free diet at least for a while!). Bear in mind that the American diet tends to be high in salt already, so this may not be necessary.

Vinegar carries herbs to the liver—try macerating liver herbs in apple cider vinegar.

Preparations for External Application

Liniments

Liniments can be used externally to help heal bruises, sprains, sore muscles, and aching joints. Macerate one to three of the following herbs—Cayenne pepper (*Capsicum annuum*), Ginger root (*Zingiber officinale*), Myrrh (*Commiphora myrrha*), Arnica (*Arnica montana*), Angelica root (*Angelica archangelica*), Wild Ginger (*Asarum canadense*), Clove (*Syzygium aromaticum*), Cumin (*Cuminum cyminum*), and Bay Laurel leaf (*Laurus nobilis, Umbellularia californica,* etc.)—in rubbing alcohol for two weeks. Strain and rub into the affected area.

Plaster

Melt beeswax and then mix in a little honey. Spread on a clean cloth, sprinkle with stimulant herbs such as Cayenne pepper and powdered Ginger, and apply as needed to relieve pain in the muscles or congestion in the chest.

Fomentation

Make a strong decoction and then soak a clean cloth in the tea. Remove the cloth and, while it is still hot, place the herbs inside the cloth, fold it up, and apply. Grated Ginger is a classic for chest conditions. A combination of Chamomile (*Matricaria recutita, Chamaemelum nobile*), Sage (*Salvia officinalis*), and Mugwort (*Artemisia vulgaris*) can be applied to sore muscles, whiplash, and so on.

Drawing Poultice

A drawing poultice is made to pull debris such as dirt or splinters, or even tiny shards of glass, from a wound. After cleaning the wound thoroughly (using hydrogen peroxide, salt water, or the like), spread the following on a cloth: fresh Comfrey (*Symphytum officinale*) root or leaf or dried Comfrey root or leaf powder (softened with a little boiling water), a pinch of Cayenne to open up the capillaries and push out the debris, Plantain (*Plantago* spp.), and a little crushed, dry Pine sap (*Pinus* spp.). Then apply to the wound.

Medicated Oils

Macerate dried, powdered herbs in oil for two days or mash fresh herbs such as Ginger, Garlic, or Onions in oil and allow them to steep overnight.

Garlic oil can be rubbed on bruises and scrapes (do not put oil on deep wounds!). It can also be taken internally for colds and flu and for sore throat; it can be placed in the ear for earache.

Chickweed oil can be rubbed into dry, flaky eczema and other dry, itchy skin conditions.

Castor oil all by itself is excellent for arthritis, sciatica, and back pain. Soak a cloth in the oil, put it on the painful part, and cover with a towel. Place a hot water bottle over the towel and leave the cloth in place for forty-five minutes to an hour, daily. Remove the cloth and wash the area with soap and water.

HERBALIST MICHAEL TIERRA'S METHOD OF FORMULA MAKING

According to this method, seventy to eighty percent of your formula should consist of one to three herbs that exhibit the *primary* action you are looking for (e.g., lung herbs for bronchitis, warming immune boosters for a cold, etc.).

Then add a small amount of a *stimulant* plant, which will cause internal secretions to move. Ginger (*Zingiber officinale*) and Cayenne pepper (*Capsicum annuum*) are good examples.

Next add a small amount of an *antispasmodic* herb to calm the organs and tissues so they are more receptive to the plants. Examples of antispasmodic herbs include Lobelia (*Lobelia inflata*), Valerian (*Valeriana officinalis*), Skullcap (*Scutellaria lateriflora*), and Peony root (*Paeonia albiflora*).

Add a small amount of a *demulcent* herb to strengthen mucous linings and ease the passage of material from and through the body. Rose hips (*Rosa* spp.), Marshmallow root (*Althaea officinalis*), Licorice (*Glycyrrhiza glabra*), and Slippery Elm (*Ulmus fulva*) are all good demulcents.

And finally, to expel excess gas, add a *carminative* such as Cumin seed (*Cuminum cyminum*), Fennel seed (*Foeniculum vulgare*), Anise seed (*Pimpinella anisum*), or Garlic (*Allium sativum*).

Discerning a Healing Crisis from an Overdose or Side Effect

When taking medicinal herbs it's important to know when you are experiencing what is known as a "healing crisis" and when you are having a reaction to (or even overdosing on) a plant.

If you begin an herbal formula and experience a reoccurrence of old symptoms for a short while (from a few hours to a day), it is a healing crisis. This indicates that the body is bringing out previously suppressed symptoms and starting to deal with them.

If a healing crisis begins, the recommendation is to stop and wait, because once the body has begun to react to a remedy, that means that its own healing forces are at play. If a healing crisis is severe, you can choose to stop the formula or, if you can tolerate it, stop and then gradually reintroduce the formula.

If there is a sudden occurrence of completely *new* symptoms, that means you are actually *reacting to the herbal formula,* not the illness. This means you are experiencing an overdose or a side effect and the formula needs to be changed.

There are a handful of herbs that are stimulant, antispasmodic, and carminative all at once; Ginger, Licorice, Fennel seed, Anise seed, and Cumin seed fit this category. Chinese herbalists like to add a bit of Licorice to most formulas. They call it the "Peacemaker." It overcomes bitter taste, prevents allergic reactions, and harmonizes the effects of other herbs (though diabetics should avoid it since it is sweeter than sugar per volume).

CONSTITUTIONAL PRESCRIBING

For deeper, longer-lasting complaints or for long-term constitutional prescribing, I suggest the use of the elegant triangle system developed by herbalist William LeSassier, who was my teacher. According to William, he was lying on the couch one day as his wife was berating him about something and he escaped her words by going within mentally. Suddenly a voice began to speak to him. It was the philosopher and mathematician Pythagoras, who showed him the "triangle system" as he lay there on the couch.

I have been teaching students to use this system for over thirty years now, and I was recently informed by herbalist Matthew Wood that I am one of only two or three herbalists in the country doing so. He said I should get it all down on paper before it's "too late" (that realization became a major impetus for me to write this book).

This is an eighteen-part formula system. It is nice to try to find just a few herbs that address all the parts. I have been able to create formulas that cover four separate organs using just four or five herbs. The simpler the formula, the clearer the message you are sending to the body.

To begin, determine which organ system is the "center of gravity" for an illness. For example, in colon cancer it would be the colon, for bronchitis or emphysema it would be the lungs, for cystitis the bladder, and so on.

Next you need to identify herbs that are "builders" (+), "cleansers" (−), and "tonics" (0) for the body systems involved. As mentioned earlier, builders are herbs that nourish organs, cleansers are herbs that clean out organs or cause them to expel materials, and tonics are herbs that perform and balance both functions. The following chapter contains a detailed chart showing which herbs are building, cleansing, or tonic to each organ.

You will also want to consider the "temperature" of each herb: Does this person need a warming formula or a cooling one? Or maybe they need a formula that is more balanced? Generally speaking, hot herbs stimulate circulation and increase metabolic activity. Cooling herbs tend to be anti-inflammatory or antibacterial. When choosing your herbs, shake the hand of the person who is about to take the formula.

- Cold hands and paleness of face usually mean the person is chilly, losing energy, yin, and in need of building and nourishment. He or she will benefit from warm or hot herbs.
- Hot hands, especially when accompanied by constipation, red skin, or skin eruptions, mean a person is full, hot, toxic, and yang. He or she will benefit from cooling or cold herbs.

For conditions with cold, watery mucus, choose warm and dry plants and mix them with honey. Put the herbed honey into a tea.

Mapping the Formula

On a piece of paper draw two triangles, an inverted smaller triangle within a larger one (see fig. 16.1).

The triangle in the center represents the "center of gravity" for the illness. Within that triangle you will list three parts of a cleansing

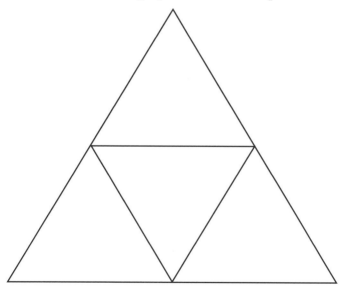

Fig. 16.1. The first step is to draw two triangles,
one inverted inside the other.

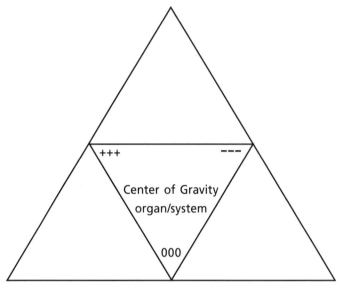

Fig. 16.2. In the inner triangle, list three parts of
a cleansing herb, three parts of a builder,
and three parts of a tonic.

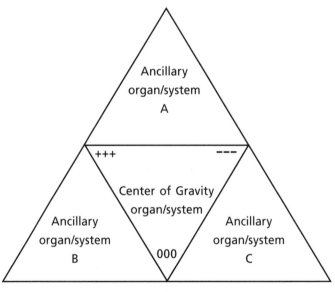

Fig. 16.3. List the ancillary organs or systems
in the three outer triangles.

herb (−), three parts of a builder (+), and three parts of a tonic herb (0) (see fig. 16.2). Your formula now has three herbs and nine parts.

Next you need to determine the concomitant or ancillary systems or organs affected. Place these in the three outer triangles. For example, a person with severe acne might have the skin as the "center of gravity" for his or her condition, and the three ancillary organs might be the liver, kidneys, and colon, (because chronic skin eruptions are often symptoms of sluggish elimination (see fig. 16.3).

Next, a "bridge herb" is selected; it needs to address both ancillary organs A and C. Select another bridge herb to address organs B and C, and a third to address A and B, for a total of three bridge herbs. Each bridge herb gets two parts in the formula (see fig. 16.4). Your formula now has fifteen parts.

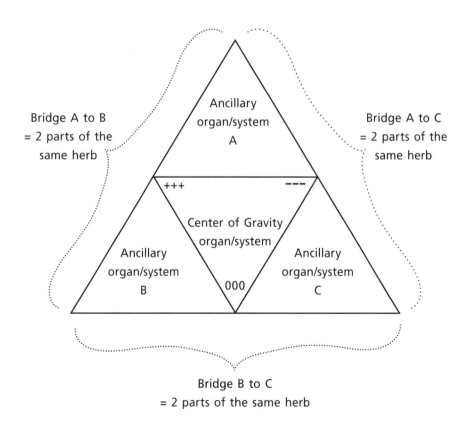

Fig. 16.4. Select three bridge herbs.

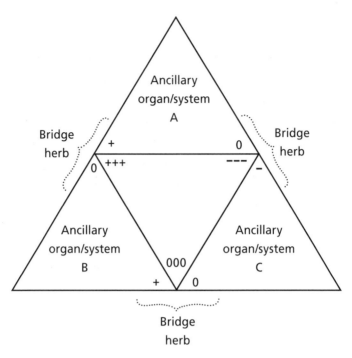

Fig. 16.5. Fill in the functions of the bridge herbs, with the goal of having each outer triangle complete with a builder, a tonic, and a cleanser.

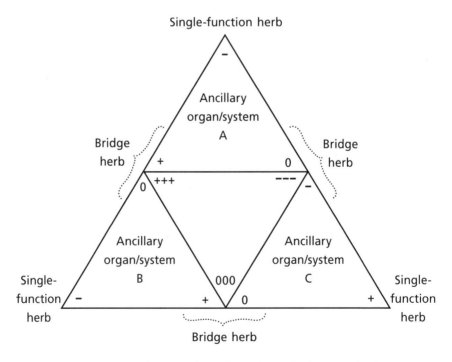

Fig. 16.6. Complete the formula with single-function herbs.

Within each outer triangle there needs to be a builder, a tonic, and a cleanser. It doesn't matter where in the triangle these occur. Begin with the bridge herbs. One bridge herb might be building to organ A and tonic for organ B. Another bridge herb could be a cleanser for organ C and a tonic for organ A. A third bridge herb could be a tonic for organ C and a builder for organ B (see fig. 16.5).

All that remains now is to complete the formula by adding a third herb at the outer corner of each outer triangle. This herb will be only one part and will ensure that each organ has a builder to nourish it, a cleanser to move waste through and out of it, and a tonic to balance it. In figure 16.5 we see that organ A is missing a cleanser, so one part of a cleansing herb is placed at the apex of that triangle. Organ B in our chart is missing a cleanser, so we place a cleansing herb at the lower left corner. Organ C is missing a builder, so we place a building herb in the lower right corner. We have now added three more herbs and brought the total parts to eighteen (see fig. 16.6).

To see what the finished eighteen-part formula looks like, turn to figure 16.7 on page 210.

The beauty of this system is that if a person is chilly, debilitated, and weak, we can simply double up on the building herbs. If a person is hot, congested, and "full," we can double up on the cleansers. Otherwise the eighteen-part formula is a balanced approach for long-term constitutional prescribing.

The way I work with this is to use the eighteen-part triangle system to address the physical body, and I add a flower essence for each client to deal with the mental/emotional sphere (as well as dietary and exercise recommendations). At the same time, it is also possible to choose herbs that affect spiritual and psychological needs. For example, flowers and leaves will help lighten a personality and make a person more flexible. Roots are more grounding, and tree parts such as barks and needles tend to be balancing (because trees have their roots in the ground and their head in the sky). The astrological signs associated with the herbs (given in chapter 9) are also a guide to how a plant will affect the mental/emotional sphere.

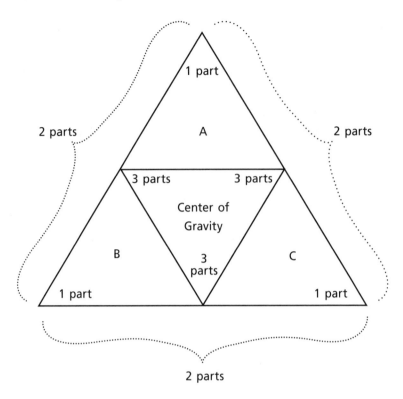

Fig. 16.7. The finished formula will have:

3 parts of a cleansing herb for the center of gravity of the illness

3 parts of a tonic herb for the center of gravity of the illness

3 parts of a building herb for the center of gravity of the illness

2 parts of a bridge herb between A and B

2 parts of a bridge herb between B and C

2 parts of a bridge herb between A and C

1 part of an herb to finish triangle A

1 part of an herb to finish triangle B

1 part of an herb to finish triangle C

17

CONSTITUTIONAL PRESCRIBING

Plants to Build, Cleanse, and Tone the Organs and Systems of the Body

This chapter consists of two tables that will guide your choices of plants as you prepare your formulas using the triangle system of constitutional prescribing described in the previous chapter.

Plants to Improve the Function of Organs and Systems of the Body 212
Plants for Some Common Conditions   275

In the first table, Plants to Improve the Function of Organs and Systems of the Body (pages 212–74), plants are grouped according to their capacity as builders, cleansers, or tonics. Please note that some plants are builders and cleansers for the same organ/system. Also note that some systems only have lists for builders and cleansers. In such cases you can make a tonic by combining a builder and a cleanser.

The second table, Plants for Some Common Conditions (pages 275–80), is a section on general and particular health concerns listing plants that can help improve overall well-being.

In the lists of plants, the information per plant is organized with the common name plus plant part (where applicable), then the scientific name, then thermal and moisture properties, followed (where applicable) by pertinent specifics and cautions regarding their application.

PLANTS TO IMPROVE THE FUNCTION
OF ORGANS AND SYSTEMS OF THE BODY

COMMON NAME AND PLANT PART	SCIENTIFIC NAME	THERMAL AND MOISTURE PROPERTIES	APPLICATION
Adrenal Glands—Builders (+)			
American Ginseng, White	Panax quinquefolius	warm	
Goldenseal	Hydrastis canadensis	dry and hot	1/10 part of a formula or less
Licorice	Glycyrrhiza glabra	warm and moist	
Red Sarsaparilla	Smilax ornata	warm and moist	
Rehmannia	Rehmannia glutinosa	cool	
Adrenal Glands—Cleansers (−)			
Burdock seeds	Arctium lappa	cold	
Damiana	Turnera aphrodisiaca	warm	
Saint-John's-Wort	Hypericum perforatum	cool and dry	
White Sage	Salvia apiana	dry and cool	
Adrenal Glands—Tonics (0)			
Nettles	Urtica dioica, U. urens	dry and hot	
Red Sarsaparilla	Smilax ornata	warm and moist	
Siberian Ginseng	Eleutherococcus senticosus	warm	
Blood—Builders (+)			
Astragalus	Astragalus hoantchy, A. membranaceus, A. mongolicus	warm	
Beets	Beta vulgaris	cool	
Cayenne	Capsicum annuum	hot	
Chives	Allium schoenoprasum	warm	
Dandelion leaf	Taraxacum officinale	cool	
Dong Quai	Angelica sinensis, A. polymorpha	warm	
Elderberries	Sambucus spp.	neutral	

COMMON NAME AND PLANT PART	SCIENTIFIC NAME	THERMAL AND MOISTURE PROPERTIES	APPLICATION
Lentils	*Lens culinaris*	warm	
Nettles	*Urtica dioica, U. urens*	dry and hot	
Raspberry fruits	*Rubus* spp.	neutral	
Rehmannia	*Rehmannia glutinosa*	cool	
White Peony	*Paeonia alba*	cold	
Yellow Dock, Curly Dock root	*Rumex crispus*	cool	
Blood—Cleansers (−)			
Angelica root	*Angelica archangelica*	warm	
Barberry root	*Berberis vulgaris*	cold	skin eruptions
Blessed Thistle	*Carbenia benedicta, Cnicus benedictus*	cool	
Burdock root	*Arctium lappa*	cool	
Calendula flowers	*Calendula officinalis*	neutral	
Centaury	*Erythraea centaurium*	cool	
Chinese Cinnamon	*Cinnamomum cassia*	dry and hot	
Cleavers, Bedstraw	*Galium aparine*	dry and cool	
Echinacea	*Echinacea angustifolia, E. pallida, E. purpurea*	dry and hot	skin eruptions, septicemia
Elderflowers	*Sambucus* spp.	cool	
Eucalyptus	*Eucalyptus globulus*	warm	
Garlic	*Allium sativum*	hot	
Gentian	*Gentiana lutea, G. officinalis*	cold	
Goat's Rue	*Galega officinalis*	cool and dry	
Goldenseal	*Hydrastis canadensis*	dry and hot	1/10 part of a formula or less
Hibiscus	*Hibiscus rosa-sinensis*	cool	
Ocotillo	*Fouquieria splendens*	cool	
Oregon Grape root	*Mahonia repens*	cold	
Pipsissewa, Prince's Pine	*Chimaphila umbellata*	dry and hot	

COMMON NAME AND PLANT PART	SCIENTIFIC NAME	THERMAL AND MOISTURE PROPERTIES	APPLICATION
Red Clover blossoms	*Trifolium pratense*	dry and cool	
Redroot, New Jersey Tea	*Ceanothus americanus*	dry and hot	slow coagulation
Red Sarsaparilla	*Smilax ornata*	warm and moist	
Sanicle	*Sanicula europaea*	dry and hot	
Shepherd's Purse	*Capsella bursa-pastoris*	neutral	elevated uric acid
Vervain	*Verbena officinalis, V. hastata*	cold	
Violet leaf	*Viola odorata*	cool	
Watercress	*Nasturtium officinale*	warm	
Wood Betony	*Betonica officinalis, Stachys officinalis*	cool	
Blood—Tonics (0)			
Amaranth	*Amaranthus hypochondriacus*	neutral	stops bleeding
American Ginseng, Red	*Panax quinquefolius*	warm	lowers blood pressure, lowers cholesterol
Bayberry, Wax Myrtle	*Myrica cerifera*	dry and hot	brings heat to the extremities
Birthroot, Trillium	*Trillium pendulum*	warm	styptic
Blessed Thistle	*Carbenia benedicta, Cnicus benedictus*	cool	
Bloodroot	*Sanguinaria canadensis*	dry and hot	brings blood to the area where applied
Blue Cohosh	*Caulophyllum thalictroides*	warm and dry	
Burdock root	*Arctium lappa*	cool	
Catnip	*Nepeta cataria*	cold and moist	lowers blood pressure
Cayenne	*Capsicum annuum*	hot	balances blood pressure, styptic
Dandelion root	*Taraxacum officinale*	cool	

COMMON NAME AND PLANT PART	SCIENTIFIC NAME	THERMAL AND MOISTURE PROPERTIES	APPLICATION
Garlic	*Allium sativum*	hot	reduces blood pressure
Goldenseal	*Hydrastis canadensis*	dry and hot	1/10 part of a formula or less
Lady's Mantle	*Alchemilla vulgaris*	neutral	stops bleeding
Motherwort	*Leonurus cardiaca*	neutral and dry	lowers blood pressure
Nettles	*Urtica dioica,* *U. urens*	dry and hot	
Oregon Grape root	*Mahonia repens*	cold	
Sage	*Salvia apiana,* *S. officinalis*	dry and cool	styptic
Siberian Ginseng	*Eleutherococcus senticosus*	warm	lowers cholesterol
Skullcap	*Scutellaria lateriflora*	dry and cool	balances blood pressure
Witch Hazel bark and leaf	*Hamamelis virginiana*	dry and hot	astringent, shrinks blood vessels
Bones—Builders (+)			
Black Walnut	*Juglans nigra*	cold	cartilage
Blessed Thistle	*Carbenia benedicta,* *Cnicus benedictus*	cool	cartilage
Chicory	*Cichorium intybus*	cold	may increase calcium absorption and bone mineral density
Comfrey leaf	*Symphytum officinale*	cool and moist	regenerates tissues
Horsetail	*Equisetum hyemale*	cool	
Raspberry leaf	*Rubus idaeus*	cool	
White Peony	*Paeonia alba*	cold	marrow
Bones—Cleansers (−)			
Elderberry	*Sambucus nigra,* *S. canadensis*	neutral	bone marrow
Brain—Builders (+)			
Black Walnut	*Juglans nigra*	cold	

COMMON NAME AND PLANT PART	SCIENTIFIC NAME	THERMAL AND MOISTURE PROPERTIES	APPLICATION
Gotu Kola	*Centella asiatica*	cool	improves rote memory
Brain—Cleansers (−)			
Angelica root	*Angelica archangelica*	warm	
Red Clover	*Trifolium pratense*	dry and cool	
Brain—Tonics (0)			
Blessed Thistle	*Carbenia benedicta, Cnicus benedictus*	cool	improves deep memory
Calamus, Sweet Flag	*Acorus calamus*	warm	improves memory
Cannabis, Da Ma tincture or tea of flowering tops, fresh or frozen raw leaf in smoothies	*Cannabis sativa*	warm and dry	insomnia, frequent waking with nightmares; acts as a sedative, regulates the brain in epilepsy
Gotu Kola	*Centella asiatica*	cool	improves rote memory
Breasts—Builders (+)			
Alfalfa	*Medicago sativa*	cool	galactagogue
Anise	*Pimpinella anisum*	warm	galactagogue
Black Cohosh	*Cimicifuga racemosa*	cool	reflex pain while breastfeeding
Blessed Thistle	*Carbenia benedicta, Cnicus benedictus*	cool	galactagogue
Borage	*Borago officinalis*	cool	galactagogue
Chasteberry, Vitex	*Vitex agnus-castus*	neutral	galactagogue
Dandelion root	*Taraxacum officinale*	cool	galactagogue
Fennel	*Foeniculum vulgare*	warm and moist	galactagogue
Fenugreek	*Trigonella foenum-graecum*	warm	galactagogue
Flax seed	*Linum usitatissimum*	neutral	galactagogue
Goat's Rue	*Galega officinalis*	cool and dry	galactagogue
Hops	*Humulus lupulus*	cool	galactagogue
Marshmallow root	*Althaea officinalis*	cool and moist	galactagogue

COMMON NAME AND PLANT PART	SCIENTIFIC NAME	THERMAL AND MOISTURE PROPERTIES	APPLICATION
Milk Thistle	*Silybum marianum*	cold	galactagogue
Nettles	*Urtica dioica, U. urens*	dry and hot	galactagogue
Osha	*Ligusticum filicinum, L. porteri*	dry and hot	galactagogue
Breasts—Cleansers (−)			
Asafoetida	*Ferula asafoetida*	dry and hot	
Bistort	*Polygonum bistorta*	cool	
Dandelion root	*Taraxacum officinale*	cool	
Echinacea	*Echinacea angustifolia, E. pallida, E. purpurea*	dry and hot	stomatitis while nursing
Guaiacum	*Guaiacum officinale*	cool	
Poke root	*Phytolacca esculenta*	dry and hot	acute mastitis; externally in poultice, internally as homeopathic remedy
Red Clover	*Trifolium pratense*	dry and cool	
Sage	*Salvia apiana, S. officinalis*	dry and cool	to wean, dry up breast milk
Circulation—Builders (+)			
Angelica root	*Angelica archangelica*	warm	
Chinese Cinnamon	*Cinnamomum cassia*	dry and hot	
Chives	*Allium schoenoprasum*	warm	
Dandelion root	*Taraxacum officinale*	cool	
Dong Quai	*Angelica sinensis, A. polymorpha*	warm	opens and drains the spleen
Gentian	*Gentiana lutea, G. officinalis*	cold	
Nettles	*Urtica dioica, U. urens*	dry and hot	
Rehmannia	*Rehmannia glutinosa*	cool	
Sassafras	*Sassafras albidum, S. variifolium*	dry and hot	

COMMON NAME AND PLANT PART	SCIENTIFIC NAME	THERMAL AND MOISTURE PROPERTIES	APPLICATION
Self-heal	*Prunella vulgaris*	cold	for infected state
Watercress	*Nasturtium officinale*	warm	
Yellow Dock, Curly Dock root	*Rumex crispus*	cool	to balance copper and iron
Circulation—Cleansers (−)			
Calendula flowers	*Calendula officinalis*	neutral	
Dong Quai	*Angelica sinensis, A. polymorpha*	warm	
Guaiacum	*Guaiacum officinale*	cool	
Oregon Grape root	*Mahonia repens*	cold	
Stillingia	*Stillingia sylvatica*	cool	
Circulation—Tonics (0)			
Blessed Thistle	*Carbenia benedicta, Cnicus benedictus*	cool	
Burdock root	*Arctium lappa*	cool	
Nettles	*Urtica dioica, U. urens*	dry and hot	
Prickly Ash	*Zanthoxylum clava-herculis, Z. americanum*	warm	
White Peony	*Paeonia alba*	cold	
Eyes—Builders (+)			
Apricots	*Prunus armeniaca*	warm and moist	food and also as a poultice
Carrots	*Daucus carota* subsp. *sativus*	neutral	food and also as a poultice
Rue	*Ruta graveolens*	warm	color blindness
Eyes—Cleansers (−)			
Chamomile	*Chamaemelum nobile, Matricaria recutita*	warm and moist	external for infections
Eyebright	*Euphrasia officinalis*	cool	
Goldenseal	*Hydrastis canadensis*	dry and hot	external for pink eye, infections

COMMON NAME AND PLANT PART	SCIENTIFIC NAME	THERMAL AND MOISTURE PROPERTIES	APPLICATION
Ground Ivy, Creeping Charlie, Gill-over-the-Ground	*Glechoma hederacea*	cool	
Horsetail	*Equisetum hyemale*	cool	
Eyes—Tonics (0)			
Cannabis, Da Ma smoke, inhaled	*Cannabis sativa*	warm and dry	glaucoma
Eyebright	*Euphrasia officinalis*	cool	
Female Reproductive System: Hormonal System—Builders (+)			
False Unicorn root	*Chamaelirium luteum*	warm	
Licorice	*Glycyrrhiza glabra*	warm and moist	
Wild Yam	*Dioscorea villosa*	warm and dry	
Female Reproductive System: Hormonal System—Cleansers (−)			
Black Cohosh	*Cimicifuga racemosa*	cool	chronic amenorrhea with congestion and irritation
Blue Cohosh	*Caulophyllum thalictroides*	warm and dry	chronic amenorrhea with congestion and irritation
Chinese Cinnamon	*Cinnamomum cassia*	hot	
Damiana	*Turnera aphrodisiaca*	warm	
False Unicorn root	*Chamaelirium luteum*	warm	amenorrhea with anemia
Water Plantain	*Alisma plantago-aquatica*	cold	
White Sage	*Salvia apiana*	dry and cool	
Female Reproductive System: Hormonal System—Tonics (0)			
Red Sarsaparilla	*Smilax ornata*	warm and moist	
Saw Palmetto berry	*Serenoa serrulata*	warm and moist	
Shatavari, Indian Asparagus root	*Asparagus racemosa*	cold and moist	balances hormones, improves fertility and vitality; for PMS, menopausal symptoms, polycystic ovary syndrome

COMMON NAME AND PLANT PART	SCIENTIFIC NAME	THERMAL AND MOISTURE PROPERTIES	APPLICATION
White Sarsaparilla	*Aralia nudicaulis*	cool and moist	
Female Reproductive System: Nervous System—Builders (+)			
Dong Quai	*Angelica sinensis, A. polymorpha*	warm	dysmenorrhea with mood swings
Ginger	*Zingiber officinale*	dry and hot	
Licorice	*Glycyrrhiza glabra*	warm and moist	
Saw Palmetto berry	*Serenoa serrulata*	warm and moist	
Siberian Ginseng	*Eleutherococcus senticosus*	warm	
Female Reproductive System: Nervous System—Cleansers (−)			
Basil	*Ocimum basilicum*	warm	
Black Haw	*Viburnum prunifolium*	cool	
Catnip	*Nepeta cataria*	cold and moist	
Cramp Bark	*Viburnum opulus*	cool	
Mugwort	*Artemisia vulgaris*	warm	
Rue	*Ruta graveolens*	warm	
Skullcap	*Scutellaria lateriflora*	dry and cool	
Vervain	*Verbena officinalis, V. hastata*	cold	
Female Reproductive System: Nervous System—Tonics (0)			
Aspen bark	*Populus* spp.	cold	chronic premestrual tension without insomnia; take for three days before the onset of menses
Chamomile	*Chamaemelum nobile, Matricaria recutita*	warm and moist	
Lady's Slipper	*Cypripedium pubescens*	neutral	hot flashes with melancholia
Motherwort	*Leonurus cardiaca*	neutral and dry	uterine stimulant, menstrual regultor; for irritability and emotional tension with and before the menses

COMMON NAME AND PLANT PART	SCIENTIFIC NAME	THERMAL AND MOISTURE PROPERTIES	APPLICATION
Oat straw	*Avena sativa*	neutral	
Passionflower	*Passiflora incarnata*	cool	premenstrual insomnia, restless in evenings
Saint-John's-Wort	*Hypericum perforatum*	cool and dry	
Slippery Elm	*Ulmus fulva*	cool and moist	
Vervain	*Verbena officinalis, V. hastata*	cold	
Female Reproductive System: Obstetric—Builders (+)			
Cayenne	*Capsicum annuum*	hot	postpartum hemorrhage with good uterine tone, miscarriage with hemorrhage or spotting
Chinese Cinnamon	*Cinnamomum cassia*	hot	postpartum hemorrhage with lack of contraction
Partridgeberry	*Mitchella repens*	warm and dry	1/5 part of a formula or less; prepartum irritability, emotional distress in last trimester, with history of miscarriage
Uva Ursi, Bearberry	*Arctostaphylos uva-ursi*	cold	sitz bath for postpartum hemorrhage with tearing or episiotomy
Female Reproductive System: Obstetric—Cleansers (−)			
Uva Ursi, Bearberry	*Arctostaphylos uva-ursi*	cold	sitz bath postpartum
Female Reproductive System: Obstetric—Tonics (0)			
Black Cohosh	*Cimicifuga racemosa*	cool	false labor pains, in last two weeks of pregnancy to prepare the uterus, uterine subinvolution

COMMON NAME AND PLANT PART	SCIENTIFIC NAME	THERMAL AND MOISTURE PROPERTIES	APPLICATION
Blue Cohosh	*Caulophyllum thalictroides*	warm and dry	delayed labor, to speed labor, fatigue, history of inflammation
Cramp Bark	*Viburnum opulus*	cool	false labor pains, impending miscarriage with cramping, history of miscarriage
Lobelia	*Lobelia inflata*	neutral	rigid cervix
Raspberry leaf	*Rubus idaeus*	cool	in last trimester to prepare the uterus
Witch Hazel	*Hamamelis virginiana*	dry and hot	external fomentation for enlarged veins in pregnancy
Yarrow	*Achillea millefolium*	neutral	external fomentation for enlarged veins in pregnancy
Female Reproductive System: Uterine Structure and Cervix—Builders (+)			
Black Cohosh	*Cimicifuga racemosa*	cool	delayed menses not from pregnancy
Black Haw	*Viburnum prunifolium*	cool	
Blue Cohosh	*Caulophyllum thalictroides*	warm and dry	painful menses
Burdock root	*Arctium lappa*	cool	uterine prolapse
Cramp Bark	*Viburnum opulus*	cool	dysmenorrhea
Damiana	*Turnera aphrodisiaca*	warm	delayed menses not from pregnancy
Dong Quai	*Angelica sinensis, A. polymorpha*	warm	taken during ovulation to increase fertility
Ginseng	*Panax* spp.	warm	delayed menses with recent growth spurt in adolescents

COMMON NAME AND PLANT PART	SCIENTIFIC NAME	THERMAL AND MOISTURE PROPERTIES	APPLICATION
Partridgeberry	*Mitchella repens*	warm and dry	1/5 part of a formula or less
Female Reproductive System: Uterine Structure and Cervix—Cleansers (−)			
Aloe	*Aloe barbadensis, A. officinalis*	cold	amenorrhea with constipation
Angelica root	*Angelica archangelica*	warm	
Birthroot, Trillium	*Trillium pendulum*	warm	expels placenta, stops bleeding
Black Cohosh	*Cimicifuga racemosa*	cool	amenorrhea with irritation, pain on walking up or down the stairs
Blue Cohosh	*Caulophyllum thalictroides*	warm and dry	amenorrhea with irritation, dysmenor-rhea, endometriosis
Calendula flowers	*Calendula officinalis*	neutral	douche, for cervicitis
Cotton root	*Gossypium herbaceum*	warm	abortive
Cramp Bark	*Viburnum opulus*	cool	leukorrhea with spasms
Dong Quai	*Angelica sinensis, A. polymorpha*	warm	amenorrhea with mood swings, cervicitis with congestion, poor circulation, dysmenorrhea, endometriosis, smelly leukorrhea, hot flashes in menopause
Echinacea	*Echinacea angustifolia, E. pallida, E. purpurea*	dry and hot	orally for cervicitis
Elecampane	*Inula helenium*	dry and hot	endometriosis with thick mucous discharge
Gentian	*Gentiana lutea, G. officinalis*	cold	

COMMON NAME AND PLANT PART	SCIENTIFIC NAME	THERMAL AND MOISTURE PROPERTIES	APPLICATION
Ginger	*Zingiber officinale*	dry and hot	cramps, spasms, helps bring on the menses
Goldenseal	*Hydrastis canadensis*	dry and hot	abortive; 1/10 part of a formula or less
Horehound	*Marrubium vulgare*	cool	expels placenta
Osha	*Ligusticum filicinum, L. porteri*	dry and hot	
Partridgeberry	*Mitchella repens*	warm and dry	1/5 part of a formula or less
Pennyroyal	*Hedeoma pulegioides, Mentha pulegium*	warm	abortive, for amenorrhea
Rue	*Ruta graveolens*	warm	abortive
Safflower	*Carthamus tinctorius*	warm	
Sassafras	*Sassafras albidum, S. variifolium*	dry and hot	after abortion to cleanse
Tansy	*Tanacetum vulgare*	warm	abortive
Yarrow flowers	*Achillea millefolium*	neutral	
Female Reproductive System: Uterine Structure and Cervix—Tonics (0)			
Black Cohosh	*Cimicifuga racemosa*	cool	
Black Haw	*Viburnum prunifolium*	cool	
Cannabis, Da Ma tincture or tea of flowering tops	*Cannabis sativa*	warm and dry	endometriosis with spasms
Chasteberry, Vitex	*Vitex agnus-castus*	neutral	premenstrual syndrome, hot flashes in menopause
Cramp Bark	*Viburnum opulus*	cool	dysmenorrhea with spasms and radiating pains, with scanty flow
Dong Quai	*Angelica sinensis, A. polymorpha*	warm	menopause
Partridgeberry	*Mitchella repens*	warm and dry	1/5 part of a formula or less

COMMON NAME AND PLANT PART	SCIENTIFIC NAME	THERMAL AND MOISTURE PROPERTIES	APPLICATION
Raspberry	*Rubus idaeus*	cool	to prepare for pregnancy, for dymenorrhea toward end of menses with bright red blood, prolonged heavy periods
Turmeric	*Curcuma longa*	warm	
Yarrow	*Achillea millefolium*	neutral	prolonged heavy periods
Gallbladder—Builders (+)			
Barberry root	*Berberis vulgaris*	cold	
Cascara Sagrada	*Cascara sagrada*	cold	
Fringe Tree	*Chionanthus virginicus*	cool	hepatitis, jaundice, gallstones
Ginger	*Zingiber officinale*	dry and hot	
Licorice	*Glycyrrhiza glabra*	warm and moist	
Oregon Grape root	*Mahonia repens*	cold	
Gallbladder—Cleansers (−)			
Blue Flag	*Iris versicolor*	cool and dry	
Parsley	*Petroselinum crispum*	neutral	
Peppermint	*Mentha piperita*	cool	
Queen of the Meadow, Joe Pye Weed, Gravel Root	*Eupatorium purpureum*	warm	
Rosemary	*Rosmarinus officinalis*	warm and hot	
Wild Yam	*Dioscorea villosa*	warm and dry	
Gallbladder—Tonics (0)			
Marshmallow root	*Althaea officinalis*	cool and moist	
Gums—Builders (+)			
Myrrh	*Commiphora myrrha*	dry and hot	
Gums—Cleansers (−)			
Bayberry, Wax Myrtle root	*Myrica cerifera*	dry and hot	

COMMON NAME AND PLANT PART	SCIENTIFIC NAME	THERMAL AND MOISTURE PROPERTIES	APPLICATION
Bloodroot	*Sanguinaria canadensis*	dry and cool in small amounts, warm in larger amounts	
Burdock root	*Arctium lappa*	cool	
Goldenseal	*Hydrastis canadensis*	dry and hot	1/10 part of a formula or less
Plantain leaf	*Plantago* spp.	cool and dry	
Heart—Builders (+)			
Blessed Thistle	*Carbenia benedicta, Cnicus benedictus*	cool	
Comfrey leaf	*Symphytum officinale*	cool and moist	regenerates tissues
Dandelion flowers	*Taraxacum officinale*	cool	
Goldenseal	*Hydrastis canadensis*	dry and hot	1/10 part of a formula or less
Hawthorn berry, also spring-gathered leaf and flower	*Crataegus* spp.	warm	
Lobelia	*Lobelia inflata*	neutral	angina with low pulse
Motherwort	*Leonurus cardiaca*	neutral and dry	
Raspberry leaf	*Rubus idaeus*	cool	
Rose hips	*Rosa* spp.	neutral	
Heart—Cleansers (−)			
American Ginseng	*Panax quinquefolius*	warm	lowers lipids
Angelica root	*Angelica archangelica*	warm	diuretic that calms the heart
Cayenne	*Capsicum annuum*	hot	
Garlic	*Allium sativum*	hot	lowers blood pressure
Mullein	*Verbascum thapsus*	warm and moist	
Heart—Tonics (0)			
Blue Cohosh	*Caulophyllum thalictroides*	warm and dry	antispasmodic

COMMON NAME AND PLANT PART	SCIENTIFIC NAME	THERMAL AND MOISTURE PROPERTIES	APPLICATION
Borage	*Borago officinalis*	cool	
Cinchona	*Cinchona officinalis*	warm	stops fibrillation, antiarrhythmic
Hawthorn young leaf and flower, berries	*Crataegus* spp.	warm	lowers blood pressure, for palpitations
Mistletoe, European	*Viscum album*	neutral	for congestive failure, heart enlargement, valvular incompetence
Passionflower	*Passiflora incarnata*	cool	for heart palpitation in evening with emotional component
Scotch Broom	*Cytisus scoparius*	warm	stimulant, edema
Walnut hull tea	*Juglans* spp.	cold	alleviates pressure and pain
Joints—Builders (+)			
Gutta-Percha Tree, Hardy Rubber Tree bark	*Eucommia ulmoides*	cool	
Horsetail	*Equisetum hyemale*	cool	
Joints—Cleansers (−)			
Devil's Claw	*Harpagophytum procumbens*	cool	anti-inflammatory, arthritis, rheumatism, gout
White Willow	*Salix alba*	cold	
Yucca	*Yucca* spp.	cool	anti-inflammatory, arthritis, rheumatism
Joints—Tonics (0)			
Cannabis, Da Ma root	*Cannabis sativa*	warm and dry	gout
Turmeric	*Curcuma longa*	warm	pain, inflammation, osteoarthritis and rheumatoid arthritis

COMMON NAME AND PLANT PART	SCIENTIFIC NAME	THERMAL AND MOISTURE PROPERTIES	APPLICATION
Kidneys—Builders (+)			
Comfrey leaf	Symphytum officinale	cool and moist	
Fenugreek	Trigonella foenum-graecum	warm	
Flax seeds	Linum usitatissimum	neutral	
Goldenseal	Hydrastis canadensis	dry and hot	1/10 part of a formula or less
Gotu Kola	Centella asiatica	cool	
Horsetail, spring gathered	Equisetum hyemale	cool	nephritis with edema
Marshmallow root	Althaea officinalis	cool and moist	
Licorice root	Glycyrrhiza glabra	warm and moist	
Oat straw	Avena sativa	neutral	
Red Sarsaparilla	Smilax ornata	warm and moist	
Siberian Ginseng	Eleutherococcus senticosus	warm	
Kidneys—Cleansers (−)			
Asparagus root	Asparagus officinalis	cold	diuretic
Bedstraw, Cleavers	Galium aparine	dry and cool	
Buchu	Agathosma betulina	dry and warm	diuretic
Burdock seeds	Arctium lappa	cold	
Calendula flowers	Calendula officinalis	neutral	
Chinese Cinnamon	Cinnamomum cassia	hot	
Damiana	Turnera aphrodisiaca	warm	diuretic
Ginger	Zingiber officinale	dry and hot	
Grindelia	Grindelia camporum	warm	diuretic
Juniper berry	Juniperus communis	warm	diuretic, chronic weakness without inflammation
Limeflower, Linden	Tilia cordata	cool and dry	
Myrrh	Commiphora myrrha	dry and hot	
Oregon Grape root	Mahonia repens	cold	
Parsley leaf or root	Petroselinum crispum	neutral	for infection only

COMMON NAME AND PLANT PART	SCIENTIFIC NAME	THERMAL AND MOISTURE PROPERTIES	APPLICATION
Pipsissewa, Prince's Pine	*Chimaphila umbellata*	dry and hot	
Queen of the Meadow, Joe Pye Weed, Gravel Root	*Eupatorium purpureum*	warm	
Saint-John's-Wort	*Hypericum perforatum*	cool and dry	
Sassafras	*Sassafras albidum, S. variifolium*	dry and hot	
Uva Ursi	*Arctostaphylos uva-ursi*	cold	
Yarrow	*Achillea millefolium*	neutral	
Yerba Santa	*Eriodictyon* spp.	warm	diuretic
Kidneys—Tonics (0)			
Aspen bark	*Populus* spp.	cold	
Astragalus	*Astragalus hoantchy, A. membranaceus, A. mongolicus*	warm	
Dandelion leaf and root	*Taraxacum officinale*	cool	
He Shou Wu, Fo-ti Tieng	*Polygonum multiflorum*	warm	
Nettles	*Urtica dioica, U. urens*	dry and hot	
Plantain leaf	*Plantago* spp.	cool and dry	
Raspberry leaf	*Rubus idaeus*	cool	
Saw Palmetto berry	*Serenoa serrulata*	warm and moist	
Self-heal	*Prunella vulgaris*		
Water Plantain	*Alisma plantago-aquatica*	cold	balances potassium
White Poplar bark	*Populus alba*	cold	
Kidneys: Nervous System—Builders (+)			
American Ginseng, White	*Panax quinquefolius*	warm	
Angelica root	*Angelica archangelica*	warm	
Chinese Cinnamon	*Cinnamomum cassia*	hot	

COMMON NAME AND PLANT PART	SCIENTIFIC NAME	THERMAL AND MOISTURE PROPERTIES	APPLICATION
Ginger	Zingiber officinale	dry and hot	
Gotu Kola	Centella asiatica	cool	
Yerba Santa	Eriodictyon spp.	warm	
Kidneys: Nervous System—Cleansers (−)			
Aspen bark	Populus spp.	cold	
Motherwort	Leonurus cardiaca	neutral and dry	
Saint-John's-Wort	Hypericum perforatum	cool and dry	
Saw Palmetto berry	Serenoa serrulata	warm and moist	
Kidneys: Nervous System—Tonics (0)			
Licorice	Glycyrrhiza glabra	warm and moist	
Nettles	Urtica dioica, U. urens	dry and hot	
Kidneys: Solid Waste—Builders (+)			
Cedar, Arborvitae, Thuja	Thuja occidentalis	cold	kidney infection
Comfrey leaf	Symphytum officinale	cool and moist	kidney infection
Flax seeds	Linum usitatissimum	neutral	
Horsetail, spring gathered	Equisetum hyemale	cool	
Marshmallow root	Althaea officinalis	cool and moist	
Oat straw	Avena sativa	neutral	
Kidneys: Solid Waste—Cleansers (−)			
Angelica root	Angelica archangelica	warm	
Bedstraw, Cleavers	Galium aparine	dry and cool	
Parsley root	Petroselinum crispum	neutral	
Queen of the Meadow, Joe Pye Weed, Gravel Root	Eupatorium purpureum	warm	
Kidneys: Solid Waste—Tonics (0)			
Nettles	Urtica dioica, U. urens	dry and hot	
Plantain leaf	Plantago spp.	cool and dry	

COMMON NAME AND PLANT PART	SCIENTIFIC NAME	THERMAL AND MOISTURE PROPERTIES	APPLICATION
Self-heal	*Prunella vulgaris*	cold	
Water Plantain	*Alisma plantago-aquatica*	cold	
Kidneys: Toxic Infection—Builders (+)			
Chinese Cinnamon	*Cinnamomum cassia*	hot	
Comfrey leaf	*Symphytum officinale*	cool and moist	
Fenugreek	*Trigonella foenum-graecum*	warm	
Marshmallow root	*Althaea officinalis*	cool and moist	strangury
Plantain leaf	*Plantago* spp.	cool and dry	
Kidneys: Toxic Infection—Cleansers (−)			
Buchu	*Agathosma betulina*	dry and warm	mucopurulent acidic urine
Cedar, Arborvitae, Thuja	*Thuja occidentalis*	cold	
Dandelion leaf and root	*Taraxacum officinale*	cool	
Goldenseal	*Hydrastis canadensis*	dry and hot	1/10 part of a formula or less
Juniper berry	*Juniperus communis*	warm	chronic nephritis without inflammation
Myrrh	*Commiphora myrrha*	dry and hot	
Oregon Grape root	*Mahonia repens*	cold	
Uva Ursi	*Arctostaphylos uva-ursi*	cold	mild nephritis, sub-acute strangury
Kidneys: Toxic Infection—Tonics (0)			
Aspen bark	*Populus* spp.	cold	
Corn silk	*Zea mays*	neutral	pyelitis, initial stage, acute or chronic, with painful urination, mucopurulent alkaline urine, strangury

COMMON NAME AND PLANT PART	SCIENTIFIC NAME	THERMAL AND MOISTURE PROPERTIES	APPLICATION
Nettles	*Urtica dioica, U. urens*	dry and hot	
Large Intestine—Builders (+)			
Arrowroot	*Maranta arundinacea*	cool and moist	demulcent, nutritive, builder
Astragalus	*Astragalus hoantchy, A. membranaceus, A. mongolicus*	warm	
Black Alder	*Alnus glutinosa*	cool	
Blackberry bark of root	*Rubus villosus*	neutral	astringent and antilaxative
Comfrey leaf	*Symphytum officinale*	cool and moist	
Fenugreek seed	*Trigonella foenum-graecum*	warm	
Flax seeds	*Linum usitatissimum*	neutral	
Marshmallow root	*Althaea officinalis*	cool and moist	as poultice for painful extruding hemorrhoids
Plantain leaf	*Plantago* spp.	cool and dry	
Slippery Elm	*Ulmus fulva*	cool and moist	
Stone Root	*Collinsonia canadensis*	warm	
Wild Cherry bark	*Prunus virginiana, P. serotina*	warm	deep lung conditions
Large Intestine—Cleansers (−)			
Aloe	*Aloe barbadensis, A. officinalis*	cold	rectal prolapse ani
Asafoetida	*Ferula asafoetida*	dry and hot	
Asparagus root	*Asparagus officinalis*	cold	
Buckthorn bark	*Rhamnus cathartica, R. frangula*	cold	
Butternut, White Walnut bark of root	*Juglans cinerea*	warm	diarrhea, burning, dyspepsia from overeating and poor food combinations

COMMON NAME AND PLANT PART	SCIENTIFIC NAME	THERMAL AND MOISTURE PROPERTIES	APPLICATION
Calamus, Sweet Flag	*Acorus calamus*	warm	constipation with light feces
Cascara Sagrada	*Cascara sagrada*	cold	
Catnip	*Nepeta cataria*	cold and moist	
Cayenne	*Capsicum annuum*	hot	stimulant
Celery seed	*Apium graveolens*	warm	
Chinese Rhubarb root	*Rheum palmatum*	cold	
Coriander leaves and seeds	*Coriandrum sativum*	neutral (seeds), cool (leaves)	
Culver's Root, Black Root	*Veronicastrum virginicum, Leptandra virginica*	warm	laxative
Dandelion root	*Taraxacum officinale*	cool	constipation with autotoxicity, yang state, mouth sores
Hazel Alder	*Alnus serrulata*	cool	diarrhea
Juniper berry	*Juniperus communis*	warm	habit forming
Oregon Grape root	*Mahonia repens*	cold	
Psyllium seeds, whole	*Plantago psyllium*	neutral	
Rose hips	*Rosa* spp.	neutral	antidiarrheal
Sanicle	*Sanicula europaea*	dry and hot	for bleeding
Senna	*Cassia acutifolia*	cold	
Wild Yam	*Dioscorea villosa*	warm and dry	
Yellow Dock, Curly Dock root	*Rumex crispus*	cool	laxative
Large Intestine—Tonics (0)			
Apple bark	*Malus domestica*	neutral	
Bayberry, Wax Myrtle	*Myrica cerifera*	dry and hot	chronic colitis
Black Alder	*Alnus glutinosa*	cool	
Blackberry bark or root	*Rubus villosus*	neutral	astringent and antilaxative
Blackberry leaves	*Rubus villosus*	neutral	

COMMON NAME AND PLANT PART	SCIENTIFIC NAME	THERMAL AND MOISTURE PROPERTIES	APPLICATION
Black Cohosh	Cimicifuga racemosa	cool	
Buckthorn bark	Rhamnus cathartica, R. frangula	cold	constipation with dry feces
Cannabis, Da Ma tincture or tea of flowering tops	Cannabis sativa	warm and dry	chronic diarrhea, hemorrhoids, rectal prolapse, colitis
Chinese Cinnamon	Cinnamomum cassia	hot	diarrhea
Crabapple bark	Malus sylvestris	cold	
Goldenseal	Hydrastis canadensis	dry and hot	ulcerative colitis, recuperation from dysentery, non-ulcerative hemorrhoids with intestinal weakness, rectal fissures, in enema; 1/10 part of a formula or less
Raspberry leaf	Rubus idaeus	cool	
Shepherd's Purse	Capsella bursa-pastoris	neutral	bleeding hemorrhoids, bleeding ulcers
Stone Root, Collinsonia	Collinsonia canadensis	warm	
Wild Cherry bark	Prunus virginiana, P. serotina	warm	
Yarrow	Achillea millefolium	neutral	
Yellow Dock, Curly Dock root	Rumex crispus	cool	
Large Intestine: Nervous System—Builders (+)			
Black Pepper	Piper nigrum	hot	
Cayenne	Capsicum annuum	hot	
Coriander seeds and leaves	Coriandrum sativum	neutral (seeds), cool (leaves)	
Fennel	Foeniculum vulgare	warm and moist	dyspepsia and gas
Ginger	Zingiber officinale	dry and hot	dyspepsia with gas
Wild Cherry bark	Prunus virginiana, P. serotina	warm	

COMMON NAME AND PLANT PART	SCIENTIFIC NAME	THERMAL AND MOISTURE PROPERTIES	APPLICATION
Large Intestine: Nervous System—Cleansers (−)			
Coriander seeds and leaves	Coriandrum sativum	neutral (seeds), cool (leaves)	
Evening Primrose oil	Oenothera biennis	moist and neutral	
Wild Cherry bark	Prunus virginiana, P. serotina	warm	
Large Intestine: Nervous System—Tonics (0)			
Comfrey leaf	Symphytum officinale	cool and moist	
Lavender flowers	Lavandula angustifolia, L. vera	hot and dry	nervous dyspepsia, nausea
Oak bark	Quercus spp.	neutral	dysentery
Slippery Elm	Ulmus fulva	cool and moist	
Liver—Builders (+)			
Aloe	Aloe barbadensis, A. officinalis	cold	
Bladderwrack, Kelp	Fucus vesiculosus	cool	
Butternut, White Walnut bark of root or inner bark of the tree	Juglans cinerea	warm	
Dandelion leaf, flower, and root	Taraxacum officinale	cool	
Gentian	Gentiana lutea, G. officinalis	cold	
Irish Moss	Chondrus crispus	cool	
Licorice root	Glycyrrhiza glabra	warm and moist	
Milk Thistle	Silybum marianum	cold	
Nettles	Urtica dioica, U. urens	dry and hot	
Rehmannia	Rehmannia glutinosa	cool	
Watercress	Nasturtium officinale	warm	
Yellow Dock, Curly Dock root	Rumex crispus	cool	

COMMON NAME AND PLANT PART	SCIENTIFIC NAME	THERMAL AND MOISTURE PROPERTIES	APPLICATION
Liver—Cleansers (−)			
Agrimony	Agrimonia eupatoria	dry and warm	
Alfalfa	Medicago sativa	cool	
Aloe	Aloe barbadensis, A. officinalis	cold	
Angelica root	Angelica archangelica	warm	
Barberry root	Berberis vulgaris	cold	
Beets	Beta vulgaris	cool	
Boldo leaves	Peumus boldus	cool	
Buckthorn bark, root bark	Rhamnus cathartica, R. frangula	cold	
Bupleurum, Chai-hu, Thorowax root	Bupleurum chinensis, B. falcatum	cool	cleans the liver and dredges out old emotions, sadness, anger
Butternut, White Walnut bark of root	Juglans cinerea	warm	
Calamus, Sweet Flag	Acorus calamus	warm	sick headache, nausea, light-colored feces, cutting pain
Centaury	Erythraea centaurium	cool	
Culver's Root, Black Root	Veronicastrum virginicum, Leptandra virginica	warm	
Dandelion leaf and root	Taraxacum officinale	cool	
Gentian	Gentiana lutea, G. officinalis	cold	
Goldenseal	Hydrastis canadensis	dry and hot	1/10 part of a formula or less
He Shou Wu, Fo-ti Tieng	Polygonum multiflorum	warm	
Horehound	Marrubium vulgare	cool	

COMMON NAME AND PLANT PART	SCIENTIFIC NAME	THERMAL AND MOISTURE PROPERTIES	APPLICATION
Mandrake, Mayapple root	*Podophyllum peltatum*	cold	toxic
Oregon Grape root	*Mahonia repens*	cold	
Pipsissewa, Prince's Pine	*Chimaphila umbellata*	dry and hot	
Red Sarsaparilla	*Smilax ornata*	warm and moist	
Sassafras bark or bark of root	*Sassafras albidum, S. variifolium*	dry and hot	
Scarlet Pimpernel	*Anagallis arvensis*	cool	toxic, use as no more than 1/6 part of a formula
Turmeric	*Curcuma longa*	warm	
Wahoo bark	*Euonymus atropurpurea*	cold	
Wild Yam	*Dioscorea villosa*	warm and dry	
Wood Betony	*Betonica officinalis, Stachys officinalis*	cool	
Liver—Tonics (0)			
Aloe	*Aloe barbadensis, A. officinalis*	cold	
Astragalus	*Astragalus hoantchy, A. membranaceus, A. mongolicus*	warm	
Barberry root	*Berberis vulgaris*	cold	
Blessed Thistle, Holy Thistle	*Carbenia benedicta, Cnicus benedictus*	cool	
Burdock root	*Arctium lappa*	warm and moist	
Dandelion root, raw	*Taraxacum officinale*	cool	
Gentian	*Gentiana lutea, G. officinalis*	cold	
He Shou Wu, Fo-ti Tieng	*Polygonum multiflorum*	warm	
Liver: Nervous System—Builders (+)			
Boldo leaves	*Peumus boldus*	cool	
Calamus, Sweet Flag	*Acorus calamus*	warm	

COMMON NAME AND PLANT PART	SCIENTIFIC NAME	THERMAL AND MOISTURE PROPERTIES	APPLICATION
Mandrake, Mayapple root	*Podophyllum peltatum*	cold	toxic
Liver: Nervous System—Cleansers (−)			
Bupleurum, Chai-hu, Thorowax	*Bupleurum chinense, B. falcatum*	cool	cleans the liver and dredges out old emotions, sadness, anger
Rosemary	*Rosmarinus officinalis*	warm and hot	
Wild Yam	*Dioscorea villosa*	warm and dry	
Wood Betony	*Betonica officinalis, Stachys officinalis*	cool	
Lungs—Builders (+)			
Apricot/Bitter Almond	*Prunus armeniaca*	warm and moist	
Astragalus	*Astragalus membranaceus*	warm	upper respiratory
Balm of Gilead	*Populus balsamifera*	warm	
Chickweed	*Stellaria media*	cool	upper respiratory and deep lung
Comfrey leaf	*Symphytum officinale*	cool and moist	upper respiratory and deep lung
Fenugreek seeds	*Trigonella foenum-graecum*	warm	upper respiratory
Honeysuckle	*Lonicera japonica*	cold	
Horsetail	*Equisetum hyemale*	cool	emphysema, to strengthen
Hyssop flowering herb	*Hyssopus officinalis*	warm and dry	for productive cough, thick mucus, spasmodic asthma, pneumonia, chronic bronchitis
Irish Moss	*Chondrus crispus*	cool	deep lung
Licorice	*Glycyrrhiza glabra*	warm and moist	upper respiratory
Marshmallow root	*Althaea officinalis*	cool and moist	
Mullein	*Verbascum thapsus*	warm and moist	acute cough, from nervousness

COMMON NAME AND PLANT PART	SCIENTIFIC NAME	THERMAL AND MOISTURE PROPERTIES	APPLICATION
Ocotillo fresh bark	*Fouquieria splendens*	dry	moist painful cough in the elderly
Pleurisy Root	*Asclepias tuberosa*	cool and moist	
Shatavari, Indian Asparagus root	*Asparagus racemosa*	cold and moist	for lung abscesses
Slippery Elm	*Ulmus fulva*	cool and moist	cough and deep lung
Lungs—Cleansers (−)			
Angelica root	*Angelica archangelica*	warm	
Balm of Gilead	*Populus balsamifera*	warm	
Black Cohosh	*Cimicifuga racemosa*	cool	influenza with aches
Bloodroot	*Sanguinaria canadensis*	dry and hot	used in very small amounts for sore throat, bronchial infection, pneumonia, colds, whooping cough, bleeding lungs and sinus conditions; added to the vaporizer to open the capillaries and ease breathing in COPD
Boneset	*Eupatorium perfoliatum*	cool	moist bronchitis with fever and aches
Calamus, Sweet Flag	*Acorus calamus*	warm	
Cayenne	*Capsicum annuum*	hot	
Chinese Cinnamon	*Cinnamomum cassia*	hot	
Echinacea	*Echinacea angustifolia, E. pallida, E. purpurea*	dry and hot	
Elecampane	*Inula helenium*	dry and hot	deep lung, wet asthma
Eucalyptus	*Eucalyptus globulus*	warm	deep lung, after pneumonia, difficult expectoration
Fennel seeds	*Foeniculum vulgare*	warm and moist	upper respiratory

COMMON NAME AND PLANT PART	SCIENTIFIC NAME	THERMAL AND MOISTURE PROPERTIES	APPLICATION
Ginger, also Wild Ginger	*Zingiber officinale, Asarum canadense*	dry and hot	upper respiratory
Grindelia	*Grindelia camporum*	warm	dry asthma, sub-acute or chronic bronchitis, dry labored breathing in emphysema, influenza
Hedge Nettle	*Stachys palustris*	warm	
Holy Basil, Tulsi	*Ocimum tenuiflorum*	warm	colds, flu, bronchitis, fevers
Horehound	*Marrubium vulgare*	cool	
Lobelia	*Lobelia inflata*	neutral	bronchitis with difficult expectoration, congestion, secretions
Lungwort	*Pulmonaria officinalis*	warm and moist	
Nettles	*Urtica dioica, U. urens*	dry and hot	
Osha	*Ligusticum filicinum, L. porteri*	dry and hot	
Pleurisy Root	*Asclepias tuberosa*	cool and moist	deep lung
Sage	*Salvia officinalis*	dry and cool	dries moist, wet lung conditions
Sanicle	*Sanicula europaea*	dry and hot	bleeding from the lungs
Skullcap	*Scutellaria lateriflora*	dry and cool	
Solomon's Seal	*Polygonatum officinale*	cool	
Star Anise	*Illicium verum, I. anisatum*	warm	
Thyme	*Thymus vulgaris*	dry and hot	upper respiratory and deep lung
White Sage	*Salvia apiana*	dry and cool	deep lung
Yerba Santa	*Eriodictyon* spp.	warm	deep lung

COMMON NAME AND PLANT PART	SCIENTIFIC NAME	THERMAL AND MOISTURE PROPERTIES	APPLICATION
Lungs—Tonics (0)			
Apple bark	*Malus* spp.	neutral	
Bayberry, Wax Myrtle bark	*Myrica cerifera*	dry and hot	deep lung
Cannabis, Da Ma tincture or tea of flowering tops	*Cannabis sativa*	warm and dry	spasmodic cough with paroxysms, spasmodic asthma, chronic cough
Coltsfoot	*Tussilago farfara*	warm and moist	bronchial, cough
Eyebright	*Euphrasia officinalis*	cool	upper respiratory and deep lung
Goldenseal	*Hydrastis canadensis*	dry and hot	1/10 part of a formula or less
Life Everlasting	*Gnaphalium obtusifolium, G. polycephalum*	warm	
Lungwort	*Pulmonaria officinalis*	warm and moist	upper respiratory and deep lung
Mullein	*Verbascum thapsus*	warm and moist	deep lung
Osha	*Ligusticum filicinum, L. porteri*	dry and hot	
Plantain leaf	*Plantago* spp.	cool and dry	
Raspberry leaf	*Rubus idaeus*	cool	
Rosemary	*Rosmarinus officinalis*	warm and hot	shallow breath
Sage	*Salvia apiana, S. officinalis*	dry and cool	
Saw Palmetto berry	*Serenoa serrulata*	warm and moist	
Solomon's Seal	*Polygonatum officinale*	cool	
Wild Cherry bark	*Prunus virginiana, P. serotina*	warm	deep lung
Lungs: Nervous System—Builders (+)			
Astragalus	*Astragalus membranaceus*	warm	
Cayenne	*Capsicum annuum*	hot	
Osha root	*Ligusticum filicinum, L. porteri*	dry and hot	

COMMON NAME AND PLANT PART	SCIENTIFIC NAME	THERMAL AND MOISTURE PROPERTIES	APPLICATION
Lungs: Nervous System—Cleansers (−)			
Apricot/Bitter Almond kernels	*Prunus armeniaca*	hot and moist	
Catnip	*Nepeta cataria*	cold and moist	
Lobelia	*Lobelia inflata*	neutral	
Wild Cherry bark	*Prunus virginiana, P. serotina*	warm	
Lungs: Nervous System—Tonics (0)			
Asafoetida	*Ferula asafoetida*	dry and hot	
Black Cohosh	*Cimicifuga racemosa*	cool	
Blue Cohosh	*Caulophyllum thalictroides*	warm and dry	
Lobelia	*Lobelia inflata*	neutral	moist, persistent cough, after pneumonia, difficult expectoration
Mullein	*Verbascum thapsus*	warm and moist	wheezing, dry cough
Nettles	*Urtica dioica, U. urens*	dry and hot	
Oat straw	*Avena sativa*	neutral and moist	
Pleurisy Root	*Asclepias tuberosa*	cool and moist	deep lung, pneumonia
Red Clover blossoms	*Trifolium pratense*	dry and cool	cough
White Sarsaparilla, Spikenard root	*Aralia nudicaulis*	warm	wheezing, dry cough, influenza
Wood Betony	*Betonica officinalis, Stachys officinalis*	cool	
Lymph and Spleen—Builders (+)			
Alfalfa	*Medicago sativa*	cool	
Apricots	*Prunus armeniaca*	warm and moist	
Astragalus	*Astragalus hoantchy, A. membranaceus, A. mongolicus*	warm	increases white blood cells
Burdock root	*Arctium lappa*	cool	

COMMON NAME AND PLANT PART	SCIENTIFIC NAME	THERMAL AND MOISTURE PROPERTIES	APPLICATION
Comfrey leaf	Symphytum officinale	cool and moist	builds and regenerates tissues
Dandelion root	Taraxacum officinale	cool	
Dong Quai	Angelica sinensis, A. polymorpha	warm	stimulant
Honeysuckle	Lonicera japonica	cold	
Licorice	Glycyrrhiza glabra	warm and moist	
Myrrh	Commiphora myrrha	dry and hot	builds and stimulates white blood cells
Plantain leaf	Plantago major	cool and dry	builds and repairs tissues
Poria, Fu Ling, Tuckahoe mushroom	Poria cocos, Wolfiporia extensa	neutral	strengthens and builds spleen energy
Red and White Clover	Trifolium pratense	cool	
Rehmannia	Rehmannia glutinosa	cool	nutritive
White Peony	Paeonia alba	cold	builds and ripens red blood cells
Lymph and Spleen—Cleansers (−)			
Aloe	Aloe barbadensis, A. officinalis	cold	
Angelica root	Angelica archangelica	warm	
Apricot/Bitter Almond kernels	Prunus armeniaca	warm and moist	
Bedstraw, Cleavers	Galium aparine	dry and cool	cleans blood via spleen
Bittersweet	Solanum dulcamara	cold	
Calamus, Sweet Flag	Acorus calamus	warm	
Calendula flowers	Calendula officinalis	neutral	cleans blood and lymph
Cedar, Arborvitae, Thuja	Thuja occidentalis	cold	lymph congestion
Dong Quai	Angelica sinensis, A. polymorpha	warm	stimulant

COMMON NAME AND PLANT PART	SCIENTIFIC NAME	THERMAL AND MOISTURE PROPERTIES	APPLICATION
Echinacea	Echinacea angustifolia, E. pallida, E. purpurea	dry and hot	
Eucalyptus	Eucalyptus globulus	warm	shrinks enlarged spleen
Guaiacum	Guaiacum officinale	cool	
Life Everlasting	Gnaphalium obtusifolium, G. polycephalum	warm	
Milk Thistle	Silybum marianum	cold	
Ocotillo	Fouquieria splendens	cool	
Oregon Grape root	Mahonia repens	cold	
Pipsissewa, Prince's Pine	Chimaphila umbellata	dry and hot	
Poke root	Phytolacca esculenta	dry and hot	
Red and White Clover blossoms	Trifolium pratense	cool	stimulates circulation through the spleen
Redroot, New Jersey Tea	Ceanothus americanus	dry and hot	cleans blood and lymph, for subacute splenitis—chronic or secondary to hepatitis
Red Sarsaparilla	Smilax ornata	warm and moist	
Sassafras	Sassafras officinale	dry and hot	for enlarged spleen
Uva Ursi, Bearberry	Arctostaphylos uva-ursi	cold	
Vervain	Verbena officinalis, V. hastata	cold	
Violet leaf	Viola odorata	cool	
White Peony	Paeonia alba	cold	
Lymph and Spleen—Tonics (0)			
Angelica root	Angelica archangelica	warm	
Apple bark	Malus spp.	neutral	
Aspen bark	Populus spp.	cold	
Blessed Thistle	Carbenia benedicta, Cnicus benedictus	cool	

COMMON NAME AND PLANT PART	SCIENTIFIC NAME	THERMAL AND MOISTURE PROPERTIES	APPLICATION
Burdock root	*Arctium lappa*	cool	
Crabapple bark	*Malus sylvestris*	cold	
Dodder	*Cuscuta chinensis, C. europea*	hot and moist	shrinks enlarged spleen, strengthens
Ginger	*Zingiber officinale*	dry and hot	balances
Ginseng	*Panax quinquefolius*	warm	
Goldenseal	*Hydrastis canadensis*	dry and hot	1/10 part of a formula or less
Oregon Grape root	*Mahonia repens*	cold	
Sassafras	*Sassafras albidum, S. variifolium*	dry and hot	
Self-heal	*Prunella vulgaris*	cold	
Uva Ursi, Bearberry	*Arctostaphylos uva-ursi*	cold	
Lymph System—Builders (+)			
Astragalus	*Astragalus hoantchy, A. membranaceus, A. mongolicus*	warm	
Bee pollen	NA	slightly cool	
Myrrh	*Commiphora myrrha*	dry and hot	builds immune system
Rehmannia	*Rehmannia glutinosa*	cool	
Lymph System—Cleansers (−)			
Apricot/Bitter Almond kernels	*Prunus armeniaca*	warm and moist	
Bedstraw, Cleavers	*Galium aparine*	dry and cool	
Bittersweet	*Solanum dulcamara*	cold	
Blessed Thistle	*Carbenia benedicta, Cnicus benedictus*	cool	
Burdock root	*Arctium lappa*	warm and moist	builds immune system, diaphoretic
Calamus, Sweet Flag	*Acorus calamus*	warm	
Calendula flowers	*Calendula officinalis*	neutral	internal infection in the lymph system

COMMON NAME AND PLANT PART	SCIENTIFIC NAME	THERMAL AND MOISTURE PROPERTIES	APPLICATION
Catnip	*Nepeta cataria*	cold and moist	promotes perspiration
Echinacea	*Echinacea angustifolia, E. pallida, E. purpurea*	dry and hot	immune suppression, inflammatory lymph nodes with fever, chronic debility, mononucleosis
Elderflowers	*Sambucus* spp.	cool	promotes perspiration, lowers fevers; mix with Mint and Yarrow flowers for stomach flu and general detox
Eucalyptus	*Eucalyptus globulus*	warm	
Ginger	*Zingiber officinale*	dry and hot	promotes perspiration
Guaiacum	*Guaiacum officinale*	cool	
Hyssop flowering herb	*Hyssopus officinalis*	warm	diaphoretic
Lemon Balm	*Melissa officinalis*	neutral	febrifuge, taken hot to decrease fever, taken cold to decrease fever
Life Everlasting	*Gnaphalium obtusifolium, G. polycephalum*	warm	
Masterwort	*Imperatoria ostruthium*	dry and hot	
Myrrh	*Commiphora myrrha*	dry and hot	depressed white blood count
Ocotillo	*Fouquieria splendens*	cool	
Peppermint	*Mentha piperita*	cold and dry	lightly promotes perspiration
Pipsissewa, Prince's Pine	*Chimaphila umbellata*	dry and hot	
Poke root	*Phytolacca esculenta*	dry and hot	

COMMON NAME AND PLANT PART	SCIENTIFIC NAME	THERMAL AND MOISTURE PROPERTIES	APPLICATION
Red Clover blossoms	*Trifolium pratense*	dry and cool	
Redroot, New Jersey Tea	*Ceanothus americanus*	dry and hot	
Red Sarsaparilla	*Smilax ornata*	warm and moist	
Saffron	*Crocus sativus*	dry and hot	removes drug residues from lymph
Saint-John's-Wort	*Hypericum perforatum*	cool and dry	diaphoretic
Sassafras	*Sassafras albidum, S. variifolium*	dry and hot	diaphoretic
Vervain	*Verbena officinalis, V. hastata*	cold	
Violet leaf	*Viola odorata*	cool	
Lymph System—Tonics (0)			
Angelica root	*Angelica archangelica*	warm	
Blessed Thistle	*Carbenia benedicta, Cnicus benedictus*	cool	
Burdock root	*Arctium lappa*	warm and moist	
Cannabis, Da Ma fresh or frozen raw leaf in smoothies	*Cannabis sativa*	warm and dry	general immune enhancer
Crabapple bark	*Malus sylvestris*	cold	
Dodder	*Cuscuta chinensis, C. europea*	hot and moist	balances immune system
Dong Quai	*Angelica sinensis, A. polymorpha*	warm	
Goldenseal	*Hydrastis canadensis*	dry and hot	1/10 part of a formula or less
Oregon Grape root	*Mahonia repens*	cold	
Pleurisy Root	*Asclepias tuberosa*	cool and moist	diaphoretic for colds, flu
Sage	*Salvia apiana, S. officinalis*	dry and cool	builds immune system
Self-heal	*Prunella vulgaris*	cold	

COMMON NAME AND PLANT PART	SCIENTIFIC NAME	THERMAL AND MOISTURE PROPERTIES	APPLICATION
Male Reproductive System—Builders (+)			
Ashwagandha root	*Withania somnifera*	warm	
Flax seeds	*Linum usitatissimum*	neutral	
Hollyhock flowers	*Althaea rosea*	cool	neck of the bladder
Marshmallow root	*Althaea officinalis*	cool and moist	
Male Reproductive System—Cleansers (−)			
Black Cohosh	*Cimicifuga racemosa*	cool	chronic prostatitis with pelvic and sacral pain
Buchu	*Agathosma betulina*	dry and warm	prostatitis with mucopurulent urine
Cedar, Arborvitae, Thuja	*Thuja occidentalis*	cold	prostatitis with incontinence
Cubeb berries	*Piper cubeba*	warm	
Horsetail	*Equisetum hyemale*	cool	prostatitis with irritable bladder and incontinence
Juniper berry	*Juniperus communis*	warm	enlarged prostate, not inflamed but with discharge
Myrrh	*Commiphora myrrha*	dry and hot	
Pareira Brava	*Chondrodendron tomentosum*	cool	
Partridgeberry	*Mitchella repens*	warm and dry	prostatitis with urethritis
Queen of the Meadow, Joe Pye Weed, Gravel Root	*Eupatorium purpureum*	warm	chronic prostatitis with pelvic and sacral pain
Male Reproductive System—Tonics (0)			
Coltsfoot	*Tussilago farfara*	warm and moist	after vasectomy
Corn silk	*Zea mays*	neutral	
Goldenseal	*Hydrastis canadensis*	dry and hot	1/10 part of a formula or less
Saw Palmetto berry	*Serenoa serrulata*	warm and moist	prostatitis from excessive sexual activity

COMMON NAME AND PLANT PART	SCIENTIFIC NAME	THERMAL AND MOISTURE PROPERTIES	APPLICATION
Male Reproductive System: Nervous System and Bladder—Builders (+)			
Damiana	*Turnera aphrodisiaca*	warm	aphrodisiac and urinary stimulant
Epimedium	*Epimedium grandiflorum*	warm	aphrodisiac
Fenugreek	*Trigonella foenum-graecum*	warm	
Male Reproductive System: Nervous System and Bladder—Cleansers (−)			
Saint-John's-Wort	*Hypericum perforatum*	cool and dry	
White Sage	*Salvia apiana*	dry and cool	
Male Reproductive System: Nervous System and Bladder—Tonics (0)			
Aspen bark	*Populus* spp.	cold	
Saw Palmetto berry	*Serenoa serrulata*	warm and moist	
Male Reproductive System: Nervous System and Prostate—Builders (+)			
Corn silk	*Zea mays*	neutral	
Damiana	*Turnera aphrodisiaca*	warm	
He Shou Wu, Fo-ti Tieng	*Polygonum multiflorum*	warm	
Horsetail	*Equisetum hyemale*	cool	
Marshmallow root	*Althaea officinalis*	cool and moist	
Saw Palmetto berry	*Serenoa serrulata*	warm and moist	
Yohimbe	*Coryanthe yohimbe, Pausinystalia yohimbe*	warm	stimulant, aphrodisiac
Male Reproductive System: Nervous System and Prostate—Cleansers (−)			
Cedar, Arborvitae, Thuja	*Thuja occidentalis*	cold	
Couchgrass	*Agropyron repens*	cool	
Cubeb berries	*Piper cubeba*	warm	

COMMON NAME AND PLANT PART	SCIENTIFIC NAME	THERMAL AND MOISTURE PROPERTIES	APPLICATION
Juniper berry	*Juniperus communis*	warm	
Parsley	*Petroselinum crispum*	neutral	
Saint-John's-Wort	*Hypericum perforatum*	cool and dry	
White Sage	*Salvia apiana*	dry and cool	
Male Reproductive System: Nervous System and Prostate—Tonics (0)			
American Ginseng, White American	*Panax quinquefolius*	warm	
Aspen bark	*Populus* spp.	cold	
Coltsfoot	*Tussilago farfara*	warm and moist	
Corn silk	*Zea mays*	neutral	
Goldenseal	*Hydrastis canadensis*	dry and hot	1/10 part of a formula or less
Hydrangea root	*Hydrangea arborescens*	cool	
Red Sarsaparilla	*Smilax ornata*	warm and moist	
Siberian Ginseng	*Eleutherococcus senticosus*	warm	
Mucous Membranes—Builders (+)			
Comfrey leaf	*Symphytum officinale*	cool and moist	regenerates tissues
Marshmallow root	*Althaea officinalis*	cool and moist	demulcent
Slippery Elm	*Ulmus fulva*	cool and moist	
White Pond Lily	*Nymphaea odorata*	cool	
Mucous Membranes—Cleansers (−)			
Calamus, Sweet Flag	*Acorus calamus*	warm	
Mucous Membranes—Tonics (0)			
Bistort	*Polygonum bistorta*	cool	taken with milk
Myrrh	*Commiphora myrrha*	dry and hot	
Plantain leaf	*Plantago* spp.	cool and moist	repairs tissues
Raspberry leaf	*Rubus idaeus*	cool	stomach oriented
Saw Palmetto berry	*Serenoa serrulata*	warm and moist	
Skullcap	*Scutellaria lateriflora*	dry and cool	

COMMON NAME AND PLANT PART	SCIENTIFIC NAME	THERMAL AND MOISTURE PROPERTIES	APPLICATION
Uva Ursi, Bearberry	*Arctostaphylos, uva-ursi*	cold	
Muscles—Builders (+)			
Black Cohosh	*Cimicifuga racemosa*	cool	rheumatic pain, pain from change of weather, sprains with muscle spasms, tendonitis
Calendula flowers	*Calendula officinalis*	neutral	
Comfrey leaf	*Symphytum officinale*	cool and moist	regenerates tissues
Goldenseal	*Hydrastis canadensis*	dry and hot	sprains without heat, synovitis; 1/10 part of a formula or less
Guaiacum	*Guaiacum officinale*	cool	chronic pain with cold hands and feet, poor circulation
Pleurisy Root	*Asclepias tuberosa*	cool and moist	rheumatic pain with dry cough and indigestion
Pubescent Angelica, Du Huo roots	*Angelica pubescens*	cool	anti-inflammatory
Yellow Dock, Curly Dock root	*Rumex crispus*	cool	
Muscles—Cleansers (−)			
Echinacea	*Echinacea angustifolia, E. pallida, E. purpurea*	dry and hot	chronic tendonitis
Sage	*Salvia apiana, S. officinalis*	dry and cool	
Muscles—Tonics (0)			
Chamomile	*Chamaemelum nobile, Matricaria recutita*	warm and moist	
Feverfew	*Tanacetum parthenium*	cool	anti-inflammatory
Nervous System—Builders (+)			
American Ginseng, White	*Panax quinquefolius*	warm	

COMMON NAME AND PLANT PART	SCIENTIFIC NAME	THERMAL AND MOISTURE PROPERTIES	APPLICATION
Angelica root	*Angelica archangelica*	warm	
Black Cohosh	*Cimicifuga racemosa*	cool	insomnia with muscular pain, agitation, nerve pain
Black Walnut hulls	*Juglans nigra*	cold	
Blessed Thistle	*Carbenia benedicta, Cnicus benedictus*	cool	
Calendula flowers	*Calendula officinalis*	neutral	
Comfrey leaf	*Symphytum officinale*	cool and moist	regenerates tissues
Gotu Kola	*Centella asiatica*	cool	
Lavender flowers	*Lavandula angustifolia, L. vera*	hot and dry	
Slippery Elm	*Ulmus fulva*	cool and moist	
Nervous System—Cleansers (−)			
Coriander seeds and leaves	*Coriandrum sativum*	neutral (seeds), cool (leaves)	
Cramp Bark	*Viburnum opulus*	cool	
Hops	*Humulus lupulus*	cool	
Lady's Slipper root	*Cypripedium pubescens*	neutral	
Mistletoe, European	*Viscum album*	neutral	
Mullein	*Verbascum thapsus*	warm and moist	
Myrrh	*Commiphora myrrha*	dry and hot	
Saint-John's-Wort	*Hypericum perforatum*	cool and dry	
Valerian	*Valeriana officinalis*	warm	insomnia—use only in combination with other herbs
White Peony	*Paeonia alba*	cold	
White Sage	*Salvia apiana*	dry and cool	
Wild Cherry bark	*Prunus virginiana, P. serotina*	warm	
Wild Lettuce, Prickly Lettuce	*Lactuca virosa, L. serriola*	cool	
Wood Betony	*Betonica officinalis, Stachys officinalis*	cool	

COMMON NAME AND PLANT PART	SCIENTIFIC NAME	THERMAL AND MOISTURE PROPERTIES	APPLICATION
Nervous System—Tonics (0)			
Arnica	*Arnica montana*	warm	externally as a pain killer
Aspen bark	*Populus* spp.	cold	
Blessed Thistle	*Carbenia benedicta, Cnicus benedictus*	cool	
Cannabis, Da Ma tincture or tea of flowering tops	*Cannabis sativa*	warm and dry	sedative, for insomnia, frequent waking with nightmares
Catnip	*Nepeta cataria*	cold and moist	
Chamomile	*Chamaemelum nobile, Matricaria recutita*	warm and moist	
Goldenseal	*Hydrastis canadensis*	dry and hot	neuralgia
Lady's Slipper root	*Cypripedium pubescens*	neutral	
Lemon Balm	*Melissa officinalis*	neutral	
Masterwort	*Imperatoria ostruthium*	dry and hot	
Oat straw	*Avena sativa*	neutral and moist	
Passionflower	*Passiflora incarnata*	cool	delirium tremens, epilepsy, petit mal, insomnia
Rosemary	*Rosmarinus officinalis*	warm and hot	
Siberian Ginseng	*Eleutherococcus senticosus*	warm	
Skullcap	*Scutellaria lateriflora*	dry and hot	epilepsy, petit mal
Star Anise	*Illicium verum, I. anisatum*	warm	abdomen oriented
Wood Betony	*Betonica officinalis, Stachys officinalis*	cool	
Nose—Builders (+)			
Witch Hazel bark and leaf	*Hamamelis virginiana*	dry and hot	astringent, shrinks blood vessels
Nose—Cleansers (−)			
Bloodroot	*Sanguinaria canadensis*	dry and hot	

COMMON NAME AND PLANT PART	SCIENTIFIC NAME	THERMAL AND MOISTURE PROPERTIES	APPLICATION
Cedar, Arborvitae, Thuja	Thuja occidentalis	cold	
Nose—Tonics (0)			
Birthroot, Trillium	Trillium pendulum	warm	styptic
Yarrow	Achillea millefolium	neutral	styptic
Pancreas—Builders (+)			
Gentian	Gentiana lutea, G. officinalis	cold	
Goat's Rue	Galega officinalis	cool and dry	
Pancreas—Cleansers (−)			
Fringe Tree	Chionanthus virginicus	cool	hepatitis, jaundice, gallstones
Thyme	Thymus vulgaris	dry and hot	
Pancreas—Tonics (0)			
Ginseng	Panax spp.	warm	to prevent hyperglycemia, also for hypoglycemia
Goldenseal	Hydrastis canadensis	dry and hot	1/10 part of a formula or less
Sinus—Builders (+)			
Angelica root	Angelica archangelica	warm	
Honeysuckle	Lonicera japonica	cold	for sinusitis with fever
Skullcap	Scutellaria lateriflora	dry and cool	for sinusitis with fever
Sinus—Cleansers (−)			
Bloodroot	Sanguinaria canadensis	dry and hot	
Boneset	Eupatorium perfoliatum	cool	fever with a moist forehead, cold with fever and aches
Calamus, Sweet Flag	Acorus calamus	warm	
Echinacea	Echinacea angustifolia, E. pallida, E. purpurea	dry and hot	acute sinusitis, as nasal spray

COMMON NAME AND PLANT PART	SCIENTIFIC NAME	THERMAL AND MOISTURE PROPERTIES	APPLICATION
Elderflowers	*Sambucus* spp.	cool	
Eyebright	*Euphrasia officinalis*	cool	acute sinusitis with runny nose and eyes
Ginger	*Zingiber officinale*	dry and hot	incipient cold with chills
Goldenseal	*Hydrastis canadensis*	dry and hot	
Ground Ivy, Creeping Charlie, Gill-over-the-Ground	*Glechoma hederacea*	cool	
Wild Ginger	*Asarum canadense*	dry and hot	warm
Sinus—Tonics (0)			
Bayberry, Wax Myrtle bark	*Myrica cerifera*	dry and hot	
Coltsfoot	*Tussilago farfara*	warm and moist	
Skin—Builders (+)			
Aloe	*Aloe barbadensis, A. officinalis*	cold	
Apricot fruit, eaten and applied as a poultice	*Prunus armeniaca*		
Calendula flowers	*Calendula officinalis*	neutral	wounds
Comfrey leaf	*Symphytum officinale*	cool and moist	regenerates tissues
Marshmallow root	*Althaea officinalis*	cool and moist	demulcent
Nettles	*Urtica dioica, U. urens*	dry and hot	external wash for itch and rash
Plantain leaf	*Plantago* spp.	cool and dry	repairs tissues
Slippery Elm	*Ulmus fulva*		apply poultice to wounds
Skin—Cleansers (−)			
Alder	*Alnus serrulata*	cool	blood cleanser, externally makes a wash for eczema and swellings

COMMON NAME AND PLANT PART	SCIENTIFIC NAME	THERMAL AND MOISTURE PROPERTIES	APPLICATION
Barberry root	Berberis vulgaris	cold	acute psoriasis episode
Bedstraw, Cleavers	Galium aparine	dry and cool	
Bistort	Polygonum bistorta	cool	
Bloodroot	Sanguinaria canadensis	dry and hot	
Burdock	Arctium lappa	warm and moist	eczema, acne, psoriasis, long-term chronic ulcers
Butternut, White Walnut bark of root	Juglans cinerea	warm	acne with constipation, gas, eczema with constipation and gas
Calendula flowers	Calendula officinalis	neutral	herpes with bacterial infection, ulcers externally
Cedar, Arborvitae, Thuja	Thuja occidentalis	cold	
Dandelion root	Taraxacum officinale	cool	acne with mouth sores
Dong Quai	Angelica sinensis, A. polymorpha	warm	for excessive gonad hormones
Echinacea root	Echinacea angustifolia, E. pallida, E. purpurea	dry and hot	eczema with sticky exudate, abrasions, internal and external abscess, external for herpes simplex, internal and external for ulcers with necrosis
Elderflowers	Sambucus spp.	cool	opens pores to allow sweating
Elecampane	Inula helenium	dry and hot	external
Ginseng	Panax quinquefolius	warm	acne from excessive cortical hormones
Goldenseal	Hydrastis canadensis	dry and hot	ulcers externally; 1/10 part of a formula or less

COMMON NAME AND PLANT PART	SCIENTIFIC NAME	THERMAL AND MOISTURE PROPERTIES	APPLICATION
Lemon Balm	Melissa officinalis	neutral	
Mugwort	Artemisia vulgaris	warm	
Myrrh	Commiphora myrrha	dry and hot	external for herpes simplex
Oak bark	Quercus spp.	neutral	
Oregon Grape root	Mahonia repens	cold	
Pleurisy Root	Asclepias tuberosa	cool and moist	obstinate eczema
Red Clover blossoms	Trifolium pratense	dry and cool	
Saffron	Crocus sativus	dry and hot	
Sanicle	Sanicula europaea	dry and hot	internal and external wounds
Sassafras	Sassafras albidum, S. variifolium	dry and hot	
Vervain	Verbena officinalis, V. hastata	cold	
Wild Carrot, Queen Anne's Lace	Daucus carota	dry and hot	
Yarrow	Achillea millefolium	neutral	
Yellow Dock, Curly Dock root	Rumex crispus	cool	pustular eczema with boil cycles; acne with pustules on back, neck, and buttocks; psoriasis with irritable bowel or colitis
Skin—Tonics (0)			
Cannabis, Da Ma tincture or tea of flowering tops	Cannabis sativa	warm and dry	pruritus with itching
Goldenseal	Hydrastis canadensis	dry and hot	sub-acute herpes simplex; 1/10 part of a formula or less
Peppermint	Mentha piperita		antiseptic and antibacterial for shingles, wounds

COMMON NAME AND PLANT PART	SCIENTIFIC NAME	THERMAL AND MOISTURE PROPERTIES	APPLICATION
Witch Hazel bark and leaf	*Hamamelis virginiana*	dry and hot	external for varicose veins, wounds, bruises, irritations; astringent, shrinks blood vessels

Small Intestine: Digestive System—Builders (+)

American Ginseng, White	*Panax quinquefolius*	warm	
Chinese Cinnamon	*Cinnamomum cassia*	hot	stimulates
Ginger	*Zingiber officinale*	dry and hot	

Small Intestine: Digestive System—Cleansers (−)

Blackberry leaves	*Rubus villosus*	neutral	
Catnip	*Nepeta cataria*	cold and moist	
Licorice	*Glycyrrhiza glabra*	warm and moist	
Raspberry leaf	*Rubus idaeus*	cool	
Slippery Elm	*Ulmus fulva*	cool and moist	
Vervain	*Verbena officinalis, V. hastata*	cold	

Small Intestine: Digestive System—Tonics (0)

Angelica root	*Angelica archangelica*	warm	
Gentian	*Gentiana lutea, G. officinalis*	cold	
Slippery Elm	*Ulmus fulva*	cool and moist	

Small Intestine: Mucous Membrane—Builders (+)

American Ginseng, White	*Panax quinquefolius*	warm	
Angelica root	*Angelica archangelica*	warm	
Aspen bark	*Populus* spp.	cold	
Comfrey leaf	*Symphytum officinale*	cool and moist	
Fenugreek	*Trigonella foenum-graecum*	warm	
Gentian	*Gentiana lutea, G. officinalis*	cold	

COMMON NAME AND PLANT PART	SCIENTIFIC NAME	THERMAL AND MOISTURE PROPERTIES	APPLICATION
Licorice	*Glycyrrhiza glabra*	warm and moist	upper bowel
Marshmallow root	*Althaea officinalis*	cool and moist	
Slippery Elm	*Ulmus fulva*	cool and moist	
Small Intestine: Mucous Membrane—Cleansers (−)			
Caraway seed	*Carum carvi*	warm	mid bowel
Catnip	*Nepeta cataria*	cold and moist	
Cayenne	*Capsicum annuum*	hot	
Chinese Cinnamon	*Cinnamomum cassia*	hot	
Chinese Rhubarb root	*Rheum palmatum*	cold	
Cumin seed	*Cuminum cyminum*	warm	
Dill	*Anethum graveolens*	warm	duodenum
Ginger	*Zingiber officinale*	dry and hot	
Psyllium seeds	*Plantago psyllium*	neutral	
Sanicle	*Sanicula europaea*	dry and hot	for bleeding
Skullcap	*Scutellaria lateriflora*	dry and cool	
Wild Yam	*Dioscorea villosa*	warm and dry	
Small Intestine: Mucous Membrane—Tonics (0)			
Bayberry, Wax Myrtle	*Myrica cerifera*	dry and hot	
Blackberry bark or root	*Rubus villosus*	neutral	astringent and anti-laxative
Blackberry leaves	*Rubus villosus*	neutral	
Fenugreek	*Trigonella foenum-graecum*	warm	
Gentian	*Gentiana lutea, G. officinalis*	cold	
Goldenseal	*Hydrastis canadensis*	dry and hot	1/10 part of a formula or less
Raspberry leaf	*Rubus idaeus*	cool	
Skullcap	*Scutellaria lateriflora*	dry and cool	
Wild Cherry bark	*Prunus virginiana, P. serotina*	warm	

COMMON NAME AND PLANT PART	SCIENTIFIC NAME	THERMAL AND MOISTURE PROPERTIES	APPLICATION
Small Intestine: Nervous System—Builders (+)			
American Ginseng, White	*Panax quinquefolius*	warm	
Angelica root	*Angelica archangelica*	warm	
Blessed Thistle	*Carbenia benedicta, Cnicus benedictus*	cool	
Calendula flowers	*Calendula officinalis*	neutral	
Cayenne	*Capsicum annuum*	hot	
Comfrey leaf	*Symphytum officinale*	cool and moist	
Cumin seed	*Cuminum cyminum*	warm	
Ginger	*Zingiber officinale*	dry and hot	
Gotu Kola	*Centella asiatica*	cool	
Lavender flowers	*Lavandula angustifolia, L. vera*	hot and dry	
Slippery Elm	*Ulmus fulva*	cool and moist	
Small Intestine: Nervous System—Cleansers (−)			
Caraway seed	*Carum carvi*	warm	mildly sedative
Catnip	*Nepeta cataria*	cold and moist	
Coriander seeds and leaves	*Coriandrum sativum*	neutral (seeds), cool (leaves)	
Cramp Bark	*Viburnum opulus*	cool	
Hops	*Humulus lupulus*	cool	
Mistletoe, European	*Viscum album*	neutral	
Mullein	*Verbascum thapsus*	warm and moist	
Rosemary	*Rosmarinus officinalis*	warm and hot	
Saint-John's-Wort	*Hypericum perforatum*	cool and dry	
Skullcap	*Scutellaria lateriflora*	dry and cool	
Valerian	*Valeriana officinalis*	warm	use only in combination with other herbs
White Peony	*Paeonia alba*	cold	
White Sage	*Salvia apiana*	dry and cool	

COMMON NAME AND PLANT PART	SCIENTIFIC NAME	THERMAL AND MOISTURE PROPERTIES	APPLICATION
Wild Cherry bark	*Prunus virginiana, P. serotina*	warm	
Wild Lettuce, Prickly Lettuce	*Lactuca virosa, L. serriola*	cool	
Wild Yam	*Dioscorea villosa*	warm and dry	
Small Intestine: Nervous System—Tonics (0)			
Arnica	*Arnica montana*	warm	external use as an herb or homepathic dilution orally
Aspen bark	*Populus* spp.	cold	
Blessed Thistle	*Carbenia benedicta, Cnicus benedictus*	cool	
Catnip	*Nepeta cataria*	cold and moist	
Chamomile	*Chamaemelum nobile, Matricaria recutita*	warm and moist	
Lady's Slipper	*Cypripedium pubescens*	neutral	
Lemon Balm	*Melissa officinalis*	neutral	
Masterwort	*Imperatoria ostruthium*	dry and hot	
Passionflower	*Passiflora incarnata*	cool	
Rosemary	*Rosmarinus officinalis*	warm and hot	
Siberian Ginseng	*Eleutherococcus senticosus*	warm	
Skullcap	*Scutellaria lateriflora*	dry and cool	
Slippery Elm	*Ulmus fulva*	cool and moist	
Star Anise	*Illicium verum, I. anisatum*	warm	abdomen oriented
Wood Betony	*Betonica officinalis, Stachys officinalis*	cool	
Stomach—Builders (+)			
Agrimony	*Agrimonia eupatoria*	dry and warm	
American Ginseng, White	*Panax quinquefolius*	warm	

COMMON NAME AND PLANT PART	SCIENTIFIC NAME	THERMAL AND MOISTURE PROPERTIES	APPLICATION
Comfrey leaf	Symphytum officinale	cool and moist	repair ulcers
Fenugreek seed	Trigonella foenum-graecum	warm	inflamed stomach
Ginger	Zingiber officinale	dry and hot	
Irish Moss	Chondrus crispus	cool	
Licorice	Glycyrrhiza glabra	warm and moist	neutralizes reaction to plants, soothes mucosa
Marshmallow root	Althaea officinalis	cool and moist	demulcent
Orange peel	Citrus sinensis	cool	stimulates HCL acid, stimulates digestion
Slippery Elm	Ulmus fulva	cool and moist	demulcent, anti-acid
Solomon's Seal	Polygonatum officinale	cool	
Stomach—Cleansers (−)			
Angelica	Angelica archangelica	warm	
Aspen bark	Populus spp.	cold	dyspepsia with gas
Calamus, Sweet Flag	Acorus calamus	warm	cleanser and tonic to mucosa; for stomach flu, flatulence with inflammation, heartburn from fats, nausea in morning after a fatty meal, dyspepsia with nausea and a headache
Caraway seeds	Carum carvi	warm	
Cardamom	Elettaria cardamomum	warm	
Catnip	Nepeta cataria	cold and moist	
Cayenne	Capsicum annuum	hot	
Chinese Cinnamon	Cinnamomum cassia	hot	hemorrhage
Coriander seeds and leaves	Coriandrum sativum	neutral (seeds), cool (leaves)	dyspepsia

COMMON NAME AND PLANT PART	SCIENTIFIC NAME	THERMAL AND MOISTURE PROPERTIES	APPLICATION
Cumin seeds	*Cuminum cyminum*	warm	
Dill	*Anethum graveolens*	warm	
Ginger	*Zingiber officinale*	dry and hot	flatulence with painful stomach/intestinal spasms
Lavender flowers	*Lavandula angustifolia, L. vera*	hot and dry	gas, nervous dyspepsia, nausea
Lobelia	*Lobelia inflata*	neutral	
Myrrh	*Commiphora myrrha*	dry and hot	cleanser and tonic to mucosa; for gas with inflammation
Raspberry leaf	*Rubus idaeus*	cool	
Rosemary	*Rosmarinus officinalis*	warm and hot	
Skullcap	*Scutellaria lateriflora*	dry and cool	
Wild Yam	*Dioscorea villosa*	warm and dry	
Stomach—Tonics (0)			
Angelica root	*Angelica archangelica*	warm	
Asafoetida	*Ferula asafoetida*	dry and hot	
Bayberry, Wax Myrtle bark or leaf	*Myrica cerifera*	dry and hot	nausea in the morning in alcoholics
Blackberry leaves	*Rubus villosus*	neutral	
Black Cohosh	*Cimicifuga racemosa*	cool	
Burdock root	*Arctium lappa*	warm and moist	
Butternut, White Walnut bark of root	*Juglans cinerea*	warm	gas from overeating, digestive abuse
Calamus, Sweet Flag	*Acorus calamus*	warm	stomach flu, cleanser and tonic to mucosa
Cannabis, Da Ma tincture or tea of flowering tops	*Cannabis sativa*	warm and dry	anorexia, loss of appetite from prolonged illness
Catnip	*Nepeta cataria*	cold and moist	dyspepsia from agitation
Centaury	*Erythraea centaurium*	cool	

COMMON NAME AND PLANT PART	SCIENTIFIC NAME	THERMAL AND MOISTURE PROPERTIES	APPLICATION
Chinese Bitter Orange peel	Citrus aurantium, Poncirus trifoliata	warm and dry	
Cinnamon	Cinnamomum cassia	hot	bleeding ulcers
Club Moss	Lycopodium clavatum	warm and dry	
Coltsfoot	Tussilago farfara	warm and moist	
Coriander seeds and leaves	Coriandrum sativum	neutral (seeds), cool (leaves)	dyspepsia from agitation
Cow Parsnip seeds	Heracleum maximum	warm	
Echinacea	Echinacea angustifolia, E. pallida, E. purpurea	dry and hot	
Fennel	Foeniculum vulgare	warm and moist	
Fenugreek	Trigonella foenum-graecum	warm	dyspepsia with gas
Garlic	Allium sativum	hot	
Gentian	Gentiana lutea, G. officinalis	cold	
Goldenseal	Hydrastis canadensis	dry and hot	1/10 part of a formula or less; nausea in the morning in alcoholics, subacute non-inflamed ulcers
Korean Ginseng, White	Panax schinseng, Panax ginseng	warm and moist	
Lady's Slipper	Cypripedium pubescens	neutral	
Lavender flowers	Lavandula angustifolia, L. vera	hot and dry	
Lemon Balm	Melissa officinalis	neutral	
Licorice	Glycyrrhiza glabra	warm and moist	
Myrrh	Commiphora myrrha	dry and hot	tonic to mucosa, chronic gastritis
Papaya	Carica papaya	warm	
Peppermint	Mentha piperita	cool	nausea after eating

COMMON NAME AND PLANT PART	SCIENTIFIC NAME	THERMAL AND MOISTURE PROPERTIES	APPLICATION
Purplestem Angelica	*Angelica atropurpurea*	warm	
Raspberry leaf	*Rubus idaeus*	cool	
Rosemary	*Rosmarinus officinalis*	warm and hot	
Saw Palmetto berry	*Serenoa serrulata*	warm and moist	
Slippery Elm	*Ulmus fulva*	cool and moist	
Spearmint	*Mentha viridis*	warm	
Stone Root	*Collinsonia canadensis*	warm	
Strawberry leaves	*Fragraria* spp.	cool	
Wild Carrot, Queen Anne's Lace	*Daucus carota*	dry and hot	
Wild Yam	*Dioscorea villosa*	warm and dry	
Willow, White or Black	*Salix alba, S. nigra*	cold	
Stomach: Hydrochloric Acid—Builders (+)			
Bitter Lime peel	*Citrus aurantifolia*	cold	
Cardamom	*Elettaria cardamomum*	warm	
Cedar, Arborvitae, Thuja	*Thuja occidentalis*	cold	
Chinese Bitter Orange peel	*Citrus aurantium, Poncirus trifoliata*	warm and dry	
Juniper berry	*Juniperus communis*	warm	
Lemon peel	*Citrus limon*	cold	
Orange peel	*Citrus reticulata*	warm	
Yarrow	*Achillea millefolium*	neutral	
Stomach: Hydrochloric Acid—Cleansers (−)			
Blackberry leaves	*Rubus villosus*	neutral	
Catnip	*Nepeta cataria*	cold and moist	dyspepsia from agitation
Fennel	*Foeniculum vulgare*	warm and moist	
Raspberry leaf	*Rubus idaeus*	cool	
Rosemary	*Rosmarinus officinalis*	warm and hot	

COMMON NAME AND PLANT PART	SCIENTIFIC NAME	THERMAL AND MOISTURE PROPERTIES	APPLICATION
Slippery Elm	*Ulmus fulva*	cool and moist	
Spearmint	*Mentha viridis*	warm	
Strawberry leaves	*Fragraria* spp.	cool	
Stomach: Hydrochloric Acid—Tonics (0)			
American Ginseng, White	*Panax quinquefolius*	warm	
Coriander seeds and leaves	*Coriandrum sativum*	neutral (seeds), cool (leaves)	dyspepsia
Gentian	*Gentiana lutea, G. officinalis*	cold	
Ginger	*Zingiber officinale*	dry and hot	
Stomach: Nervous System—Builders (+)			
Angelica root	*Angelica archangelica*	warm	flatulence with inflammation
Cayenne	*Capsicum annuum*	hot	flatulence without inflammation
Gentian	*Gentiana lutea, G. officinalis*	cold	
Ginger	*Zingiber officinale*	dry and hot	flatulence with painful intestinal spasms
Ginseng	*Panax quinquefolius*	warm	
Stomach: Nervous System—Cleansers (−)			
Bayberry, Wax Myrtle	*Myrica cerifera*	dry and hot	flatulence with inflammation
Calamus, Sweet Flag	*Acorus calamus*	warm	flatulence with inflammation
Catnip	*Nepeta cataria*	cold and moist	dyspepsia from agitation
Cayenne	*Capsicum annuum*	hot	flatulence without inflammation
Chamomile	*Chamaemelum nobile, Matricaria recutita*	warm and moist	dyspepsia from agitation
Coriander seeds and leaves	*Coriandrum sativum*	neutral (seeds), cool (leaves)	dyspepsia from agitation

COMMON NAME AND PLANT PART	SCIENTIFIC NAME	THERMAL AND MOISTURE PROPERTIES	APPLICATION
Lobelia	*Lobelia inflata*	neutral	
Peppermint	*Mentha piperita*	cool	dyspepsia from agitation
Slippery Elm	*Ulmus fulva*	cool and moist	
Valerian	*Valeriana officinalis*	warm	flatulence with emotional depression; use only in combination with other herbs
Stomach: Nervous System—Tonics (0)			
Goldenseal	*Hydrastis canadensis*	dry and hot	1/10 part of a formula or less
Wild Yam	*Dioscorea villosa*	warm and dry	
Teeth—Builders (+)			
Alfalfa	*Medicago sativa*	cool	
Bedstraw, Cleavers	*Galium aparine*	dry and cool	
Comfrey leaf	*Symphytum officinale*	cool and moist	regenerates tissues
Nettles	*Urtica dioica, U. urens*	dry and hot	
Parsley	*Petroselinum crispum*	neutral	
Raspberry leaf	*Rubus idaeus*	cool	
Red Clover blossoms	*Trifolium pratense*	dry and cool	
Watercress	*Nasturtium officinale*	warm	
Teeth—Cleansers (−)			
Borage	*Borago officinalis*	cool	
Chamomile	*Chamaemelum nobile, Matricaria recutita*	warm and moist	
Coltsfoot	*Tussilago farfara*	warm and moist	
Horsetail	*Equisetum hyemale*	cool	
Myrrh	*Commiphora myrrha*	dry and hot	mouthwash
Plantain leaf	*Plantago* spp.	cool and dry	repairs tissues
Shepherd's Purse	*Capsella bursa-pastoris*	neutral	

COMMON NAME AND PLANT PART	SCIENTIFIC NAME	THERMAL AND MOISTURE PROPERTIES	APPLICATION
Teeth—Tonics (0)			
Chicory	*Cichorium intybus*	cold	may increase calcium absorption and bone mineral density
Dandelion root	*Taraxacum officinale*	cool	
Throat—Builders (+)			
Comfrey leaf	*Symphytum officinale*	cool and moist	coughs, regenerates tissues
Hollyhock	*Althaea rosea*	cool	
Marshmallow root	*Althaea officinalis*	cool and moist	laryngitis
Plantain leaf	*Plantago* spp.	cool and dry	builds and repairs tissue
Yarrow	*Achillea millefolium*	warm and dry	heals mucous membranes
Throat—Cleansers (−)			
Calamus, Sweet Flag	*Acorus calamus*	warm	sore throat, hoarseness in speakers
Echinacea root	*Echinacea angustifolia, E. pallida, E. purpurea*	dry and hot	pneumonia, strep throat, sore throat
Hazel Alder	*Alnus serrulata*	cool	colds, sore throat, cough, sore mouth
Hyssop flowering herb	*Hyssopus officinalis*	warm	
Myrrh	*Commiphora myrrha*	dry and hot	sore throat, gargle, tonic to mucosa
Nettles	*Urtica dioica, U. urens*	dry and hot	increase circulation, warming to the blood
Osha	*Ligusticum filicinum, L. porteri*	dry and hot	sore throat, upper respiratory
Sage	*Salvia apiana, S. officinalis*	dry and hot	
Sanicle	*Sanicula europaea*	dry and hot	cleans mucosa

COMMON NAME AND PLANT PART	SCIENTIFIC NAME	THERMAL AND MOISTURE PROPERTIES	APPLICATION
Skunk Cabbage root	*Symplocarpus foetidus*	cool	antispasmodic, coughs
Usnea lichen	*Usnea barbata*	neutral	strep throat, pharyngitis, oral inflammation
Wild Garlic	*Allium vineale*	hot	antibiotic, antiseptic, cleanser
Throat—Tonics (0)			
Amaranth	*Amaranthus hypochondriacus*	neutral	gargle for sore throat
Apricot pits, boiled	*Prunus armeniaca*	warm and moist	antispasmodic for coughs
Bayberry, Wax Myrtle	*Myrica cerifera*	dry and hot	sore throat
Burdock root	*Arctium lappa*	cool	tonsillitis
Burdock seeds	*Arctium lappa*	cold	sore throat
Calendula flowers	*Calendula officinalis*	neutral	sore throat, cancer of the larynx
Coltsfoot	*Tussilago farfara*	warm and moist	syrups for coughs, upper respiratory
Comfrey leaf	*Symphytum officinale*	cool and moist	coughs, regenerates tissues
Echinacea root	*Echinacea angustifolia, E. pallida, E. purpurea*	dry and hot	
Elecampane	*Inula helenium*	dry and hot	for wet coughs
Fenugreek	*Trigonella foenum-graecum*	warm	soothing to throat, vocal cords
Garlic	*Allium sativum*	hot	asthma, whooping cough, sore throat
Goldenseal	*Hydrastis canadensis*	dry and hot	gargle for sore throat, tonsillitis
Grindelia	*Grindelia camporum*	warm	whooping cough, sedative, expectorant
Licorice root	*Glycyrrhiza glabra*	warm and moist	

COMMON NAME AND PLANT PART	SCIENTIFIC NAME	THERMAL AND MOISTURE PROPERTIES	APPLICATION
Life Everlasting	Gnaphalium obtusifolium, G. polycephalum	warm and moist	upper respiratory astringent tonic, demulcent for sore throat
Lungwort	Pulmonaria officinalis	warm and moist	chronic upper respiratory cough and spasm
Marshmallow root	Althaea officinalis	cool and moist	demulcent
Mullein	Verbascum thapsus	warm and moist	coughs with thick sticky mucus
Prickly Ash	Zanthoxylum, clava-herculis, Z. americanum	warm	promotes mucous discharge
Red Clover	Trifolium pratense	cool	antitussive
Rose hips	Rosa spp.	neutral	tonsillitis, soothing to throat
Saw Palmetto berry	Serenoa serrulata	warm and moist	tones mucosa
Skullcap	Scutellaria lateriflora	dry and hot	tones mucous passages
Slippery Elm	Ulmus fulva	cool and moist	demulcent, for sore throats
Thyme	Thymus vulgaris	dry and hot	whooping cough
White Sarsaparilla, Spikenard root	Aralia nudicaulis	warm	sore throat
Yellow Root	Xanthorhiza simplicissima	cool	sore throat
Thyroid Gland—Builders (+)			
Bladderwrack, Kelp	Fucus vesiculosus	cool	obesity and edema
Licorice	Glycyrrhiza glabra	warm and moist	
Thyroid Gland—Cleansers (−)			
Burdock root	Arctium lappa	warm and moist	
Mullein	Verbascum thapsus	warm and moist	
Saint-John's-Wort	Hypericum perforatum	cool and dry	

COMMON NAME AND PLANT PART	SCIENTIFIC NAME	THERMAL AND MOISTURE PROPERTIES	APPLICATION
Thyroid Gland—Tonics (0)			
Black Walnut hulls	*Juglans nigra*	cold	hypothyroid
Bugleweed	*Lycopus virginicus*	cool and dry	hyperthyroid
Calamus, Sweet Flag	*Acorus calamus*	warm	hyperthyroid, hypothyroid
Cayenne	*Capsicum annuum*	hot	stimulant
Lemon Balm	*Melissa officinalis*	cool and moist	
Motherwort	*Leonurus cardiaca*	cool	
Passionflower	*Passiflora incarnata*	cool	hypothyroid
Poke root	*Phytolacca esculenta*	dry and hot	stimulant
Red Sarsaparilla	*Smilax ornata*	warm and moist	
Siberian Ginseng	*Eleutherococcus senticosus*	warm	
Tissue Regenerators—Builders (+)			
Aloe	*Aloe barbadensis, A. officinalis*	cold	
Arnica	*Arnica montana*	warm	external in liniments
Black Walnut	*Juglans nigra*	cold	
Calendula flowers	*Calendula officinalis*	neutral	
Comfrey leaf	*Symphytum officinale*	cool and moist	regenerates tissues
Gotu Kola	*Centella asiatica*	cool	
Horsetail	*Equisetum hyemale*	cool	
Plantain leaf	*Plantago* spp.	cool and dry	repairs tissues
Raspberry leaf	*Rubus idaeus*	cool	
Saint-John's-Wort	*Hypericum perforatum*	cool and dry	
Tissue Regenerators—Cleansers (−)			
Goldenseal	*Hydrastis canadensis*	dry and hot	1/10 part of a formula or less
Myrrh	*Commiphora myrrha*	dry and hot	
Sanicle	*Sanicula europaea*	dry and hot	internal and external wounds

COMMON NAME AND PLANT PART	SCIENTIFIC NAME	THERMAL AND MOISTURE PROPERTIES	APPLICATION
Tissue Regenerators—Tonics (0)			
Ginger	*Zingiber officinale*	dry and hot	
Urinary Tract—Builders (+)			
Arrowroot	*Maranta arundinacea*	cool and moist	demulcent, nutritive, builder
Bistort	*Polygonum bistorta*	cool	
Comfrey leaf	*Symphytum officinale*	cool and moist	regenerates tissues
Corn silk	*Zea mays*	neutral	cystitis, urethritis, incontinence, pain generally
Dandelion root	*Taraxacum officinale*	cool	
Fenugreek	*Trigonella foenum-graecum*	warm	
Hollyhock	*Althaea rosea*	cool	neck of the bladder
Horsetail	*Equisetum hyemale*	cool	inflammation and irritation, incontinence while sleeping from cystitis
Marshmallow root	*Althaea officinalis*	cool and moist	cystitis, urethritis, pain generally
Plantain leaf	*Plantago* spp.	cool and dry	repairs tissues
Yarrow	*Achillea millefolium*	neutral	soothing and healing of mucosa
Urinary Tract—Cleansers (−)			
Alder, Buckthorn	*Rhamnus cathartica*	cold	diuretic
Amaranth	*Amaranthus hypochondriacus*	neutral	diuretic
Bladderwrack, Kelp	*Fucus vesiculosus*	cool	diuretic
Blue Cohosh	*Caulophyllum thalictroides*	warm and dry	slightly diuretic
Borage	*Borago officinalis*	cool	slightly diuretic
Buchu	*Agathosma betulina*	warm	antiseptic
Calamus, Sweet Flag	*Acorus calamus*	warm	
Cedar, Arborvitae, Thuja	*Thuja occidentalis*	cold	

COMMON NAME AND PLANT PART	SCIENTIFIC NAME	THERMAL AND MOISTURE PROPERTIES	APPLICATION
Couchgrass	*Agropyron repens*	cool	
Cubeb berries	*Piper cubeba*	warm	chronic cystitis with mucus at menses
Dandelion root	*Taraxacum officinale*	cool	
Elecampane	*Inula helenium*	dry and hot	diuretic
Goldenseal	*Hydrastis canadensis*	dry and hot	1/10 part of a formula or less
Guaiacum	*Guaiacum officinale*	cool	
Juniper berry	*Juniperus communis*	warm	chronic cystitis with mucus, without inflammation
Nettles	*Urtica dioica, U. urens*	dry and hot	diuretic, drying to mucosa
Osha	*Ligusticum filicinum, L. porteri*	dry and hot	stimulates
Pareira Brava	*Chondrodendron tomentosum*	cool	
Parsley leaf	*Petroselinum crispum*	neutral	
Plantain leaf	*Plantago* spp.	cool and dry	
Queen of the Meadow, Joe Pye Weed, Gravel Root	*Eupatorium purpureum*	warm	dark or milky urine
Saint-John's-Wort	*Hypericum perforatum*	cool and dry	
Sanicle	*Sanicula europaea*	dry and hot	
Sassafras	*Sassafras albidum, S. variifolium*	dry and hot	
Stone Root	*Collinsonia canadensis*	warm	diuretic
Thyme	*Thymus vulgaris*	dry and hot	antiseptic
Uva Ursi, Bearberry	*Arctostaphylos uva-ursi*	cold	antiseptic, purulent scanty urine
Urinary Tract—Tonics (0)			
Aspen bark	*Populus* spp.	cold	spasms after urination

COMMON NAME AND PLANT PART	SCIENTIFIC NAME	THERMAL AND MOISTURE PROPERTIES	APPLICATION
Balm of Gilead	*Populus balsamifera*	warm	
Bistort	*Polygonum bistorta*	cool	
Cannabis, Da Ma tincture or tea of flowering tops	*Cannabis sativa*	warm and dry	cystitis, urethritis with irritability more than pain
Cedar, Arborvitae, Thuja	*Thuja occidentalis*	cold	incontinence in aged males with enlarged prostate
Coltsfoot	*Tussilago farfara*	warm and moist	
Coriander seeds and leaves	*Coriandrum sativum*	neutral (seeds), cool (leaves)	
Marshmallow root	*Althaea officinalis*	cool and moist	demulcent, diuretic
Plantain leaf	*Plantago* spp.	cool and dry	balancer
Prickly Ash	*Zanthoxylum clava-herculis, Z. americanum*	warm	promotes mucous discharge
Skullcap	*Scutellaria lateriflora*	dry and hot	tones passages

PLANTS FOR SOME COMMON CONDITIONS

COMMON NAME AND PLANT PART	SCIENTIFIC NAME	THERMAL AND MOISTURE PROPERTIES	APPLICATION
Allergies			
Eyebright herb or homeopathic dilution	*Euphrasia officinalis*	cool	anti-inflammatory for watery catarrh of nose, sinus, and middle ear
Fevers			
Basil	*Ocimum basilicum*	warm	fever with indigestion, vomiting, stomach cramps
Blue Vervain	*Verbena hastata*	cold	fevers, colds, flu
Boneset	*Eupatorium perfoliatum*	cool	moist fever with deep pain in the bone, aching in the muscles
Bupleurum, Chai-hu, Thorowax root	*Bupleurum chinense, B. falcatum*	cool	lowers fevers, cleans the liver, and dredges out old emotions, sadness, anger
Cannabis, Da Ma tincture or tea of flowering tops	*Cannabis sativa*	warm and dry	fever with delirium, wakes frequently
Catnip	*Nepeta cataria*	cold and moist	calming and relaxing for insomnia, fever
Chrysanthemum flowers	*Chrysanthemum morifolium*	cool	fevers, colds, flu, headaches
Echinacea	*Echinacea angustifolia, E. pallida, E. purpurea*	dry and hot	general fever remedy, for septic conditions, necrosis
Elderflowers	*Sambucus nigra, S. canadensis*	cool	colds, flu, fever; opens skin pores and increases sweating; mix with Mint and Yarrow for stomach flu and general detox
Feverfew	*Tanacetum parthenium*	cool	colds, flu, fever, and digestive problems
Gentian	*Gentiana lutea, G. officinalis*	cold	fever, poor digestion
Ginger	*Zingiber officinale*	dry and hot	induces sweating; for nausea, vomiting, fevers

COMMON NAME AND PLANT PART	SCIENTIFIC NAME	THERMAL AND MOISTURE PROPERTIES	APPLICATION
Holy Basil, Tulsi	Ocimum tenuiflorum	warm	colds, flu, bronchitis, fevers
Horsemint	Monarda punctata	cool	colds, flu, fever with stomach upset
Horsetail	Equisetum hyemale	cool	fever, diarrhea, dysentery
Kudzu root	Pueraria lobata	cool	colds, flu, headache, muscular tension, diarrhea; also a tonic for diabetes and hypoglycemia; a valuable edible and medicinal plant so misunderstood in the USA
Lemon Balm	Melissa officinalis	neutral	fever, nervousness, insomnia, depression, bronchial catarrh
Mulberry leaves	Morus alba	cold	colds, flu, fever
Peppermint	Mentha piperita	cool	colds, flu, fever with mild digestive upset; mix with Yarrow and Elderflowers for stomach flu and general detox
Pleurisy Root	Asclepias tuberosa	cool	colds, fever, flu, lung conditions
White Willow	Salix alba	cold	fever, insomnia, restlessness, sore muscles, headache
Yarrow	Achillea millefolium	neutral	fever, colds, flu, digestive upset; mix with Peppermint and Elderflowers for stomach flu and general detox
Imbalanced Metabolism			
Cayenne	Capsicum annuum	hot	debility, lack of secretions with dryness
Echinacea	Echinacea angustifolia, E. pallida, E. purpurea	dry and hot	to counter immunosuppression from cancer drugs

COMMON NAME AND PLANT PART	SCIENTIFIC NAME	THERMAL AND MOISTURE PROPERTIES	APPLICATION
Ginseng	*Panax quinquefolius*	warm	chilly person, cold fingers, poor appetite with normal stools and dry skin
Poke root	*Phytolacca esculenta*	dry and hot	cancer with lymph involvement
Red Clover blossoms	*Trifolium pratense*	dry and cool	metastatic cancers
Yellow Dock, Curly Dock root	*Rumex crispus*	cool	debility with chronic skin disorders, ulcerations
Nutrition Deficiencies			
Alfalfa	*Medicago sativa*	cool	promotes appetite in people who are nervous, after major illness, after surgery
Bladderwrack, Kelp	*Fucus vesiculosus*	cool	for mineral deficiencies
Calamus, Sweet Flag	*Acorus calamus*	malabsorption from too rapid dietary changes	
Gentian	*Gentiana lutea, G. officinalis*	cold	malabsorption in the aged
Goldenseal	*Hydrastis canadensis*	dry and hot	malabsorption in the aged; 1/10 part of a formula or less
Guarana	*Paullinia cupana, P. crysan, P. sorbilis*	warm	appetite suppressant for obesity; has a high caffeine content
Hops	*Humulus lupulus*	faulty digestion of starches	
Maravilla, Wild Four o'Clock root	*Mirabilis multiflora*	cool	strong decoction of the root or the powdered root baked into bread taken before meals to curb the appetite; root tea or poultice used as a wash for rheumatic swellings; antiseptic wash for wounds in horses and as a mouthwash for humans

COMMON NAME AND PLANT PART	SCIENTIFIC NAME	THERMAL AND MOISTURE PROPERTIES	APPLICATION
Red Clover	*Trifolium pratense*	dry and cool	promotes appetite in people who are nervous, after major illness, after surgery
Yellow Dock	*Rumex crispus*		malabsorption with greasy face, acne, ileocecal inflammation
Pain			
Goldenseal	*Hydrastis canadensis*	dry and hot	as a recuperative after inflammations; 1/10 part of a formula or less
Guarana	*Paullinia cupana, P. crysan, P. sorbilis*	warm	painful hangover with headache, headache with confusion, worse for motion, migraines from vasoconstriction
Hops	*Humulus lupulus*	cool	chronic headache with dyspepsia
Passionflower	*Passiflora incarnata*	cool	chronic migraine in the evening, headache with ringing in the ears
Skullcap	*Scutellaria lateriflora*	dry and hot	pain with fear and agitation
White Willow	*Salix alba*	cold	fever, restlessness, insomnia, headache, sore muscles, tooth pain
Pediatric Ailments			
Note: Herbs can be safely delivered to infants if the mother takes the remedy and passes it along through her breast milk. For children who are not breastfeeding consider making herbal glycerites.			
Anise	*Pimpinella anisum*	warm	colic with gas
Blackberry fruit, berry juice, root tea	*Rubus villosus*	neutral	diarrhea
Blue Vervain	*Verbena officinalis*	cold	agitated, hysterical fever with upset stomach and teething
Cannabis, Da Ma tincture or tea of flowering tops	*Cannabis sativa*	warm and dry	violent, spasmodic cough

COMMON NAME AND PLANT PART	SCIENTIFIC NAME	THERMAL AND MOISTURE PROPERTIES	APPLICATION
Caraway seeds	Carum carvi	warm	colic with gas
Catnip	Nepeta cataria	cold and moist	colic with gas, crying, hysteria, fever
Chamomile	Chamaemelum nobile, Matricaria recutita	warm and moist	fever with upset stomach, teething with agitation, vomiting with green diarrhea
Chinese Cinnamon	Cinnamomum cassia	dry and hot	diarrhea
Corn silk	Zea mays	neutral	cystitis, urethritis, to strengthen the bladder
Drosera, Sundew	Drosera rotundifolia	warm	cough with measles, whooping cough, bronchitis
Fennel	Foeniculum vulgare	warm and moist	colic with gas
Ginger	Zingiber officinale	dry and hot	nausea, vomiting, car sickness
Lavender flowers	Lavandula angustifolia, L. vera	hot and dry	colic with pain, nausea, bad breath, acidic vomit
Lemon Balm	Melissa officinalis	neutral	fever, nervousness, insomnia, depression, bronchial catarrh
Lobelia	Lobelia inflata	neutral	spasmodic cough, cough with laryngitis, wheezing, measles with dry cough
Mullein	Verbascum thapsus	warm and moist	incontinence
Passionflower	Passiflora incarnata	cool	teething with agitation and gastric upset
Peppermint	Mentha piperita	cool	diarrhea, fever, nausea, to prevent vomiting
Plantain leaf	Plantago spp.	cool and dry	incontinence
Privet berry	Ligustrum lucidum	neutral	thrush
Wild Ginger	Asarum canadense	dry and hot, warm	colic with gas

COMMON NAME AND PLANT PART	SCIENTIFIC NAME	THERMAL AND MOISTURE PROPERTIES	APPLICATION
Psychological Imbalances			
Cannabis, Da Ma	*Cannabis sativa*	warm and dry	mild anorexia nervosa in adolescence, depression from painful spasmodic illnesses
Goldenseal	*Hydrastis canadensis*	dry and hot	general tonic for depression; as a recuperative after inflammations; 1/10 part of a formula or less
Lobelia	*Lobelia inflata*	neutral	convulsions with hysteria
Passionflower	*Passiflora incarnata*	cool	premenstrual depression, depression from abuse of psychoactive drugs
Valerian	*Valeriana officinalis*	warm	apathy, depression, poor digestion, depression with hysteria; use only in combination with other herbs

GLOSSARY OF HERBAL CONTRAINDICATIONS

Please note—this is not an exhaustive list and new drug and herb interactions are being discovered daily. Please look for the most current information online if you are taking allopathic medications and want to ingest herbs!

Here is a thumbnail sketch of some herbal contraindications and precautions.

Agrimony may cause photosensitivity to UV light if used for an extended period.

Alfalfa is contraindicated in those who are gaining weight, in pregnancy, in nursing mothers, and in cases of lupus.

Aloe should be avoided in pregnancy, if there is profuse menstruation, by nursing mothers, by children under twelve, in cases of stomach or intestinal inflammation, kidney disorders, appendicitis, or laxative abuse. Avoid extended use (more than ten days). It may reduce absorption of oral drugs due to decrease in bowel transit time.

Angelica may worsen peptic ulcers due to increased hydrochloric acid production. It can cause photosensitivity and may worsen acid reflux.

Arnica is for external use only and not to be used on broken skin; it is toxic in even very low doses. However, the homeopathic dilution is very safe for internal consumption.

Ashwagandha root is contraindicated in pregnancy because it may be abortive. Do not use with other sedatives.

Astragalus may actually worsen hot conditions, infections, and fevers;

it should not be used if there is an engorgement of blood in body tissues or by those who have difficulty sweating (it seems to close the pores). It can help restore the immune system after immunosuppressants and may enhance the potency of interferon. This herb should be used in combination with others and not be taken alone.

Barberry root should be used with caution when there is severe liver disease, bile duct or pancreatic cancer, septic gallbladder, or bile duct obstruction. Avoid during pregnancy. It should not be taken before the menstrual period or by those with hemorrhoids.

Bayberry or Wax Myrtle should be avoided if there is severe inflammation of an acute nature in the intestinal tract.

Black Alder or Buckthorn bark is contraindicated in cases of intestinal obstruction or inflammation, such as irritable bowel syndrome (IBS), colitis, or appendicitis, and also in pregnancy, nursing mothers, and children under twelve. Do not take for more than two weeks. The bark must be aged one year before using. It may reduce absorption of oral drugs due to decreased bowel transit time.

Blackberry should be avoided if there is constipation.

Black Cohosh in large amounts may cause a frontal headache, vertigo, impaired vision, dilated pupils, nausea, vomiting, feeble circulation, or even a condition resembling delirium tremens in some persons. High in tannins, it can interfere in iron absorption. A phytoestrogen, it should be avoided in pregnancy, by nursing mothers, and by those taking estrogen-replacement therapy. It should be avoided by those with high blood pressure.

Black Haw should not be used as more than one-fifth part of a formula and should not be used alone. A diuretic, it can be irritating to the urinary tract. Those with weak kidneys or kidney disease should avoid it.

Bladderwrack or Kelp is high in salt and iodine; it should be avoided if there is high blood pressure, during pregnancy and nursing, by those using lithium salts, and by those on blood thinners or before surgery, due to its antithrombin effect. It is not for persons with weak, cold digestion, hyperthyroidism, iodine-induced goiter, or iodine-induced thyroid deficiency. Prolonged use can lead to acne.

Blessed Thistle should not be used by women who experience enlarged, sore breasts during their menstrual cycle. It may be emetic for some and causes diarrhea in overdose. Avoid during pregnancy and lactation or in cases of allergy to the Aster family of plants.

Blue Cohosh is contraindicated if there is heavy bleeding. It is an emmenagogue and abortifacient (use only in the last five weeks of pregnancy). It should be avoided by those with heart disease or high blood pressure.

Blue Flag may cause contact dermatitis, gastrointestinal irritation, and potassium loss if there is overuse of the herb as a laxative. It should be avoided in pregnancy and by nursing mothers.

Borage fresh leaf can cause contact dermatitis in some individuals. Do not use with seizure medications, anticonvulsants, hepatotoxic herbs or drugs, anabolic steroids, or tricyclic antidepressants. This herb may interact with oral anticoagulants. It is not recommended for prolonged use. Avoid topical use on broken skin, and avoid when there is a history of liver disease.

Buchu is contraindicated if there is acute genitourinary tract inflammation or acute kidney inflammation or disease. Avoid in pregnancy; it is a mucosal irritant and uterine stimulant. It is not recommended for long-term use due to hepatotoxic components. It may darken or add aroma to the urine.

Bugleweed should be avoided during pregnancy and lactation and in cases of acute nephritis, acute urinary tract infections, or any other acute inflammatory condition, and if there is low thyroid activity. It may interfere with thyroid hormones.

Burdock root is a drying agent (it is both diuretic and diaphoretic), so it should be used for moist conditions. It may actually worsen dry itchy skin conditions, even as it increases oily skin secretions. Insulin may need to be adjusted by diabetic users. The root may cause contact dermatitis in some individuals. Avoid in pregnancy.

Butternut Tree or White Walnut should be dried before use. Leaves may cause contact dermatitis or gastrointestinal irritation. The bark should be avoided by those who abuse laxatives. It is not for habitual use.

Calendula may seal in infection when applied externally to infected deep wounds. An emmenagogue, it is contraindicated in early pregnancy, and it may cause contact dermatitis in some individuals.

Cannabis or Da Ma (Chinese) chronic usage may cause amotivational syndrome, aimlessness, and poor communication. Withdrawal symptoms may include anorexia, insomnia, anxiety, and depression. Smoking it during pregnancy may result in miscarriage or an underweight fetus. Other cautions: it may cause dysphoria, tachycardia, or orthostatic hypotension, and it may abruptly trigger latent schizophrenia.

Cascara Sagrada is contraindicated in cases of intestinal inflammation, colitis, IBS, intestinal obstruction or ulcers, appendicitis, Crohn's disease, abdominal pain, heavy menstruation, and acute diarrhea, and in children under twelve, pregnant or nursing mothers, and debilitated subjects. Do not use with steroids, diuretics, corticosteroids, or Licorice root.

Catnip should be avoided in pregnancy and can interfere with central nervous system medications. Do not use with antidepressant, antianxiety, or sleep medications.

Cayenne may aggravate hot or dry conditions with extended use. Inhalation may aggravate asthma. Avoid contact with the eyes. Some persons may be allergic to Cayenne preparations, leading to urticaria. No additional heat applications should be used. Avoid if peptic ulcers are present. It is a good clotting agent, but do not apply to very deep, open wounds.

Cedar, Arborvitae, or Thuja may cause gastrointestinal irritation; avoid during pregnancy and lactation and in cases of epilepsy or gastritis (except in a homeopathic dose); it's not for prolonged use. Avoid getting in the eyes. The volatile oil may be toxic; use with medical supervision.

Celery seeds should not be used by pregnant women as they are abortive. Pregnant women should also avoid the daily use of celery juice. The seeds are contraindicated in kidney inflammation, kidney failure, and diabetes and if using UV light therapy or tanning.

Chamomile may cause contact dermatitis (especially to the eyes), respiratory allergy, and allergic conjunctivitis in persons who are also sensitive to Ragweed, Yarrow, Tansy, Arnica, Mugwort, or Birch pollen. Do not use in early pregnancy.

Chasteberry (Vitex) may increase progesterone and worsen depression. Do not take with progesterone-containing drugs. Vitex is contraindicated in pregnancy and in spasmodic dysmenorrhea.

Chinese Rhubarb—see Rhubarb.

Cinnamon should be avoided in pregnancy and if there is allergic hypersensitivity to Peruvian Balsam or to Cinnamon. Prolonged use may irritate tissues; it is contraindicated in cases of stomach ulcers, intestinal ulcers, and acid reflux disease.

Clover (Red and White) should be avoided in pregnancy and in children under two; it may cause birth defects or delayed puberty. Clover is contraindicated with estrogen-replacement therapy and with anticoagulant medications such as warfarin.

Coltsfoot can have high levels of pyrrilizidine alkaloids and should not be used for more than a few weeks (Eastern Coltsfoot is slightly safer than Western Coltsfoot). Avoid in pregnancy and during lactation, if there is a history of liver disease, or if there is mucus in the chest. Coltsfoot may cause contact dermatitis in some individuals. Do not use for more than four weeks a year, total.

Comfrey leaf contains pyrrilizidine alkaloids that could cause liver disease such as cirrhosis if taken continually. This risk is most serious for children and unborn fetuses. When applied externally to infected deep wounds and serious burns, Comfrey can potentially seal in the infection. It is contraindicated if bones are growing too fast (as in Osgood-Schlatter disease) and should be avoided by nursing mothers and those with a history of liver disease. It is not for prolonged use (more than five weeks). The root is probably too dangerous for internal use.

Coriander should be avoided by those with low blood sugar.

Corn silk is purgative when improperly dried, lowers blood sugar and blood pressure, and can interfere with anticoagulant medications.

Cotton root is a "controlled substance" and illegal to own, sell, or transport across state lines in the United States at this time. It can cause nausea, cramping, pain for up to four months after use, and genitourinary tract inflammation. It produces significant side effects and drug interactions with corticosteroids, thiazide diuretics, and grapefruit juice. It may interfere with iron absorption and so should not be used by anemics.

Cramp Bark fresh berry is poisonous but edible after cooking. A diuretic, it can be irritating, so avoid when there is genitourinary tract inflammation.

Damiana must be used for two weeks to achieve results. Cautions: it lowers blood sugar, overuse can cause headache and insomnia, and it stimulates the nervous system.

Dandelion, a bitter, may increase digestive tract pain if hypersecretion of gastric acid already exists. A liver herb, it may cause release of negative emotions stored in the liver. Taken for prolonged periods, it may permanently cool the constitution. Do not use with other diuretics. It may be toxic to children if grown in polluted areas, may cause diarrhea. It is contraindicated in acid reflux, bipolar disease (can increase lithium toxicity), intestinal spasms, jaundice, acute liver disease, allergic sensitivity to latex (rare), liver cancer, acute stomach inflammation, IBS, stomach ulcers, digestive weakness, bile duct obstruction, gallstones, pancreatic cancer, septic gallbladder, and intestinal obstruction. Large doses can be emetic.

Devil's Claw should be avoided if there is stomach inflammation, ulcers, or gallstones. Do not use with warfarin or other blood thinners.

Dodder will take on the properties of its host plant so pay attention to what this herb is growing on.

Dong Quai may increase menstrual bleeding and can exacerbate heat symptoms.

Dragon's Blood should be avoided during pregnancy and lactation.

Echinacea may exacerbate autoimmune conditions, may increase antibody production, and increases white blood cell count. Overuse may cause joint pain; prolonged use may lead to deeper, more persistent infections or exhaustion and chronic fatigue. It is contraindicated in leukemia, AIDS, multiple sclerosis, lupus, rheumatoid arthritis and other autoimmune conditions, tuberculosis, and leukosis. It should not be used for more than eight weeks (when using it be sure to add iron-rich foods such as lentils, chives, and beets to the diet). Avoid if allergic to the Aster family.

Elder is not for use for longer than twelve weeks. The leaves, stems, and uncooked and unripe fruits are unsafe and can produce nausea, vomiting, and diarrhea. The berries must be cooked or tinctured before ingesting. Avoid the berries in pregnancy and while breastfeeding (the flowers are safe for infants). Autoimmune diseases such as multiple sclerosis, lupus, rheumatoid arthritis, or other conditions may actually worsen if Elderberries are consumed.

Elecampane may cause contact dermatitis in some and can worsen eczema if used as a poultice for several days in some individuals.

False Unicorn root should be avoided by those with gastrointestinal irritation and in pregnancy (especially early pregnancy); in large doses it can be emetic.

Fennel should be avoided in pregnancy; the essential oil may be toxic to infants and small children; it is a phytoestrogen that could cause cancer over prolonged use and may cause allergic sensitivity to the skin or lungs. Do not use when there is acid reflux or in epilepsy. It may cause photodermatitis and interferes with the pharmacokinetic profile of some medications.

Fenugreek should be avoided in pregnancy; it may interfere with the absorption of some medications. Do not take with diabetic medications as it could precipitate a hypoglycemic crisis.

Feverfew may cause menstrual pain in some migraine patients.

Flax is contraindicated on open wounds (as the seeds may adhere to the wound), in intestinal obstruction, in inadequate fluid intake, in early pregnancy, in stricture of the esophagus, in stricture of stomach or intestinal sphincters, and in acute inflammation of the same. Avoid in iron-deficiency anemia, osteoporosis, and chronic mineral malnutrition.

Fringe Tree should be avoided in pregnancy and lactation, bile duct obstruction or impaction, cholangitis, hepatic cancer, bile duct cancer, and pancreatic cancer.

Garlic is a very heating and drying herb that can cause tissue destruction topically, so it is contraindicated in the dry person. It may cause nausea and vomiting if overused and must be taken raw to derive the full benefits; avoid if there is acute or chronic stomach inflammation or irritation, in early pregnancy, in low thyroid function, and in acid reflux. Garlic prolongs the clotting time of blood, so avoid it for two weeks before surgery.

Gentian taken in excess will produce nausea. Avoid when there is stomach inflammation or irritability, duodenal ulcers, or stomach ulcers.

Ginger should be used with caution in pregnancy (take no more than 250 mg daily for morning sickness or the root may be abortive). It is contraindicated in gallstones; it inhibits blood clotting, so stop taking it two weeks before elective surgery; regular exposure may cause contact dermatitis.

Ginseng (Panax **spp.***)* should be discontinued or reduced when normal energy is achieved. Overuse may cause neck tension and insomnia. It may also exacerbate pain or cough, stimulate menses, and worsen fibrocystic breasts; it may cause nosebleed and hypertension; and it should not be used to mask symptoms of chronic fatigue due to diet or lifestyle. American Ginseng has milder effects than Asian Ginseng but it may still increase the intensity of a cough. Do not use Ginseng for acute asthma (it can be used in combinations for chronic asthma) or acute infections (it may be used in combinations to increase resistance over time). Avoid if there are heavy menses or hemophilia, and stop taking it two weeks before surgery.

Goldenseal overuse may lead to constipation, vomiting, bleeding mucosa, and deranged digestion. If used as one-tenth part of a formula or less it is a tonic; more than that makes it an antibiotic. It is contraindicated in diabetes, high blood pressure, purulent discharge from the ear, kidney disease, acute stomach inflammation, and jaundice in newborns. After a course of this herb intestinal flora must be rebuilt; try miso soup, sauerkraut, garlic, plain yogurt, or raw apple cider.

Gotu Kola should be avoided in early pregnancy, as it is an emmenagogue. Do not use during lactation, or if there is an allergy to carrots. Use it with caution in conjunction with anticoagulants or in cases of epilepsy.

Ground Ivy, Creeping Charlie, or Gill-over-the-Ground should be avoided in pregnancy and lactation. If there is active bleeding, do not use concurrently with other anticoagulants.

Guaiacum is not intended for long-term use.

Guarana has the same side effects as caffeine: insomnia, anxiety, restlessness, upset stomach, and quickened heartbeat. Long-term use may result in tolerance and psychological dependence. It is not recommended for children or for pregnant or lactating women.

Gutta-Percha Tree or Hardy Rubber Tree should be avoided by those with a latex allergy.

Hawthorn may potentiate the effects of other heart medications, leading to a rapid and steep drop in blood pressure. (I have personally witnessed this three times.)

Hops is a depressant and sedative and should be avoided by those with depression issues. Do not use for extended periods of time; long-term use leads to tolerance. A pillow of Hops may be placed near a child's head, but the pillow should be removed once the child is asleep. Some persons may experience contact dermatitis or allergic hypersensitivity when inhaling the pollen.

Horsetail should be spring gathered—in the fall it builds toxic elements. Children can be poisoned by chewing the stems. It is not for long-term use. Avoid during pregnancy and lactation.

Hydrangea root should only be taken for a few days. Overuse can lead to vertigo, nausea, vomiting, diarrhea, dizziness, and chest tightness.

Hyssop is contraindicated in pregnancy and lactation. It should be used in small doses only and as a part of a larger formula, not by itself.

Juniper berries should be avoided if there is kidney inflammation, infection, or failure, and also in pregnancy. Prolonged use (over four weeks) can cause kidney damage.

Lady's Slipper root may cause contact dermatitis in some individuals.

Lavender should not be combined with Catnip or Valerian. Avoid in early pregnancy.

Lemon Balm should be avoided in pregnancy: it is abortive and an emmenagogue, and it may interfere with fetal development. It is contraindicated in low thyroid conditions, glaucoma, and swollen prostate.

Licorice overuse can lead to hypertension and fluid retention, and it may suppress testosterone in men and women. Avoid if there are swollen ovaries or ovarian cysts, high blood pressure, weak kidneys, tendency to water retention, history of cancer in female relatives, or cardiac edema. It is not for prolonged use (more than four weeks).

Avoid in pregnancy, liver cirrhosis, bile stasis, chronic hepatitis, alcoholism, obesity, diabetes, catarrhal respiratory conditions (it increases mucous production), or decreased libido.

Limeflower or Linden should be avoided in pregnancy and breast-feeding. Use caution with heart conditions as it may worsen those.

Lobelia is a traditional emetic that can cause nausea in some persons. Lobelia sedates the respiratory system and cough reflex and should be avoided in congestive heart failure. This herb should not be used by the elderly or the very young, or by those who are emotionally unstable or have low or high blood pressure or low energy. Avoid in nervous prostration, shock, paralysis, dyspnea from heart disease, enlarged or fatty heart, pneumonia, dry irritable cough, or pregnancy, and if there is tobacco sensitivity.

Mandrake or Mayapple root overdose could be fatal; use only with medical supervision. Avoid in pregnancy, if there are gallstones or intestinal obstruction, and in debilitated subjects; avoid topical use near eyes, on birthmarks or warts, and by diabetics. This herb is a skin irritant and use for over one hour or on more than several inches of skin could prove toxic. Homeopathic potencies are very safe.

Marshmallow root should not be used if there is profuse catarrh or mucous discharge.

Milk Thistle is a very benign plant that may cause headaches in some individuals.

Mistletoe berries are poisonous. The leaves and twigs are the parts used but they are contraindicated in pregnancy and lactation, hyperthyroidism, and in serious progressive conditions such as tuberculosis or AIDS. Eating raw, unprocessed European Mistletoe or American Mistletoe can cause vomiting, seizures, a slowing of the heart rate, and even death. American Mistletoe is toxic and not suitable for medical use.

Motherwort can alter the duration of the menstrual cycle. Avoid during pregnancy, especially in the early stages, in menorrhagia, and with concurrent use of digitaloids or anticoagulants.

Mugwort should be avoided in pregnancy and it may cause allergic hypersensitivity, especially in those allergic to Chamomile.

Mullein is contraindicated when there is profuse catarrh.

Myrrh should be avoided for internal use in pregnancy, and in case of acute internal inflammation, fever, bleeding, lymphoma, or collagen-associated autoimmune disease such as lupus erythematosus, poly-arteritis, scleroderma, or rheumatoid arthritis. It may accelerate the pulse and worsen excessive uterine bleeding.

Nettles are both diuretic and drying and so should be avoided by those who have dry mucosa or dry scalp. Nettles may worsen dry eczema and dandruff. Nettles harvested late in the year may lead to kidney irritation, so it's best to gather them in the early spring. Persons with sensitive stomachs may have difficulties with this plant and large amounts can be purgative. Avoid in pregnancy and in heart- or kidney-centered edema. Some persons may be hypersensitive to the sting and should avoid the fresh or dry leaves. (Gather with rubber kitchen gloves on the hands; rinsing nettles for a few seconds in cold water completely removes the stinging acid on the leaves.)

Oak should be avoided as a bath or wash for large areas of skin due to the tannins. Avoid internal use if there is constipation, iron deficiency anemia, or malnutrition. It may reduce the absorption of other herbs and medications.

Orange peel is contraindicated if there are stomach ulcers.

Oregon Grape root may worsen hypersecretion in the digestive organs. It has caused jaundice in babies born to women taking this liver herb. Avoid during pregnancy, in bile duct obstruction or inflammation, in bile duct or pancreatic cancer, in hemolytic anemia or hyperbilirubinemia in newborns, and in acute or severe liver disease, gallstones, septic gallbladder, and intestinal spasm.

Osha can irritate a dry cough if taken alone (add other herbs such as Licorice to counteract this). Avoid in pregnancy except during labor to expel the placenta.

Parsley can actually cause stones if overeaten. Avoid when there is heart- or kidney-centered edema or kidney inflammation. The seeds and root are abortive and should be avoided in pregnancy. Do not exceed more than two cups of the seed tea per day.

Partridgeberry should not be more than one-fifth part of a formula; do not use alone.

Passionflower can be narcotic and accumulative; do not take for more than two weeks. It is contraindicated in pregnancy, nursing women, and depression. Large amounts can be harmful.

Pennyroyal in large doses can cause or worsen nervousness and nerve weakness. Avoid in pregnancy and nursing (it could be fatal to an infant), kidney disease, or liver disease. Overuse on a cat's collar will cause it to vomit.

Peppermint causes a worsening of heartburn in some people; using it as part of a larger formula can mitigate this effect. Avoid in pregnancy, gallstones, hiatal hernia, and acid reflux. Do not apply the essential oil to the face or nose of a small child or infant; menthol can cause spasm of the glottis.

Pine is a potential abortifacient, so avoid it during pregnancy.

Pipsissewa or Prince's Pine leaves may cause contact dermatitis in some individuals.

Plantain is contraindicated when there is profuse catarrh or mucus congestion; do not use internally during pregnancy.

Pleurisy Root affects the overall circulation. Do not use if there is a full pulse; use only when the pulse is faint and weak. Avoid in pregnancy.

Poke root should not be used if there is gastrointestinal irritation or acute inflammation. A uterine stimulant and laxative, it should be avoided in pregnancy and in lactation. This herb is toxic and only one or two drops of tincture should be taken internally per day, for no more than two days. Slightly larger amounts may be added to external poultices for tumors, mastitis, and so on. The homeopathic potency is very safe.

Prickly Ash is contraindicated in acute stomach and intestinal ulcers or inflammation, in pregnancy, and in breastfeeding.

Psyllium seeds should not be used when there is bowel obstruction, in diabetes, or in iron deficiency. Lithium salts should be taken one hour before or after taking this herb (it may reduce the absorption of oral medications).

Queen of the Meadow, Joe Pye Weed, or Gravel Root is not for prolonged use due to pyrrilizidine alkaloids. Avoid in pregnancy, while breastfeeding, topical use on abraded skin, and if there is a history of liver disease.

Raspberry leaf should be used only in the last five weeks of pregnancy. Avoid if there is a history of miscarriage; it may affect fetal development.

Red Clover may cause blood-thinning and bleeding problems when taken alone for prolonged periods.

Redroot or New Jersey Tea may cause spleen swelling; avoid in conditions such as sickle cell anemia, mononucleosis, or leukemia with enlarged spleen.

Rehmannia is contraindicated in diarrhea, in anorexia, and if there is excessive menstrual flow. Avoid use if there is weak digestion or a tendency to gas and abdominal bloating.

Rhubarb or Chinese Rhubarb root should be avoided in pregnancy and lactation, by children under twelve, and if there is severe fever or inflammation, acute intestinal inflammation such as colitis, IBS, Crohn's disease, ulcerative colitis, intestinal obstruction, diarrhea, laxative abuse, hemorrhoids, appendicitis, history of kidney stones, or abdominal pains of unknown origin. It is not for extended use; do not use for more than two weeks.

Rose may slow the absorption of herbal components.

Rue essential oil should not be taken internally—it could lead to death. Avoid the herb during pregnancy; it is abortive. It may cause photosensitivity when taken internally or cause contact dermatitis when the leaf or juices are handled. Avoid this herb if there is kidney weakness of any kind. Goldenseal is the supposed antidote if too large a dose is taken.

Sage essential oil, with prolonged use, can lead to epileptiform cramps. Do not use this plant if your libido is low. Taken for long periods of time, this herb can cause liver irritation and swelling (combine with tonic and building liver herbs to counteract this). Do not use in pregnancy, as it can be abortive. It should not be used while breastfeeding unless the objective is to dry up the breast milk.

Saint-John's-Wort affects the liver biotransformation of drugs and hormones, so it could lead to overdose or underdose if taken with pharmaceuticals. When taken for several months, this plant can lead to photosensitivity in animals and humans (I have personally observed this). To avoid the rash caused by sunlight I recommend only taking this plant in the dark half of the year and stopping a full month before sun exposure is likely to occur. In the light half of the year I recommend Damiana (*Turnera aphrodisiaca*) and Kava Kava (*Piper methysticum*) as antidepressants. Other effects include anxiety or panic attacks when taken with antidepressant medications or after those pharmaceuticals have been discontinued. Avoid in pregnancy, AIDS, severe depression, and elective surgery (it may interfere with anesthetic agents). It interferes with immunosuppressants used with organ transplants.

Sassafras is a possible hepatocarcinogen with prolonged use (daily for about a year). The root should be used for a few days only. Do not use with an IUD, in summer, or in early pregnancy.

Saw Palmetto berries may cause breast swelling and tenderness in men or women. Do not use if you have bad skin.

Scarlet Pimpernel in large amounts can be toxic; do not use as more than one-sixth part of a formula.

Shatavari or Indian Asparagus root should not be used in cold and damp disorders such as excess mucus, phlegm, and diarrhea. It is contraindicated with the use of lithium because as a diuretic it could end up concentrating large amounts of lithium salts in the body. Avoid if allergic to asparagus and in kidney disorders, heart disease, edema, lung congestion, fibrocystic breasts, and estrogen-related problems. It may cause breast tenderness and premenstrual distress.

Shepherd's Purse is contraindicated in pregnancy.

Siberian Ginseng overuse can lead to anxiety, heart palpitations, and rash on the face and nose. Extreme doses have led to mania. Do not use for long periods of time without periodic breaks of one to three months. Avoid in high blood pressure or acute infections.

Skullcap should not be used with sedatives (including alcohol) or tranquilizers. This herb is often adulterated with Germander (*Teucrium* spp.), which can be hepatotoxic, therefore long-term use and use by those with weak livers should be discouraged.

Slippery Elm slows or reduces the absorption of other herbs and medications.

Tansy is toxic and can cause breast lumps. Misuse may lead to paralysis or uterine contractions lasting for months. Do not use if you have allergic sensitivity to the Aster family. Avoid self-prescribing; use with medical advice. The poisoning symptoms are identical to rabies symptoms; overuse of the oil or tea could prove fatal.

Turmeric may cause stomach upset, nausea, and dizziness in some individuals. It is safe as a food but should be avoided as a supplement in pregnancy and lactation. Avoid if there are gallstones, bile duct obstruction, bleeding disorders, diabetes, gastroesophageal reflux disease, hormone-sensitive cancers (such as breast, uterine, ovarian cancers), endometriosis, fibroids, infertility issues, or iron deficiency. It may cause extra bleeding, so stop using it two weeks before surgery.

Usnea is safe used externally but should only be used for a short time internally. Liver damage symptoms such as nausea, weakness, fatigue, abdominal pain, and yellowing of the skin have occurred in as little as two weeks.

Uva Ursi is not for prolonged use. Avoid in pregnancy and lactation, kidney disorders, and children under twelve. It may cause stomach upset.

Valerian is generally a sedative, but some people experience insomnia, anxiety, depression, and vivid dreams while using this plant; it may also cause headache, nausea, giddiness, slurred speech, dizziness, or agitation. Best used by those with pale face and cold skin, the plant may be contraindicated in hot, red-faced individuals. Use may become addictive after two weeks; never use alone, only as part of a larger formula. It may irritate the liver, leading to nausea; avoid if there is low blood pressure or hypoglycemia.

Vervain should be avoided in pregnancy and lactation and by young children.

Wahoo or Spindle Tree bark should be avoided in gall duct obstruction, impacted gallstones, bile duct inflammation, bile duct cancer, pancreatic cancer, jaundice, severe or acute liver disease, septic gallbladder inflammation, intestinal spasm, and liver cancer.

Watercress enhances the absorption of vitamins and minerals but could also increase the absorption of medications. Use with caution.

White Willow is contraindicated if there are stomach ulcers, allergy to aspirin, or gout and kidney problems. It may slow or reduce the absorption of herbal components and medications.

Wild Cherry bark should not be collected after the first frost because it will contain cyanide. Avoid prolonged use and use in pregnancy. The leaves can kill a horse or a cow.

Wild Lettuce or Prickly Lettuce should not be used for a prolonged period as an antitussive. It is a sedative and should not be used by those with depression. Use with medical supervision.

Wild Yam in large doses can be diuretic and emetic. Avoid if there are impacted gallstones, bile duct inflammation, liver cancer, internal spasms, septic gallbladder, acute liver disease, jaundice from hemolytic anemia, hyperbilirubinemia, bile duct obstruction, or bile duct or pancreatic cancer.

Witch Hazel should not be used for long periods internally due to concentrated tannins.

Yarrow should not be used in pregnancy or if there is allergic hypersensitivity to the Aster family. It reduces sperm count.

Yellow Dock may cause diarrhea; if it does, cut the dose in half until the proper dosage is determined. Avoid if there are kidney stones; do not use with other laxatives because it may cause potassium loss if overused as a laxative. It may lead to gastrointestinal irritation and can slow the absorption of other herbs and medications; do not use with other drugs for the GI tract.

Yucca overdose could cause purging. Counteract this by adding Ginger root and Prickly Ash bark (use two parts each of Ginger and Prickly Ash to six parts of Yucca).

SOURCES
AND RESOURCES

1. THE SIGNATURES OF PLANTS— LEARNING NATURE'S ALPHABET

Bjerklie, David. "The Doctrine of Signatures: Isn't Mother Nature Amazing?" *Time*, October 2003.

Clarke, John Henry. "A Dictionary of Practical Materia Medica, Lobelia Cardinalis." www.homeoint.org/clarke/l/lob_card.htm (accessed December 2, 2013).

"Find a Vitamin or Supplement: Liverwort." WebMD, www.webmd.com/vitamins -supplements/ingredientmono-37-liverwort.aspx?activeIngredientId=37&active IngredientName=liverwort&source=1 (accessed August 4, 2015).

Grieve, Margaret. *A Modern Herbal*. New York: Dover Publications Inc., 1971.

Harris, Ben Charles. *Compleat Herbal*. New York: Larchmont Books, 1982.

"Herbal History." http://herbwisdom.tripod.com/herb_history.html (accessed November 29, 2013).

Tierra, Michael. *Planetary Herbology*. Santa Fe, N.Mex.: Lotus Press, 1988.

Wolfson, P., and D. L. Hoffmann. "An Investigation into the Efficacy of Scutellaria Lateriflora in Healthy Volunteers." *Alternative Therapies in Health and Medcine* 9, no. 2 (March–April 2003): 74–78.

2. HERBS OF SPRING

Crooked Chimney. "Sycamore Syrup." www.crookedchimneysyrup.com/?page _id=320 (accessed March 2014).

Hard, Lindsay-Jean. "Stinging Nettles and the Best Ways to Eat Them." Food 52, food52.com/blog/9935-stinging-nettles-and-the-best-ways-to-eat-them (accessed March 2014).

Hopman, Ellen. *A Druid's Herbal for the Sacred Earth Year*. Rochester, Vt.: Destiny Books, 1995.

———. *A Druid's Herbal of Sacred Tree Medicine.* Rochester, Vt.: Destiny Books, 2008.

Lust, John. *The Herb Book.* New York: Bantam Books, 1974.

Nardozzi, Charlie. "Edible of the Month: Violets." Edible Landscaping, www.garden .org/ediblelandscaping/?page=edible-month-violets (accessed April 25, 2014).

Provident Homemaker. "[Garden-]Jungle Medicine." theprovidenthomemaker .com/1/category/edible%20weeds/1.html (accessed May 27, 2014).

Rudalevige, Christine B. "Birch Syrup: Maple's Sassier Cousin from New England." Zester Daily, zesterdaily.com/cooking/birch-syrup-maples-sassier-plate-mate -new-england/ (accessed March 2014).

Wong, Tama Matsuoka. "Foraged Flavor: How to Tap Maple Trees (And What to Do with the Sap)." www.seriouseats.com/2014/03/foraged-flavor-how-to-tap -maple-trees-what-to-do-with-sap.html (accessed March, 2014).

3. HERBS OF SUMMER

Hopman, Ellen. *A Druid's Herbal for the Sacred Earth Year.* Rochester, Vt.: Destiny Books, 1995.

———. *A Druid's Herbal of Sacred Tree Medicine.* Rochester, Vt.: Destiny Books, 2008.

Lust, John. *The Herb Book.* New York: Bantam Books, 1974.

4. HERBS OF FALL

"Acorns: The Inside Story." Eat the Weeds and Other Things, Too, www.eattheweeds .com/acorns-the-inside-story/ (accessed November 11, 2014).

"Hickory Nut Preparation." Preparetosurvivenow, sites.google.com/site/prepareto survivenow/hickory-nut-preparation (accessed November 10, 2014).

Hopman, Ellen. *A Druid's Herbal for the Sacred Earth Year.* Rochester, Vt.: Destiny Books, 1995.

———. *A Druid's Herbal of Sacred Tree Medicine.* Rochester, Vt.: Destiny Books, 2008.

Lee, Robert. "Goldenrod: A Miracle Wild Food Source." Eating Wild, eatingwild .blogspot.com/2011/03/goldenrod-miracle-wild-food-source.html (accessed October 1, 2013).

Lust, John. *The Herb Book.* New York: Bantam Books, 1974.

Olson, Danielle Prohom. "Let Us Eat Acorn Cake! A Lazy Cook's Guide." Gather, gathervictoria.com/2014/11/04/let-us-eat-acorn-cake-a-lazy-cooks-guide/ (accessed November 10, 2014).

5. WINTER COLD AND FLU CARE, NATURALLY!

Castleman, Michael. "Preventing and Treating Winter Colds." Mother Earth Living, www.motherearthliving.com/health-and-wellness/preventing-treating -winter-colds (accessed November 20, 2014).

Masé, Guido. "Herbal Support for Influenza." A Radicle, aradicle.blogspot.com /search/label/influenza (accessed September 30, 2009).

Mayo Clinic. "Drugs and Supplements: Zinc." Patient Care and Health Info, www.mayoclinic.org/drugs-supplements/zinc/dosing/hrb-20060638 (accessed November 20, 2014).

Meininger, Kathryn. "Dosage for Astragalus Root." Livestrong.com, www.livestrong .com/article/445773-astragalus-root-herb-dosage (accessed November 20, 2014).

Mountain Rose Blog. "Craft Your Own Fire Cider!" mountainroseblog.com/fire -cider/ (accessed December 29, 2013).

Rose, Stephanie. "All Natural Vapor Rub Recipe." Garden Therapy, gardentherapy .ca/vicks-vapo-rub-recipe/ (accessed January 1, 2014).

Vukovic, Laurel. "How to Boost Your Immune System with Herbs." Mother Earth Living, www.motherearthliving.com/health-and-wellness/how-to-boost-your -immune-system-with-herbs (accessed January 1, 2014).

6. BUG STUFF— PLANTS TO REPEL MOSQUITOES, TICKS, AND FLEAS

Adams, Kathy. "Homemade Lemon Spray for Flea Control." http://homeguides .sfgate.com/homemade-lemon-spray-flea-control-75930.html (accessed May 2, 2014).

Dharmananda, Subhuti. "Chrysanthemum and Chamomile: Flower Teas." http:// www.itmonline.org/articles/chrysanthemum/chrysanthemum.htm (accessed November 1, 2014).

Ehman, Mandi. "Homemade Tick and Mosquito Spray." Life Your Way: Intentional and Creative Living, http://lifeyourway.net/homemade-tick-mosquito-spray/ (accessed May 22, 2014).

Gilmer, Maureen. "Fleabane Plants Really Do Repel Dog Fleas." Mo Plants, http:// www.moplants.com/fleabane-plants-really-do-repel-dog-fleas/ (accessed October 30, 2014).

Olkowski, William, Sheila Darr, and Helga Olkowski. "Pyrethrum-Based Insecticides from Chrysanthemums." Vegetable Gardener, http://www .vegetablegardener.com/item/5456/pyrethrum-based-insecticides-from -chrysanthemums (accessed November 1, 2014).

Roth, Harold A. "Erigeron speciosus, Showy Fleabane." http://www.alchemy-works .com/erigeron.html (accessed October 30, 2014).

Spengler, Teo. "Is There a Homemade Mixture to Spray Your Yard That Will Kill Fleas and Ticks?" http://homeguides.sfgate.com/there-homemade-mixture -spray-yard-kill-fleas-ticks-83466.html (accessed May 2, 2014).

7. MAGIC OF THE DRAGON AND THE HAG— DRACAENA AND MULLEIN

"Ancient Ink Formula Recipe: How to Make and How to Use Dragon's Blood Ink." Magical Recipes, www.magicalrecipesonline.com/2012/04/ancient-ink -formula-recipe-dragons.html (accessed September 5, 2013).

Beyerl, Paul. *A Compendium of Herbal Magick*. Custer, Wash.: Phoenix Publishing, 1998.

Dawson, Debbie. "Magickal Herbs—The Uses of Dragon's Blood." suite101.com/a /magickal-herbs-the-uses-of-dragons-blood-a291227 (accessed August 29, 2013).

Grieve, Maude. "Dragon's Blood." Botanical.com, A Modern Herbal, botanical .com/botanical/mgmh/d/dragon20.html (accessed August 29, 2013).

Hopman, Ellen Evert. *A Druid's Herbal for the Sacred Earth Year*. Rochester, Vt.: Destiny Books, 1995.

Lust, John. *The Herb Book*. New York: Bantam Books, 1974.

McDonald, Jim. "Mullein." herbcraft.org/mullein.html (accessed May 17, 2013).

Rose, Kiva. "A Golden Torch: Mullein's Healing Light." The Medicine Woman's Roots, http://bearmedicineherbals.com/a-golden-torch-mullein.html (accessed May 17, 2013).

Wigington, Patti. "What Is Dragon's Blood?" About Religion, paganwiccan.about .com/od/othermagicspells/ss/What-Is-Dragons-Blood.htm (accessed August 29, 2013).

Yronwode, Catherine. "Mojo Hand and Root Bag." Hoodoo in Theory and Practice, www.luckymojo.com/mojo.html (accessed September 5, 2013).

8. ANIMAL SPIRIT MEDICINES

Erichsen-Brown, Charlotte. *Medicinal and Other Uses of North American Plants: A Historical Survey with Special References to the Eastern Indian Tribes*. New York: Dover Publications Inc., 1989.

Moerman, Daniel E. *Native American Medicinal Plants: An Ethnobotanical Dictionary*. Portland, Oreg.: Timber Press Inc., 2009.

"Rabbit Tobacco (Pseudognaphalium Obtusifolium)." Wildflowers of the Southeastern U.S., 2bnthewild.com/plants/H64.htm (accessed May 24, 2014).

Sams, Jamie, and David Carson. *Medicine Cards: The Discovery of Power through the Ways of Animals*. Santa Fe, N.Mex.: Bear and Company, 1988.

Trine, Morgaine. "Fernleaf Biscuitroot." The Oregon Encyclopedia, www.oregonen cyclopedia.org/articles/fernleaf_biscuitroot_lomatium_dissectum_/ (accessed April 20, 2014).

Vogel, Virgil J. *American Indian Medicine*. Norman, Okla.: University of Oklahoma Press, 1970.

Wood, Matthew. *The Book of Herbal Wisdom: Using Plants as Medicines*. Berkeley, Calif.: North Atlantic Books, 1997.

———. "Medicine Plants and Medicine Animals." *Plant Healer Magazine,* Fall 2014.

9. HERBAL ASTROLOGY

"Astrology and the Use of Herbs." Humanity Healing University, humanityhealing .net/2012/08/astrology-and-the-use-of-herbs/ (accessed January 16, 2015).

"Astrology: Ruling Planet and Plants and Herbs." Planetary Astrology, www .astromap.co/Astrology_planets_Herbs_Plants.htm (accessed January 15, 2015).

Beyerl, Paul. *A Compendium of Herbal Magick*. Custer, Wash.: Phoenix Publishing, 1998.

Hopman, Ellen Evert. *A Druid's Herbal for the Sacred Earth Year*. Rochester, Vt.: Destiny Books, 1995.

Potterton, David, ed. *Culpepper's Color Herbal*. New York: Sterling, 1983.

Whitmore, Nathaniel. "Herbs and Astrology." Traditional Herbal Medicine, www .nathanielwhitmore.com/herbs--astrology.html (accessed January 15, 2015).

10. WORKING WITH PLANT SPIRITS

Birch, John. "Celtic Prayers and Blessings." Faith and Worship—Christian Prayers and Resources, www.faithandworship.com/Celtic_Blessings_and_Prayers.htm (accessed November 21, 2014).

Buhrman, Sarasvati. "Yoga and Ayurveda: Helping Humanity for Thousands of Years." Ayurvedic Medicine and Classical Yoga Therapy, ayurvedicsolutions .com/inspirations.html (accessed November 21, 2014).

"Native American Prayers" World Healing Prayers, www.worldhealingprayers .com/2.html (accessed November 21, 2014).

"What Does Sanjeevani Mean?" Sanjeevani Retreat, www.sanjeevani-retreat.com /en/what-does-sanjeevani-mean/ (accessed November 21, 2014).

11. BEE MEDICINE—THE SPLENDORS OF HONEY

Beith, Mary. *Healing Threads*. Edinburgh: Polygon, 1995.

Bricklin, Mark. *The Practical Encyclopedia of Natural Healing*. Emmaus, Pa.: Rodale Press, 1976.

"Egyptian Temple Incense—Kyphi." Magickwyrd, magickwyrd.wordpress.com

/how-to-topics/ritual-incense-recipes/egyptian-temple-incense-kyphi/ (accessed November 1, 2013).

"Golden Honey: The Strongest Known Natural Antibiotic." Health and Love Page, www.healthandlovepage.com/golden-honey-strongest-antibiotic/ (accessed November 3, 2014).

Hill, J. "Kyphi." Ancient Egypt Online, www.ancientegyptonline.co.uk/kyphi.html (accessed November 1, 2013).

"Honey in Egypt." Health Benefits of Honey, http://www.honey-health.com /honey-egypt/ (accessed November 1, 2013).

Hopman, Ellen Evert. *Scottish Herbs and Fairy Lore*. Los Angeles: Pendraig Publishing, 2010.

———. *Walking the World in Wonder: A Children's Herbal*. Rochester, Vt.: Healing Arts Press, 2000.

Matheny, Monica. "Natural Fruit and Honey Syrups." The Yummy Life, www .theyummylife.com/Fruit_Herb_Honey_Syrups (accessed November 15, 2013).

———. "Natural Honey Citrus Syrups for Coughs and Sore Throats." The Yummy Life, www.theyummylife.com/Honey_Citrus_Syrups (accessed September 27, 2013).

Meredith, Leda. "Cooking with Roses: How to Use Rose Petals, Leaves and Hips." Mother Earth News, www.motherearthnews.com/real-food/cooking-with -roses-zbcz1311.aspx (accessed November 11, 2013).

Molan, Peter. "The Antibacterial Activity of Honey and Its Role in Treating Diseases." Academia.edu, www.academia.edu/2189571/Pdf_6 (accessed September 1, 2015).

Quelch, Mary Thorne. *Herbal Remedies and Recipes and Some Others*. London: Faber and Faber, 1945.

Treadwell, Terry. "Honey's Healing History." *Wounds* 19, no. 9 (September, 2007): www.woundsresearch.com/article/7749.

12. SOME KITCHEN MEDICINES

Cook, Katsi. "Using the Berry Plants for Nutrition and Medicine." www .indigenouspeople.net/berry.htm (accessed November 12, 2013).

Foster, Steven, and James A. Duke. *Eastern/Central Medicinal Plants and Herbs*. New York: Houghton Mifflin, 1990.

Hopman, Ellen Evert. *The Secret Medicines of Your Kitchen*. London: mPowrPublishing, 2012.

Kulisić, T., A. Krisko, V. Dragović-Uzelac, M. Milos, and G. Pifat. "The Effects of Essential Oils and Aqueous Tea Infusions of Oregano (*Origanum vulgare*

L. spp. *hirtum*), Thyme (*Thymus vulgaris* L.) and Wild Thyme (*Thymus serpyllum* L.) on the Copper-Induced Oxidation of Human Low-Density Lipoproteins." *International Journal of Food Sciences and Nutrition* 58, no. 2 (March 2007): 87–93.

Lust, John. *The Herb Book.* New York: Bantam Books, 1974.

Mercola, Joseph. "What Are the Health Benefits of Oregano?" Mercola.com, articles.mercola.com/sites/articles/archive/2014/02/01/oregano-health-benefits.aspx (accessed October 12, 2014).

Osborn, David K. "Your Kitchen Medicine Cabinet." Greek Medicine.net, www.greekmedicine.net/therapies/Your_Kitchen_Medicine_Cabinet.html (accessed June 1, 2014).

13. HEDGEROWS ARE FOOD, MEDICINE, AND MAGIC

Beyerl, Paul. *A Compendium of Herbal Magick.* Custer, Wash.: Phoenix Publishing, 1998.

"Juneberries: A New Berry Crop for the Northeast US." Cornell University Cooperative Extension, www.juneberries.org (accessed August 31, 2013).

Lust, John. *The Herb Book.* New York: Bantam Books, 1974.

14. DECIDUOUS TREES FOR HEALING

Baker, Margaret. *Discovering the Folklore of Plants.* Bucks, UK: Shire Publications, 1975.

Bergner, Paul. "Tree Medicine from Tommie Bass." *Medical Herbalism* 13, no. 1 (Fall 2002): 15–17. medherb.com/bi/home.htm (accessed January 1, 2015).

Foster, Steven, and James A. Duke. *Eastern/Central Medicinal Plants and Herbs.* New York: Houghton Mifflin, 1990.

Friedrich, Paul. *Proto-Indo-European Trees.* Chicago: The University of Chicago Press, 1970.

Hopman, Ellen Evert. *A Druid's Herbal of Sacred Tree Medicine.* Rochester, Vt.: Destiny Books, 2008.

———. *Tree Medicine Tree Magic.* Custer, Wash.: Phoenix Publishing, 1992.

Lust, John. *The Herb Book.* New York: Bantam Books, 1974.

Moerman, Daniel E. *Native American Medicinal Plants: An Ethnobotanical Dictionary.* Portland, Oreg.: Timber Press Inc., 2009.

15. CONIFERS FOR HEALING

"Conifer Tree Potions (Solstice Medicine—or How to Use Your Christmas Tree)." Plant Journeys, plantjourneys.blogspot.com/2012/12/conifer-tree-potions-solstice-medicine.html (accessed December 11, 2013).

Cook, Katsi. "Using the Berry Plants for Nutrition and Medicine." www
.indigenouspeople.net/berry.htm (accessed November 12, 2013).

"The Edible Christmas Tree." Along the Grapevine, alongthegrapevine.wordpress
.com/2013/12/17/the-edible-christmas-tree/ (accessed February 24, 2014).

"Fairy Gingerbread with Black Pepper and Pine." Hunger and Thirst,
hungerandthirstforlife.blogspot.com/2012/12/fairy-gingerbread-with-black
-pepper-and.html (accessed January 7, 2014).

"Getting to Know White Pine." By Earth, Root and Flower: An Herbal Blog, www
.hawthornehillherbs.com/content/getting-know-white-pine (accessed November
27, 2013).

"Junipers." Eat the Weeds and Other Things, Too, http://www.eattheweeds.com/
junipers/ (accessed October 21, 2014).

"Juniper Snickerdoodles." Hunger and Thirst, hungerandthirstforlife.blogspot
.com/2012/10/juniper-snickerdoodles.html (accessed October 29, 2014).

Lust, John. *The Herb Book*. New York: Bantam Books, 1974.

McNeill, F. Marian. *The Silver Bough,* vol. 3: *A Calendar of Scottish National
Festivals, Halloween to Yule*. Glasgow: William MacLellan, 1961.

Moerman, Daniel E. *Native American Medicinal Plants: An Ethnobotanical
Dictionary*. Portland, Oreg.: Timber Press Inc., 2009.

Moore, Michael. *Medicinal Plants of the Mountain West*. Sante Fe, N.Mex.: Museum
of New Mexico Press, 1979.

"November: Alligator Juniper: Juniperus deppeana." Santa Fe Botanical Garden,
www.santafebotanicalgarden.org/november-2013/ (accessed October 21, 2014).

"Pine Pitch Salve" The Medicine Woman's Roots, bearmedicineherbals.com/pine
-pitch-salve.html (accessed October 19, 2014).

"Plant Journeys, A Journal of Healing Plants." http://mad.ly/d7a9c1 (accessed
December 11, 2013).

"Using Venice Turpentine." The Chronicle of the Horse, www.chronofhorse.com
/forum/showthread.php?185274-Using-Venice-Turpentine (accessed October 8,
2013).

"Wild and Edible Medicinal Plants 117—Juniper." Wild and Edible Medicinal
Plants—Using What Nature Provides in Plants, keys2liberty.wordpress.com
/tag/juniper-edible-berries/ (accessed November 13, 2013).

17. CONSTITUTIONAL PRESCRIBING— PLANTS TO BUILD, CLEANSE, AND TONE THE ORGANS AND SYSTEMS OF THE BODY

Alfs, Matthew. *300 Herbs: Their Indications and Contraindications*. New Brighton,
Minn.: Old Theology Book House, 2003.

Moore, Michael, with Daniel Gagnon. *Herbal Repertory in Clinical Practice.* Santa Fe, N.Mex.: The Institute of Traditional Medicine, 1982.

Thomsen, Michael, and Hanni Gennat. *Phytotherapy Desk Reference: A Clinical Handbook,* 4th ed. Hobart, Australia: Global Natural Medicine, 2009.

Tierra, Michael. *Planetary Herbology.* Santa Fe, N.Mex.: Lotus Press, 1988.

GLOSSARY OF HERBAL CONTRAINDICATIONS

Bergner, Paul. "The Adverse Effects of Herbs Part III." *Medical Herbalism* 13, no. 1 (Fall 2002): medherb.com/bi/home.htm (accessed January 1, 2015).

———. "Adverse Effects of the Top Medicinal Herbs Part II." *Medical Herbalism* 12, no. 4 (Spring 2002): medherb.com/bi/home.htm (accessed January 1, 2015).

———. "Side Effects of the Top Medicinal Herbs Part I." *Medical Herbalism* 12, no. 3 (Fall 2001): medherb.com/bi/home.htm (accessed January 1, 2015).

Brinker, Francis. *Herb Contraindications and Drug Interactions,* 3rd ed. Sandy, Oreg: Eclectic Medical Publications, 2001.

Chu, Joe Hing Kwok. "Da Ma, Cannabis Sativa, Cannabis Plant, Marijuana." Complementary and Alternative Healing University, alternativehealing.org /da_ma.htm (accessed January 1, 2015).

Philip, Richard B. *Herbal-Drug Interactions and Adverse Effects,* 1st ed. New York: McGraw-Hill, 2004.

"Vitamins and Supplements Lifestyle Guide: Guarana." WebMD, www.webmd .com/vitamins-and-supplements/lifestyle-guide-11/supplement-guide-guarana (accessed January 1, 2015).

INDEX OF PLANTS BY COMMON NAME

Numbers in *italics* preceded by *pl.* indicate colored plate numbers.

Adam's Needle, 85, *pl.1*

Agrimony, 134, 236, 261, 281, *pl.2*

Alder, 7, 166–67, 255, 272

Alfalfa, 216, 236, 242, 267, 277, 281

Alligator Juniper, 183

Aloe, 11, 12, 223, 232, 235, 236, 237, 243, 255, 271, 281

Aloe Yucca, 85

Amaranth, 214, 269, 272

American Basswood, 176

American Beech, 168, *pl.9*

American Bittersweet, 102, *pl.3*

American Ginseng, 86–87, 212, 214, 226, 229, 250, 251, 258, 260, 261, 266

American Holly, 173

American Licorice, 81, *pl.4*

American Spikenard, 81

American Wake Robin, 35–36

Andrographis, 52

Angelica, 81, 98–99, 201, 213, 216, 217, 223, 229, 236, 239, 243, 244, 247, 252, 254, 258, 260, 262, 263, 266, 281, *pl.5*

Anise, 141–42, 203, 216, 278

Annual Sunflower, 84

Apothecary's Rose, 156–57

Apple, 138, 167–68, 233, 241, 244

Apricot, 218, 238, 242, 243, 245, 255, 269

Arborvitae, 194–95, 265, 272, 274, 284, *pl.23*

Arnica, 201, 253, 261, 271, 281

Arrowleaf Balsam Root, 81–82

Arrowroot, 232, 272

Asafoetida, 217, 232, 242, 263

Ash, 164–65, 168

Ashe's Juniper, 183

Ashwagandha, 52, 248, 281

Asian Red Sage, 58

Aspalathos, 129

Asparagus, 57, 228, 232

Aspen, 220, 229, 231, 244, 249, 250, 253, 258, 261, 262, 273

Asthma Weed, 17

Astragalus, 13, 52, 53, 54, 55, 212, 229, 232, 237, 238, 241, 242, 245, 281–82

Baikal Skullcap, 58

Balm of Gilead, 238, 239, 274

Balsam of Peru, 11

Banana Yucca, 85

Barberry, 12, 60, 157, 213, 225, 236, 237, 256, 282, *pl.6*

Barley, 16

Basil, 12, 52, 65, 138, 139, 142, 220, 275

Bayberry, 214, 225, 233, 241, 255, 259, 263, 266, 269, 282, *pl.7*

Bay Laurel, 142–43, 201, *pl.8*

Bearberry, 7, 10, 89, 221, 244, 245, 273, *pl.84*

Bedstraw, 7, 8, 63–64, 100–101, 213, 228, 243, 245, 256, 267, *pl.27*

Bee Balm, 12, 39, 99, 174, *pl.92*

Beech, 168, *pl.9*

Bee Pollen, 245

Beet, 9, 212, 236

Benzoin, 11

Birch, 10, 168–69, *pl.10*

Birthroot, 214, 223, 254

Bistort, 217, 250, 256, 272, 274

Bitter Almond, 238, 242, 243, 245

Bitter Lime, 265

Bitternut, 49

Bittersweet, 10, 213, 245

Bittersweet Vine, 102, *pl.3*

Black Alder, 166–67, 232, 233, 282, *pl.11*

Blackberry, 10, 11, 138, 157, 232, 233, 258, 259, 263, 265, 278, 282, *pl.12*

Black Bugbane, 89, *pl.13*

Black Cohosh, 89, 216, 219, 221, 222, 223, 224, 234, 239, 242, 248, 251, 252, 263, 282, *pl.13*

Black Elder, 169

Black Haw, 220, 222, 224, 282

Blackjack Oak, 106

Black Locust, 24

Black Oak, 106

Black Pepper, 52, 57, 59, 143, 147, 191, 234

Blacksamson Echinacea, 91

Blackseed Plantain, 95

Black Snake Root, 89, 94–95, *pl.13*

Black Walnut, 179, 215, 252, 271

Bladderwrack, 235, 270, 272, 277, 282

Blessed Thistle, 11, 213, 214, 215, 216, 218, 226, 237, 245, 247, 252, 253, 260, 261, 283

Bloodroot, 21, 214, 226, 239, 253, 254, 256, *pl.14*

Blueberry, 31–32, 138

Blueberry Juniper, 183

Blue Cohosh, 8, 214, 219, 222, 223, 226, 242, 272, 283

Blue Flag, 225, 283

Blue Oak, 106

Blue Vervain, 97, 275, 278, *pl.15*

Blue Violet, 29

Blue Wild Indigo, 91

Boldo, 236, 237

Boneset, 7, 13, 17, 58, 239, 254, 275

Borage, 216, 227, 267, 272, 283, *pl.16*

Brewer's Angelica, 98

Bryony, 10

Buchu, 228, 231, 248, 272, 283

Buckthorn, 232, 234, 236, 282

Bugleweed, 271, 283

Bulrush, 21, 42

Bupleurum, 236, 238, 275

Burdock, 9, 12, 13, 18, 41–42, 52, 212, 213, 214, 218, 222, 226, 228, 237, 242, 245, 247, 263, 269, 270, 283, *pl.17*

Burr Oak, 106

Butternut, 179, 232, 235, 236, 256, 263, 283

Button Eryngo, 92, *pl.18*

Calamus, 104–5, 216, 233, 236, 237, 239, 243, 245, 250, 254, 262, 263, 266, 268, 271, 272, 277, *pl.19*

Calendula, 18, 39, 174, 213, 218, 223, 228, 243, 246, 251, 252, 255, 256, 260, 269, 271, 283–84, *pl.20*

California Bay Laurel, 143

California Juniper, 183–84

California Nettle, 103

California Scrub Oak, 106

California White Oak, 106–7

Camel Grass, 129

Camellia, 154

Camphor, 60

Canada Horsebalm, 105

Canada Snakeroot, 89–90

Canadian Black Snake Root, 94

Cannabis, 216, 219, 224, 227, 234, 241, 247, 253, 257, 263, 274, 275, 278, 280, 284, *pl.21*

Caraway, 143, 259, 260, 262, 279
Cardamom, 59, 138, 143, 262, 265
Cardinal Flower, 14–15
Cascara Sagrada, 225, 233, 284
Catnip, 58, 149, 214, 220, 233, 242,
　　246, 253, 258, 259, 260, 261, 262,
　　263, 265, 266, 275, 279, 284, *pl.22*
Cattail, 21, 42
Cayenne, 52, 132, 143–44, 199, 201,
　　202, 212, 214, 221, 226, 233, 234,
　　239, 241, 259, 260, 262, 266, 271,
　　276, 284
Cedar, 193, 194–95, 231, 243, 248, 249,
　　254, 256, 265, 272, 274, 284, *pl.23*
Celandine, 12
Celery, 57, 144, 233, 284
Centaury, 16, 213, 236, 263
Chai-hu, 236, 238, 275
Chamomile, 18, 37–38, 139, 194, 201,
　　218, 220, 251, 253, 261, 266, 267,
　　279, 284, *pl.24*
Chasteberry, 216, 224, 285
Checkerboard Juniper, 183
Cherry, 10, 59, 138
Cherrybark Oak, 107
Cherrystone Juniper, 185
Chickweed, 21, 238
Chicory, 13, 21–22, 215, 268, *pl.25*
Chili Peppers, 51–52
Chinese Bitter Orange, 161, 264, 265
Chinese Cinnamon, 213, 217, 219, 221,
　　228, 229, 231, 234, 239, 258, 259,
　　262, 279
Chinese Dogwood, 15
Chinese Rhubarb, 233, 259, 293
Chinkapin Oak, 107
Chives, 212, 217
Chrysanthemum, 53, 63, 275, *pl.26*
Chuckley Pear, *pl.75*
Cinchona, 227
Cinnabar, 69
Cinnamon, 16, 59, 129, 138, 144–45,
　　264, 285
Cinquefoil, 8, 10

Citronella, 65
Cleavers, 7, 8, 63–64, 100–101, 213,
　　228, 243, 245, 256, 267, *pl.27*
Clove, 65, 135, 138, 145, 151, 201
Clover, 8, 65
Club Moss, 264
Coastalplain Saint-John's-Wort, 93
Colic Root, 17
Collinsonia, 234
Coltsfoot, 12, 241, 248, 250, 255, 264,
　　267, 269, 274, 285
Comfrey, 8, 9, 12, 13, 170–71, 174,
　　201–2, 215, 226, 228, 231, 232,
　　235, 238, 243, 250, 251, 252, 255,
　　258, 260, 262, 267, 268, 269, 271,
　　272, 285, *pl.28*
Common Boneset, 90
Common Juniper, 184
Common Plantain, 95–96
Common Saint-John's-Wort, 93
Common Viper's Bugloss, 90
Coriander, 233, 234, 235, 252, 260,
　　262, 264, 266, 274, 285
Corn Silk, 231, 248, 249, 250, 272, 279,
　　285
Cotton Root, 223, 285–86
Couchgrass, 249, 273
Cough Herb, 17
Cow Parsnip, 264
Crabapple, 234, 245, 247
Cramp Bark, 220, 222, 223, 224, 252,
　　260, 286, *pl.29*
Cranesbill, 32
Creeping Charlie, 23, 219, 255, 288,
　　pl.42
Creeping Juniper, 184–85
Cubeb, 248, 249, 273
Cucumber Tree, 169
Culver's Root, 233, 236
Cumin, 145, 201, 203, 259, 260, 263
Curly Dock, 30, 87–88, 213, 218, 233,
　　234, 235, 251, 257, 277, *pl.96*
Currant, 11
Cusick's Sunflower, 84

Cyperus Grass, 129

Daisy, 39, 134
DaMa, 115, 216, 219, 224, 227, 234,
   241, 247, 253, 257, 263, 274, 275,
   278, 280, 284
Damiana, 212, 219, 222, 228, 249, 286,
   294
Dandelion, 8, 12, 13, 18, 19, 22, 29, 39,
   212, 216, 217, 226, 229, 231, 233,
   235, 236, 237, 243, 256, 268, 272,
   273, 286, *pl.30*
Date, 16
Daylily, 22, 38, 39
Desert Indianwheat, 96
Desert Juniper, 186
Desert White Cedar, 183–84
Devil's Claw, 227, 286
Dill, 57, 145, 259, 263
Dodder, 245, 247, 286
Dog Grass, 10
Dong Quai, 212, 217, 218, 220, 222,
   223, 224, 243, 247, 256, 286
Downy Rattlesnake Plantain, 92–93
Dracaena, 68–71
Dragon's Blood, 68–71, 286, *pl.31*
Drosera, 279
Dwarf Nettle, 103
Dysentery Bark, 17

Eastern Purple Coneflower, 92
Eastern Red Cedar, 186–87
Echinacea, 53–54, 60, 74, 91–92, 97,
   132, 199, 213, 217, 223, 239, 244,
   246, 251, 254, 256, 264, 268, 269,
   275, 276, 286, *pl.32*
Elder (Elderberry and Elderflower),
   7, 10, 32, 39, 53–55, 58, 59, 61,
   72–73, 132, 169–70, 193, 199, 212,
   215, 287, *pl.33*
Elecampane, 7, 13, 54, 55, 59, 89, 174,
   223, 239, 256, 269, 273, 287
Elm, 170–71
English Elm, 170

English Holly, 157–58, 173, *pl.34*
English Ivy, 34–35, 174
Epimedium, 249
Eucalyptus, 7, 60, 64–65, 171, 213, 239,
   244, 246, *pl.35*
Evening Primrose, 235
Eyebright, 10, 17, 218, 219, 241, 255,
   275

False Hellebore, 45
False Rhubarb, 87
False Solomon's Seal, 42–43
False Spikenard, 42–43
False Unicorn, 219, 287
Fendler's Bedstraw, 100
Fennel, 12, 33, 146, 203, 216, 234, 239,
   264, 265, 279, 287
Fenugreek, 216, 228, 231, 232, 238, 249,
   258, 259, 262, 264, 269, 272, 287
Fernleaf Biscuitroot, 82–83
Fernleaf Licorice Root, 83, *pl.65*
Feverfew, 251, 275, 287, *pl.36*
Feverwort, 17
Fewleaf Sunflower, 84
Figwort, 18
Flax, 11, 216, 228, 232, 248, 287
Fleabane, 63–64
Forsythia, 23
Fo-ti Tieng, 229, 236, 237
Fragrant Bedstraw, 100
Frankincense, 128, 129, 193
Fringe Tree, 172, 225, 254, 287
Fu Ling, 243

Gambel's Oak, 107
Garlic, 8, 51–52, 56, 57, 58, 64, 133,
   146–47, 203, 213, 215, 226, 264,
   269, 287–88
Gentian, 13, 16, 18, 59, 213, 217, 223,
   235, 236, 237, 254, 258, 259, 264,
   266, 275, 277, 288, *pl.37*
Geranium, 64–65
Germander Speedwell, 134, 294
Giant Solomon's Seal, 111

Gill-over-the-Ground, 23, 219, 255, 288, *pl.42*

Ginger, 11, 16, 51–52, 54, 55, 58, 59, 132, 135, 137, 138, 139, 147–48, 201, 202, 220, 224, 225, 228, 234, 240, 245, 246, 255, 258, 259, 260, 262, 263, 266, 275, 279, 288

Ginseng, 10, 16, 52, 56, 59, 222, 245, 254, 256, 266, 277, 288, *pl.38*

Goat's Rue, 213, 216, 254

Goji Berries, 55

Goldenrod, 33, 43–44, *pl.39*

Goldenseal, 247, 248, 250, 251, 253, 254, 255, 256, 257, 259, 264, 267, 269, 271, 277, 278, 280

Gold Thread, 8, 17

Gold Wire, 93

Gotu Kola, 216, 228, 252, 260, 271, 288

Grape, 10, 14, 31–32

Grapefruit, 52

Gravel Root, 105, 225, 229, 248, 273, 292, *pl.41*

Greater Burdock, 83

Great Saint-John's-Wort, 94

Green Tea, 56

Grindelia, 228, 240, 269

Ground Ivy, 23, 134, 219, 255, 288, *pl.42*

Guaiacum, 217, 218, 244, 246, 251, 273, 288

Guarana, 277, 278, 288–89

Gutta-Percha Tree, 227, 289

Hairy Angelica, 98

Hairy Solomon's Seal, 111

Hardhack, 11, 105

Hardy Rubber Tree, 227, 289

Harvest Lice, 110

Hawthorn, 11, 12, 15, 158, 165, 172–73, 226, 227, 289, *pl.43*

Hazel Alder, 167, 233, 268

Hazel Nut, 134

Heal-all, 17

Heartleaf Plantain, 96

Heartsease, 17

Heather, 130, 136–37, 149, *pl.44*

Hedge Nettle, 240

Hellebore, 19

Hemlock, 23, 195

Henderson's Angelica, 98

He Shou Wu, 229, 236, 237, 249

Hibiscus, 154–55, 213

Hippophae, 159–60, *pl.72*

Holly, 173

Hollyhock, 10, 11, 39, 248, 268, 272, *pl.45*

Holy Basil, 240, 276

Holy Wood, 193

Honeysuckle, 58, 134, 238, 243, 254, *pl.46*

Hops, 10, 11, 194, 216, 252, 260, 277, 278, 289

Horehound, 10, 12, 35, 59, 224, 236, 240

Horse Chestnut, 173–74, *pl.47*

Horsefly Weed, 91

Horsemint, 276

Horseradish, 51–52, 148

Horsetail, 7, 8, 215, 219, 227, 228, 238, 248, 249, 267, 271, 272, 276, 289, *pl.48*

Houseleek, 135

Huckleberry, 31–32

Hydrangea, 250, 289

Hyssop, 19, 58, 59, 238, 246, 268, 289

Indian Asparagus, 219, 294

Indian Turnip, 35–36

Interior Live Oak, 107

Irish Moss, 8, 11, 235, 238, 262

Jack in-the-Pulpit, 7, 35–36

Jamaican Dogwood, 75

Japanese Knotweed, 23

Jewelweed, 34

Joe Pye Weed, 13, 225, 229, 248, 273, 292, *pl.41*

Johnny-jump-up, 29, 39

Juneberry, 160–61, *pl.75*
Juniper, 7, 12, 129, 148–49, 181–87, 228, 233, 248, 250, 265, 273, 289, *pl.49*

Kava Kava, 294
Kelp, 235, 270, 272, 277, 282
Kidneywort, 17
King of Bitters, 58
Korean Ginseng, 264
Kudzu, 276

Lady's Mantle, 215
Lady's Slipper, 8, 220, 252, 253, 261, 264, 289
Lamb's-quarter, 23–24
Larch, 175, *pl.50*
Largebracted Plantain, 96
Largeleaf Wild Indigo, 91
Lavender, 37–38, 39, 60, 64–65, 138, 149, 158, 174, 193, 194, 235, 252, 260, 263, 264, 279, 289, *pl.51*
Lemon, 12, 15, 31, 51–52, 65, 132, 133, 135, 137, 138, 147, 151, 161, 265
Lemon Balm, 37–38, 39, 138, 246, 253, 257, 261, 264, 271, 276, 279, 289, *pl.52*
Lemongrass, 64–65
Lentils, 213, 286
Lesser Burdock, 83
Lesser Rattlesnake Plantain, 93
Licorice, 10, 58, 60, 203, 212, 219, 220, 225, 228, 235, 238, 243, 258, 259, 262, 264, 269, 270, 289–90
Licorice Bedstraw, 100
Life Everlasting, 12, 241, 244, 246, 270
Limeflower, 228, 290
Linden Tree, 176, 228, 290
Live Oak, 107
Liverwort, 9, 17
Lobelia, 74, 199, 202, 222, 226, 240, 242, 263, 267, 279, 280, 290, *pl.53*
Locust, 24
Longbract Wild Indigo, 91

Lungmoss, 17
Lungwort, 10, 11, 72–73, 240, 241, 270
Lyre-Leaved Sage, 152

Maidenhair Fern, 135
Maitake, 56
Majestic Giant, 29
Mallow, 10, 11, 12, 24
Mandrake, 10, 237, 238, 290
Maple, 176
Maravilla, 277
Marjoram, 12, 149
Marshmallow Root, 44, 72–73, 203, 216, 225, 228, 231, 232, 238, 248, 249, 250, 255, 259, 262, 268, 270, 272, 274, 290, *pl.54*
Maryland Sanicle, 95
Masterwort, 246, 253, 261
Mastic, 11, 129
Mayapple, 237, 238, 290
Mexican Plantain, 96
Milk Thistle, 217, 235, 244, 290, *pl.55*
Milkweed, 24
Mint, 7, 12, 18, 39, 55, 64, 129, 132, 138, 139
Mintleaf Bee Balm, 99
Mistletoe, 227, 252, 260, 290, *pl.56*
Mockernut, 49–50
Mock Orange, 156
Motherwort, 11, 215, 226, 271, 290
Mountain Ash, 158–59, 178, *pl.57*
Mountain Cedar, 183
Mugwort, 16, 193, 201, 220, 257, 290, *pl.58*
Mulberry, 276
Mullein, 10, 11, 71–75, 226, 238, 241, 242, 252, 260, 270, 279, 290, *pl.59*
Mushrooms, 56
Mustard, 149–50
Myrrh, 11, 129, 193, 201, 225, 228, 231, 243, 245, 246, 248, 250, 252, 257, 263, 264, 267, 268, 271, 291

Narrowleaf Plantain, 96

Narrowleaf Yucca, 85
Nasturtium, 38, *pl.60*
Nettles, 11, 24–25, 55, 212, 213, 215, 217, 218, 229, 232, 235, 240, 242, 255, 267, 268, 273, 291, *pl.61*
New Jersey Tea, 156, 214, 244, 247, 293, *pl.62*
Northern Bedstraw, 100
Northern Pin Oak, 107
Northern Red Oak, 107–8, *pl.63*
Norway Maple, 26, *pl.64*
Nosebleed, 17
Nutmeg, 130, 150
Nuttall's Sunflower, 84

Oak, 11, 106–9, 163–64, 174, 176–77, 235, 257, 291
Oat, 135, 221, 228, 242, 253
Ocotillo, 213, 239, 244, 246
Ohio Buckeye, 174
Old Man's Beard, 172
Oneflower Bedstraw, 101
Oneseed Juniper, 185
Onion, 8, 51–52, 57, 135
Orange, 52, 138, 194
Orangegrass, 94
Orange Jessamine, 156
Orange Peel, 193, 262, 265, 291
Oregano, 52, 150
Oregon Grape, 8, 12, 16, 60, 87, 167, 212, 213, 215, 218, 224, 225, 226, 228, 231, 233, 234, 236, 237, 241, 244, 245, 247, 257, 288, 291, *pl.40*
Oregon White Oak, 108
Osha, 55, 80, 83, 217, 224, 240, 241, 268, 273, 291, *pl.65*
Ostrich Fern, 26
Oswego Tea, 99

Pacific Blacksnakeroot, 95
Paleleaf Woodland Sunflower, 84
Pale Purple Coneflower, 92
Papaya, 264
Papyrus Grass, 129

Pareira Brava, 248, 273
Parsley, 7, 52, 57, 225, 228, 250, 267, 273, 291
Parsnip, 9
Partridgeberry, 221, 223, 224, 248, 291
Passionflower, 221, 227, 253, 261, 271, 278, 279, 280, 292
Pau D'Arco, 55
Peach, 138, 177
Peelbark Saint-John's-Wort, 94
Pennyroyal, 65, 224, 292
Peony, 202
Peppercorn, 59
Peppergrass, 7
Peppermint, 7, 58, 59, 60, 61, 65, 151, 171, 194, 225, 246, 257, 264, 267, 276, 279, 292
Periwinkle, 135
Pilewort, 17
Pine, 11, 12, 129, 174, 188–94, 202, 292
Pink Locust, 24
Pin Oak, 108
Pipsissewa, 213, 229, 237, 244, 246, 292
Plantain, 8, 26, 34, 92–93, 95–97, 135, 171, 174, 202, 226, 229, 231, 232, 241, 243, 250, 255, 267, 268, 271, 272, 273, 274, 279, *pl.66*
Pleurisy Root, 58, 239, 240, 242, 247, 251, 257, 276, 292
Poison Ivy, 34
Poison Sanicle, 95
Poke, 10, 13, 26, 87–88, 217, 244, 246, 271, 277, 292, *pl.67*
Poplar, 177
Poria, 243
Post Oak, 108
Prairie Sunflower, 84
Prickly Ash, 16, 218, 261, 270, 274, 292
Prickly Lettuce, 11, 252, 296
Prince's Pine, 213, 229, 237, 244, 246, 292
Privet, 279
Psyllium, 233, 259, 292
Pubescent Angelica, 251

Puke Weed, 17
Purple Loosestrife, 36
Purple Sanicle, 95
Purplestem Angelica, 83, 98, 265
Purslane, 26, 36

Quaking Aspen, 177
Queen Anne's Lace, 9, 257, 265, *pl.93*
Queen of the Meadow, 105, 225, 229,
    230, 248, 273, 292, *pl.41*
Quinoa, 23–24

Rabbit Tobacco, 102
Raspberry, 9, 10, 11, 12, 31–32, 36, 138,
    213, 215, 222, 225, 226, 229, 234,
    241, 250, 258, 259, 263, 265, 267,
    271, 293, *pl.68*
Rattle Root, 89, *pl.13*
Rattlesnake Master, 92
Red Alder, 167
Redbud, 26
Red Clover, 12, 13, 38, 39, 214, 216,
    217, 242, 243, 244, 247, 257, 267,
    270, 277, 278, 285, 293, *pl.69*
Red Ginseng, 214
Red Osier Dogwood, 77, 81
Red Pepper, 16
Red Raspberry, 36
Redroot, 156, 214, 244, 247, 293, *pl.62*
Red Sarsaparilla, 212, 214, 219, 228,
    237, 244, 247, 250, 271
Red Willow, 77, 81
Redwood, 187–88, *pl.74*
Reeds, 9
Rehmannia, 16, 212, 213, 217, 235, 243,
    245, 293
Reishi, 56
Rhubarb, 19, 293
Richweed, 105
Rocky Mountain Juniper, 185–86
Rocky Mountain Red Cedar, 185–86
Rose, 10, 12, 15, 29, 37–38, 39, 40, 52,
    54, 55, 132, 193, 194, 203, 226,
    233, 270, 293

Rose Geranium, 38–39
Rose Mallow, 154–55
Rosemary, 12, 39, 60, 64, 65, 138, 193,
    225, 238, 241, 253, 260, 261, 263,
    265
Rough Bedstraw, 101
Rowan, 158–59, 178, *pl.57*
Rue, 218, 220, 224, 293

Safflower, 224
Saffron, 247, 257
Sage, 12, 64, 74, 139, 152, 193, 201, 215,
    217, 240, 241, 247, 251, 268, 293
Saint-John's-Wort, 8, 10, 75, 93–94,
    212, 221, 229, 247, 249, 250, 252,
    260, 270, 271, 273, 293–94, *pl.70*
Saint-Peter's-Wort, 94
Salsify, 9
Sanicle, 214, 233, 240, 257, 259, 268,
    272, 273
Saskatoon, 31–32, 160–61, *pl.75*
Sassafras, 7, 27, 178–79, 217, 224, 229,
    237, 244, 245, 247, 257, 273, 294,
    pl.71
Savin Juniper, 186
Savory, 12
Saw Palmetto, 219, 220, 229, 230, 241,
    248, 249, 250, 265, 270, 294
Sawtooth Sunflower, 85
Scabwort, 17
Scarlet Pimpernel, 237, 294
Schizandra, 52
Scotch Broom, 227
Scouler's Saint-John's-Wort, 94
Sea Buckthorn, 159–60, *pl.72*
Seashore Plantain, 96
Self-heal, 11, 18, 218, 229, 231, 245, 247,
    pl.73
Senna, 19, 233
Septfoil, 8
Sequoia, 120, 187–88, *pl.74*
Serviceberry, 160–61, *pl.75*
Shadbush, 160–61, *pl.75*
Shagbark Hickory, 27, 49–50

Shatavari, 219, 239, 294
Shellbark Hickory, 49–50
Shepherd's Purse, 7, 37, 214, 234, 267,
    294, *pl.76*
Shiitake, 56
Shingle Oak, 108
Shining Bedstraw, 101
Showy Sunflower, 85
Siberian Ginseng, 52, 54, 55, 58, 215,
    220, 228, 250, 253, 261, 271, 294
Skippy XL Plum-Gold, 29
Skullcap, 10, 17, 18, 202, 215, 220, 240,
    250, 253, 254, 259, 260, 261, 263,
    270, 274, 278, 294
Skunk Cabbage, 7, 44–45, 269, *pl.77*
Slippery Elm, 11, 36, 56, 58, 74, 170,
    203, 221, 232, 235, 239, 250, 252,
    255, 258, 259, 260, 261, 262, 265,
    266, 267, 270, 294, *pl.78*
Small Soapweed, 85–86
Smooth Alder, 167
Snakeweed, 95–97
Snowdrop Tree, 172
Soapweed Yucca, 86
Solomon's Seal, 111, 240, 241, 262,
    pl.79
South African Geranium, 56
Southern Red Cedar, 186–87
Southern Red Oak, 108
Spearmint, 265, 266
Spicebush, 27–28
Spikenard, 37, 98, 242, *pl.90*
Spindle Tree, 295
Spreading Dog Bane, 110
Staghorn Sumac, 97
St. Andrew's Cross, 94
Star Anise, 139, 240, 253, 261, *pl.80*
Starwort, 21
Stickywilly, 101
Stiff Marsh Bedstraw, 101
Stillingia, 218
Stinging Nettle, 103–4
Stinking Arrach, 12
Stone Root, 89, 232, 234, 265, 273

Storksbill, 32
Strawberry, 11, 28, 138, 265, 266
Striped Maple, 176
Sugar Maple, 176
Sumac, 10, 11, 189, *pl.81*
Sundew, 7, 11
Sunflower, 7, 84–85
Swamp Verbena, 97, *pl.15*
Swamp White Oak, 108
Sweet Everlasting, 102
Sweet Fern, 34
Sweet Flag, 7, 104–5, 129, 216, 236, 237,
    239, 243, 245, 250, 254, 262, 263,
    266, 268, 271, 272, 277, *pl.19*
Sweet Goldenrod, 43–44
Sweet-Scented Joe Pye Weed, 105
Sycamore, 28, *pl.82*

Taheebo Tea, 55
Tall Hairy Agrimony, 110
Tansy, 65, 224, 295
Tarragon, 152
Tea Tree, 151
Thai Basil, 33, 142
Thinkleaf Sunflower, 85
Thistle, 37
Thorowax, 236, 238, 275
Threepetal Bedstraw, 101
Thuja, 194–95, 265, 272, 274, 284,
    pl.23
Thyme, 8, 12, 19, 52, 59, 64, 139,
    152–53, 240, 254, 270, 273
Tolu Balsam, 11
Tormentil, 8
Tragacanth, 11
Trifoliate Orange, 161
Trillium, 214, 223, 254
True Solomon's Seal, 42–43
Tulip, 28
Tulip Poplar, 179, *p.83*
Tuliptree, 179, *pl.83*
Tulsi, 240, 276
Turmeric, 52, 58, 133, 153, 225, 227,
    237, 295

Usnea, 269, 295
Utah Juniper, 186
Uva Ursi, 221, 229, 231, 244, 245, 251, 273, 295, *pl.84*

Valerian, 8, 202, 252, 260, 267, 280, 295
Verdolagas, 36
Vervain, 7, 13, 214, 220, 221, 244, 247, 257, 258, 295
Violet, 19, 29, 39, 134, 214, 244, 247, *pl.85*
Virginia Juniper, 186–87
Virginia Snakeroot, 90
Vitex, 216, 224, 285

Wahoo, 237, 295
Walnut, 10, 170–80, 227, *pl.86*
Wasabi, 148
Watercress, 214, 218, 235, 267, 295
Water Hemlock, 13, *pl.87*
Water Plantain, 219, 229, 231
Wavyleaf Oak, 109
Wax Myrtle, 214, 225, 233, 241, 255, 259, 263, 266, 269, 282, *pl.7*
Werewolf Root, 110
Western Juniper, 187
Western Larch, 175
Western Rattlesnake Plantain, 93
Western Sunflower, 85
White Aspen, *pl.88*
White Clover, 243, 244, 285
White Oak, 46–49, 109, 168
White Peony, 213, 215, 218, 243, 244, 252, 260
White Pine, 189–90, *pl.89*
White Pond Lily, 250
White Poplar, 177, 229
White Sage, 212, 219, 240, 249, 250, 252, 260
White Sarsaparilla, 37, 174, 220, 242, 270, *pl.90*
White Walnut, 179, 232, 235, 236, 256, 283

White Willow, 227, 276, 278, 295–96, *pl.91*
Wild Bergamot, 99, 100, *pl.92*
Wild Carrot, 9, 257, 265, *pl.93*
Wild Celery, 98
Wild Cherry, 59, 232, 234, 235, 241, 242, 252, 259, 261, 296
Wild Four o'Clock, 277
Wild Garlic, 269
Wild Ginger, 18, 89–90, 201, 255, 279
Wild Lettuce, 11, 252, 261, 296
Wild Onion, 29
Wild Spinach, 23–24
Wild Thyme, 135
Wild Yam, 219, 225, 233, 237, 238, 259, 261, 263, 265, 267, 296
Willow, 7, 132, 180, 265
Willowherb, 36
Willow Oak, 109
Wintergreen, 90
Wisteria, 30
Witch Hazel, 39–40, 215, 222, 253, 258, 296
Wolf berries, 55
Wood Betony, 214, 237, 238, 242, 252, 253, 261
Woodbine, 10
Woodland Angelica, 98, *pl.94*
Wood Sorrel, 30
Woolly Angelica, 99
Woolly Plantain, 96–97

Yarrow, 8, 30, 61, 132, 222, 224, 225, 229, 234, 254, 257, 265, 268, 272, 276, 296, *pl.95*
Yellow Dock, 30, 45, 87–88, 213, 218, 233, 234, 235, 251, 257, 277, 278, 296, *pl.96*
Yellow Root, 270
Yerba Santa, 229, 230, 240
Yohimbe, 249
Yucca, 85–86, 227, 296

Zucchini, 39

INDEX OF PLANTS BY SCIENTIFIC NAME

Numbers in *italics* preceded by *pl.* indicate colored plate numbers.

Abies canadensis, 195

Acacia spp., 11

Acer pensylvanicum, 176

Acer platanoides, 26, *pl.64*

Acer saccharum, 176

Acer spp., 176

Achillea millefolium, 8, 17, 30, 61, 132, 222, 224, 225, 229, 234, 254, 257, 265, 268, 272, 276, *pl.95*

Acorus calamus, 7, 104–5, 129, 216, 233, 236, 237, 239, 243, 245, 250, 254, 262, 263, 266, 268, 271, 272, 277, *pl.19*

Aesculus glabra, 174

Aesculus hippocastanum, 173–74, *pl.47*

Agathosma betulina, 228, 231, 248, 272

Agrimonia eupatoria, 134, 236, 261, *pl.2*

Agrimonia gryposepala, 110

Agrimonia parviflora, 110

Agropyron repens, 10, 249, 273

Alcea spp., 11, 39

Alchemilla vulgaris, 215

Alisma plantago-aquatica, 219, 229, 231

Allium canadense, 8, 51–52, 58

Allium cepa, 8, 51–52, 135

Allium sativum, 8, 51–52, 56, 58, 64, 146–47, 203, 213, 215, 226, 264, 269

Allium schoenoprasum, 212, 217

Allium spp., 29

Allium vineale, 269

Alnus glutinosa, 166–67, 232, 233, *pl.11*

Alnus rubra, 167

Alnus serrulata, 7, 167, 233, 255, 268

Alnus spp., 166–67

Aloe barbadensis, 223, 232, 235, 236, 237, 243, 255, 271

Aloe officinalis, 223, 232, 235, 236, 237, 243, 255, 271

Aloe spp., 11–12

Althaea officinalis, 44, 72–73, 203, 216, 225, 228, 230, 231, 232, 238, 248, 249, 250, 255, 259, 262, 268, 270, 272, 274, *pl.54*

Althaea rosea, 248, 268, 272, *pl.45*

Amaranthus hypochondriacus, 214, 269, 272

Amelanchier arborea, *pl.75*

Amelanchier spp., 160–61

Anagallis arvensis, 237

Andrographis paniculata, 52, 58

Anemone hepatica, 17

Anethum graveolens, 145, 259, 263

Angelica archangelica, 201, 213, 216, 217, 223, 226, 229, 230, 236, 239, 243, 244, 247, 252, 254, 258, 260, 262, 263, 266

Angelica atropurpurea, 81, 83, 98, 265, *pl.5*

Angelica lucida, 98

Angelica polymorpha, 212, 217, 218, 220, 222, 223, 224, 243, 256

Angelica pubescens, 251

Angelica sinensis, 212, 217, 218, 220, 222, 223, 224, 243, 256

Angelica sylvestris, 98, *pl.94*

Angelica tomentosa, 98, 99

Angelica venenosa, 98

Apium graveolens, 144, 233

Apocynum androsaemifolium, 110

Aralia nudicaulis, 37, 174, 220, 242, 270, *pl.90*

Aralia racemosa, 81, 98

Arctium lappa, 9, 12, 13, 18, 41–42, 52, 83, 212, 213, 214, 218, 222, 226, 228, 237, 242, 245, 247, 256, 263, 269, 270, 272, *pl.17*

Arctium minus, 83

Arctostaphylos uva-ursi, 7, 10, 89, 221, 229, 231, 244, 245, 251, 273

Arisaema triphyllum, 7, 35–36

Aristolochia serpentaria, 90

Armoracia rusticana, 51–52, 148

Arnica montana, 201, 253, 261, 271

Artemisia dracunculus, 152

Artemisia vulgaris, 16, 201, 220, 257, *pl.58*

Asarum canadense, 89–90, 201, 240, 255, 279

Asarum spp., 18

Asclepias syriaca, 24

Asclepias tuberosa, 239, 240, 242, 247, 251, 257, 276

Asparagus officinalis, 228, 232

Asparagus racemosa, 219, 239

Asplenium spp., 135

Astragalus adscendens, 11

Astragalus brachycalyx, 11

Astragalus gummifer, 11

Astragalus hoantchy, 229, 232, 237, 242, 245

Astragalus membranaceus, 13, 52, 53, 55, 229, 232, 237, 238, 241, 242, 245

Astragalus mongolicus, 229, 232, 237, 242, 245

Astragalus spp., 212

Astragalus tragacanthus, 11

Avena sativa, 135, 221, 228, 230, 242, 253

Balsamorhiza sagittata, 81–82

Baptisia alba, 91

Baptisia australis, 91

Baptisia bracteata, 91

Baptisia tinctoria, 91

Bellis perennis, 39

Berberis vulgaris, 12, 60, 157, 213, 225, 236, 237, 256, *pl.6*

Beta vulgaris, 9, 212, 236

Betonica officinalis, 214, 237, 238, 242, 252, 253, 261

Betula pendula, pl.10

Betula spp., 10, 168–69

Borago officinalis, 216, 227, 267, 272, *pl.16*

Boswellia spp., 128, 129

Brassica hirta, 149–50

Brassica nigra, 149–50

Bryonia dioica, 10

Bupleurum chinensis, 236, 238, 275

Bupleurum falcatum, 236, 238

Calendula officinalis, 18, 39, 174, 213, 218, 223, 228, 246, 251, 252, 255, 256, 260, 269, 271, *pl.20*

Calluna vulgaris, pl.44

Camellia japonica, 154

Camellia reticulata, 154

Camellia sasanqua, 154

Camellia sinensis, 55, 56

Cannabis sativa, 216, 219, 224, 227, 234, 241, 247, 253, 257, 263, 274, 275, 278, 280, *pl.21*

Capsella bursa-pastoris, 7, 37, 214, 234, 267, *pl.76*

Capsicum annuum, 16, 51–52, 132, 143–44, 199, 201, 202, 212, 214, 221, 226, 233, 234, 239, 241, 259, 260, 262, 266, 271, 276

Carbenia benedicta, 214, 213, 215, 216, 218, 226, 237, 245, 247, 252, 253, 260, 261

Carica papaya, 264
Carthamus tinctorius, 224
Carum carvi, 143, 259, 260, 262, 279
Carya cordiformis, 49
Carya laciniosa, 49–50
Carya ovata, 27, 49–50
Carya tomentosa, 49–50
Cascara sagrada, 225, 233
Cassia acutifolia, 19, 233
Cassia angustifolia, 19
Caulophyllum thalictroides, 8, 214, 219, 222, 223, 226, 242, 272
Ceanothus americanus, 156, 214, 244, 247, *pl.62*
Celastrus scandens, 102, *pl.3*
Centaurium umbellatum, 16
Centella asiatica, 216, 228, 230, 252, 260, 271
Cercis canadensis, 26
Chamaelirium luteum, 219
Chamaemelum nobile, 18, 37–38, 74, 139, 201, 218, 219, 220, 251, 253, 261, 266, 267, 279, *pl.24*
Chelidonium majus, 12
Chenopodium album, 23–24
Chenopodium olidum, 12
Chichorium intybus, 13, 21–22, *pl.25*
Chimaphila umbellata, 213, 229, 237, 244, 246
Chionanthus virginicus, 172, 254
Chondrodendron tomentosum, 248, 273
Chondrus crispus, 8, 11, 235, 238, 262
Chrysanthemum cinerariaefolium, 63
Chrysanthemum indicum, 53
Chrysanthemum morifolium, 53, 275, *pl.26*
Cichorium intybus, 215, 268
Cicuta spp., 13
Cicuta virosa, *pl.87*
Cimicifuga racemosa, 89, 216, 219, 221, 222, 223, 224, 234, 239, 242, 248, 251, 252, 263, *pl.13*
Cinchona officinalis, 227
Cinnamomum camphora, 60

Cinnamomum cassia, 16, 59, 129, 217, 219, 221, 228, 229, 231, 234, 239, 258, 259, 262, 264, 279
Cinnamomum officinalis, 213
Cinnamomum verum, 16, 59, 129, 144–45
Cirsium spp., 37
Citrus aurantifolio, 265
Citrus aurantium, 264
Citrus limon, 12, 15, 51–52, 265
Citrus paradisi, 52
Citrus reticulata, 265
Citrus sinensis, 52, 262
Cnicus benedictus, 11, 213, 214, 215, 216, 218, 226, 237, 245, 247, 252, 253, 260, 261
Collinsonia canadensis, 89, 105, 232, 234, 265, 273
Commiphora myrrha, 11, 129, 201, 225, 228, 231, 243, 245, 246, 248, 250, 252, 257, 263, 264, 267, 268, 271
Comptonia peregrina, 34
Coptis greenlandica, 8, 17
Coriandrum sativum, 233, 234, 235, 252, 262, 264, 266, 274
Cornus officinalis, 15
Cornus sericea, 81
Coryanthe yohimbe, 249
Corylis avellana, 134
Cotyledon umbilicus, 17
Crataegus oxyacantha, *pl.43*
Crataegus spp., 11, 15, 158, 172–73, 226, 227
Crocus sativus, 247, 257
Croton draco, 69
Cucurbita pepo, 39
Cuminum cyminum, 145, 201, 203, 259, 260, 263
Curcuma longa, 52, 58, 133, 153, 225, 227, 237
Cuscuta chinensis, 245, 247
Cymbopogon schoenanthus, 129
Cyperus spp., 129
Cypripedium calceolus, 8

Cypripedium pubescens, 8, 220, 252, 253, 261, 264

Cytisus scoparius, 227

Daucus carota, 9, 140, 218, 257, 265, *pl.93*

Dioscorea villosa, 17, 219, 225, 233, 237, 238, 259, 261, 263, 265, 267

Dracaena cinnabari, 69

Dracaena draco, 68–71, *pl.31*

Dracaena terminalis, 69

Drosera anglica, 7, 11

Drosera linearis, 7, 11

Drosera rotundifolia, 7, 11, 279

Echinacea angustifolia, 53–54, 60, 74, 91, 97, 132, 199, 213, 217, 223, 239, 244, 246, 251, 254, 256, 264, 268, 269, 275, 276

Echinacea pallida, 92, 132, 199, 217, 223, 239, 244, 246, 251, 254, 256, 264, 268, 269, 275, 276

Echinacea purpurea, 53–54, 60, 74, 92, 132, 199, 217, 223, 239, 244, 246, 251, 254, 256, 264, 268, 269, 275, 276, *pl.32*

Echinacea spp., 53–54

Echium vulgare, 90

Elettaria cardamomum, 59, 138, 143, 262, 265

Eleutherococcus senticosus, 52, 54, 55, 58, 212, 215, 220, 228, 250, 253, 261, 271

Epimedium grandiflorum, 249

Equisetum arvense, pl.48

Equisetum hyemale, 7, 8, 35, 215, 219, 227, 228, 230, 238, 248, 249, 267, 271, 272, 276

Erigeron speciosus, 63–64

Eriodictyon spp., 229, 230, 240

Erodium cicutarium, 32

Eryngium aquaticum, 92

Eryngium yuccifolium, 92, *pl.18*

Erythraea centaurium, 16, 17, 213, 236, 263

Eucalyptus globulus, 7, 213, 239, 244, 246, *pl.35*

Eucalyptus spp., 60, 171

Eucommia ulmoides, 227

Euonymus atropurpurea, 237

Eupatorium perfoliatum, 7, 13, 17, 58, 90, 105, 225, 230, 239, 254, 275

Eupatorium purpureum, 13, 229, 248, 273, *pl.41*

Euphrasia officinalis, 10, 17, 218, 219, 241, 255, 275

Eutrema japonica, 148

Fagus grandifolia, 168, *pl.9*

Ferula asafoetida, 217, 232, 242, 263

Foeniculum vulgare, 12, 33, 146, 203, 216, 234, 239, 264, 265, 279

Forsythia spp., 23

Fouquieria splendens, 213, 239, 244, 246

Fragaria ananassa, 28

Fragraria spp., 11, 265, 266

Fragraria virginiana, 28

Fraxinus spp., 168

Fucus vesiculosus, 235, 270, 272, 277

Galega officinalis, 213, 216, 254

Galium aparine, 7, 8, 63–64, 101, 213, 228, 230, 243, 245, 256, 267, *pl.27*

Galium asprellum, 101

Galium boreale, 100

Galium circaezans, 100

Galium concinnum, 101

Galium fendleri, 100

Galium tinctorium, 101

Galium trifidum, 101

Galium triflorum, 100

Galium uniflorum, 101

Ganoderma lucidum, 56

Ganoderma sichuanense, 56

Ganoderma tsugae, 56

Gaultheria procumbens, 90

Gentiana lutea, 13, 15, 18, 59, 213, 217, 223, 235, 236, 237, 254, 258, 259, 264, 266, 275, 277, *pl.37*

Gentiana officinalis, 213, 217, 223, 235, 236, 237, 254, 258, 259, 264, 266, 275, 277, *pl.37*

Geranium terebinthinaceum, 38–39

Gigartina mamillosa, 8

Glechoma hederacea, 23, 219, 255, *pl.42*

Glycyrrhiza glabra, 10, 58, 60, 134, 203, 212, 219, 220, 225, 228, 230, 235, 238, 243, 258, 259, 262, 264, 269, 270

Glycyrrhiza lepidota, 81, *pl.4*

Gnaphalium obtusifolium, 12, 241, 244, 246, 270

Gnaphalium polycephalum, 12, 241

Goodyera oblongifolia, 93

Goodyera pubescens, 92–93

Goodyera repens, 93

Gossypium herbaceum, 223

Grifola frondosa, 56

Grindella camporum, 228, 240, 269

Guaiacum officinale, 217, 218, 244, 246, 251, 273

Hamamelis virginiana, 215, 222, 253, 258

Harpagophytum procumbens, 227

Hedeoma pulegioides, 224

Hedera helix, 34–35, 174

Helianthus annuus, 7, 84

Helianthus anomalus, 85

Helianthus cusickii, 84

Helianthus decapetalus, 85

Helianthus grosseserratus, 85

Helianthus niveus, 85

Helianthus nuttallii, 84

Helianthus occidentalis, 84

Helianthus petiolaris, 84

Helianthus strumosus, 84

Hemerocallis fulva, 22, 38, 39

Hepatica spp., 9

Heracleum maximum, 264

Hibiscus rosa-sinesis, 154–55, 213

Hippophae rhamnoides, 159–60, *pl.72*

Hordeum vulgare, 16

Humulus lupulus, 10, 11, 216, 252, 260, 277, 278

Hydrangea arborescens, 250

Hydrastis canadensis, 8, 12, 15, 87, 212, 213, 215, 224, 226, 228, 231, 234, 236, 241, 247, 248, 250, 251, 253, 254, 255, 256, 257, 259, 264, 267, 269, 271, 273, 277, 278, 280, *pl.40*

Hypericum ascyron, 94

Hypericum brachyphyllum, 93

Hypericum concinnum, 93

Hypericum crux-andreae, 94

Hypericum fasciculatum, 94

Hypericum gentianoides, 94

Hypericum hypericoides, 94

Hypericum multicaule, 94

Hypericum perforatum, 8, 10, 93, 212, 221, 229, 230, 247, 249, 250, 252, 260, 270, 271, 273, *pl.70*

Hypericum scouleri, 94

Hypericum spp., 93-94

Hyssopus officinalis, 19, 58, 59, 238, 246

Ilex aquifolium, 157–58, 173, *pl.34*

Ilex opaca, 173

Ilex spp., 173

Illicium anisatum, 240, 253, 261, *pl.80*

Illicium verum, 139, 240, 253, 261, *pl.80*

Impatiens aurea, 34

Imperatoria ostruthium, 246, 253

Inula helenium, 7, 13, 17, 54, 55, 59, 89, 174, 223, 239, 256, 269, 273

Iris versicolor, 225

Juglans cinerea, 179, 232, 235, 236, 256, 263

Juglans nigra, 179, 215, 252, 271

Juglans regia, *pl.86*

Juglans spp., 10, 170–80, 227

Juniperus ashei, 183

Juniperus californica, 183–84

Juniperus communis, 7, 148–49, 184, 228, 231, 233, 248, 250, 265, 273, *pl.49*

Juniperus deppeana, 183

Juniperus horizontalis, 184–85
Juniperus monosperma, 185
Juniperus occidentalis, 187
Juniperus osteosperma, 186
Juniperus phoenicea, 129
Juniperus sabina, 186
Juniperus scopulorum, 185–86
Juniperus silicicola, 186–87
Juniperus spp., 12, 181–87
Juniperus virginiana, 186–87

Lactuca serriola, 11, 261
Lactuca virosa, 11, 252, 261
Larix decidua, 175, *pl.50*
Larix europaea, 175, *pl.50*
Larix laricina, 175, *pl.50*
Larix occidentalis, 175
Laurus nobilis, 142–43, 201, *pl.8*
Lavandula angustifolia, 37–38, 39, 60, 138, 158, 174, 235, 252, 260, 263, 264, 279, *pl.51*
Lavandula vera, 37–38, 39, 60, 158, 174, 235, 252, 260, 263, 264, 279, *pl.51*
Lens culinaris, 213
Lentinula edodes, 56
Leonurus cardiaca, 11, 215, 220, 226, 230, 271
Lepidium viginicum, 7
Leptandra virginica, 7, 233, 236
Leucanthemum vulgare, 39, 134
Ligusticum filicinum, 55, 80, 83, 217, 224, 240, 241, 268, 273, *pl.65*
Ligusticum porteri, 55, 80, 83, 217, 224, 240, 241, 268, 273, *pl.65*
Ligustrum lucidum, 279
Lindera benzoin, 27–28
Linum usitatissimum, 11, 216, 228, 230, 232, 248
Liriodendron tulipifera, 179, *pl.83*
Lobaria pulmonaria, 17
Lobelia cardinalis, 13–14
Lobelia inflata, 17, 74, 199, 202, 222, 226, 240, 242, 263, 267, 279, 280, *pl.53*

Lomatium dissectum, 82–83
Lonicera japonica, 238, 243, 254
Lonicera periclymenum, 10, 134, *pl.46*
Lonicera spp., 58
Lycium barbarum, 55
Lycium chinense, 55
Lycopodium clavatum, 264
Lycopus virginicus, 271
Lythrum salicaria, 36

Magnolia acuminata, 169
Mahonia repens, 60, 213, 215, 218, 225, 228, 231, 233, 237, 244, 245, 247, 257
Maianthemum racemosum, 42–43
Malus domestica, 233
Malus spp., 167–68, 241, 244
Malus sylvestris, 234, 245, 247
Malva neglecta, 24
Malva rotundifolia, 10, 11, 12
Mandragora officinarum, 10
Maranta arundinacea, 232, 272
Marrubium vulgare, 10, 12, 59, 224, 236, 240
Matricaria recutita, 18, 37–38, 74, 139, 201, 218, 220, 251, 253, 261, 266, 267, 279, *pl.24*
Matteuccia struthiopteris, 26
Medicago sativa, 216, 236, 242, 267, 277
Melissa officinalis, 37–38, 39, 138, 246, 253, 257, 261, 264, 271, 276, 279, *pl.52*
Mentha balsamea, 7, 58, 59, 60, 61, 151
Mentha piperita, 7, 58, 59, 60, 61, 151, 225, 246, 257, 264, 267, 276, 279
Mentha pulegium, 12, 224
Mentha spp., 7, 10, 12, 18, 39, 55, 60, 64, 129, 139
Mentha viridis, 265, 266
Mirabilis multiflora, 277
Mitchella repens, 221, 224, 248
Monarda fistulosa, 12, 99, 100, *pl.92*
Monarda punctata, 276
Monarda spp., 39, 99–100, 174

Morus alba, 276
Murraya paniculata, 156
Myrica cerifera, 214, 225, 233, 241, 255, 259, 263, 266, 269, pl.7
Myristica fragrans, 150
Myroxylon balsamum pereirae, 11

Nasturtium officinale, 214, 218, 235, 267
Nepeta cataria, 58, 214, 220, 233, 242, 246, 253, 258, 259, 260, 261, 262, 263, 265, 266, 275, 279, pl.22
Nymphaea odorata, 250

Ocimum basilicum, 52, 139, 142, 220, 275, 276
Ocimum spp., 12
Ocimum tenuiflorum, 240
Oenothera biennis, 235
Origanum marjorana, 12, 52, 149
Origanum vulgare, 150
Oxalis spp., 30

Paeonia alba, 213, 215, 218, 243, 244, 252, 260
Paeonia albiflora, 202
Panax quinquefolius, 10, 16, 52, 56, 59, 86–87, 212, 214, 226, 229, 245, 250, 251, 256, 258, 260, 261, 266, 277, pl.38
Panax schinseng, 264
Panax spp., 222, 254
Passiflora incarnata, 221, 227, 253, 271, 278, 279, 280
Pastinaca sativa, 9
Paullinia cupano, 277, 278
Pausinystalia yohimbe, 249
Pelargonium graveolens, 38–39
Pelargonium sidoides, 56
Pelargonium terebinthinaceums, 38–39
Petroselinum crispum, 7, 52, 225, 228, 230, 250, 267, 273
Peumus boldus, 236, 237
Phoenix dactylifera, 16

Phragmites communis, 9
Phytolacca americana, 10, 13, 26, 87–88, pl.67
Phytolacca esculenta, 244, 246, 271, 277
Pimpinella anisum, 12, 141–42, 203, 216, 278
Pinus canadensis, 195
Pinus spp., 11, 12, 129, 174, 188–94, 202
Pinus strobus, 189–90, pl.89
Piper cubeba, 248, 249, 273
Piper nigrum, 52, 59, 143, 234
Piscidia piscupula, 75
Pistacia lentiscus, 11, 129
Plantago aristata, 96
Plantago australis, 96
Plantago cordata, 96
Plantago lanceolata, 96
Plantago macrocarpa, 96
Plantago major, 8, 95–96, 243, pl.66
Plantago ovata, 96
Plantago patagonica, 96–97
Plantago psyllium, 259
Plantago rugelii, 95
Plantago spp., 26, 34, 135, 171, 174, 202, 226, 229, 230, 231, 232, 233, 241, 250, 255, 267, 268, 271, 272, 273, 274, 279
Platanus occidentalis, 28, pl.82
Podophyllum peltatum, 237, 238
Polygonatum biflorum, 111
Polygonatum multiflorum, 42–43, 111, pl.79
Polygonatum officinale, 240, 241, 262
Polygonatum pubescens, 111
Polygonum bistorta, 217, 250, 256, 272, 274
Polygonum cuspidatum, 23
Polygonum multiflorum, 229, 236, 237, 249
Poncirus trifoliata, 161
Populus alba, 177, 229
Populus balsamifera, 178, 238, 239
Populus candicans, 178

Populus spp., 177, 220, 229, 230, 231, 244, 249, 250, 253, 258, 261, 262, 273, 274
Populus tremula, pl.88
Populus tremuloides, 177
Poria cocos, 243
Portulaca oleracea, 26, 36
Potentilla reptans, 8, 10
Potentilla tormentilla, 8
Prunella vulgaris, 11, 18, 218, 229, 231, 245, 247, *pl.73*
Prunus armeniaca, 218, 238, 242, 243, 245, 255, 269
Prunus persica, 177
Prunus serotina, 59, 232, 234, 235, 241, 242, 252, 259, 261
Prunus serriola, 252
Prunus spp., 10
Prunus virginiana, 59, 232, 234, 235, 241, 242, 252, 259, 261
Pseudognaphalium obtusifolium, 102
Pueraria lobata, 276
Pulmonaria officinalis, 10, 11, 72–73, 240, 241, 270

Quercus agrifolia, 107
Quercus alba, 46–49, 109
Quercus bicolor, 108
Quercus douglasii, 106
Quercus dumosa, 106
Quercus ellipsoidalis, 107
Quercus falcata, 108
Quercus gambelii, 107
Quercus garryana, 108
Quercus imbricaria, 108
Quercus lobata, 106–7
Quercus macrocarpa, 106
Quercus marilandica, 106
Quercus muehlenbergii, 107
Quercus pagoda, 107
Quercus palustris, 108
Quercus pauciloba, 109
Quercus phellos, 109
Quercus rubra, 107–8, *pl.63*

Quercus spp., 11, 174, 176–77, 235, 257
Quercus stellata, 108
Quercus velutina, 106
Quercus virginiana, 107
Quercus wislizeni, 107

Ranunculus ficaria, 17
Rehmannia glutinosa, 16, 212, 213, 217, 235, 243, 245
Rhamnus cathartica, 232, 234, 236, 272
Rhamnus frangula, 232, 234, 236
Rheum palmatum, 19, 233, 259
Rheum rhaponticum, 87
Rhus hirta, 97, 189
Rhus typhina, 10, 11, 189, *pl.81*
Ribes spp., 11
Robinia neomexicana, 24
Robinia pseudoacacia, 24
Robinia spp., 24
Rosa gallica, 156–57
Rosa officinalis, 156–57
Rosa spp., 10, 12, 15, 29, 37–38, 39, 40, 52, 54, 55, 203, 226, 233, 270
Rosemarinus officinalis, 12, 39, 60, 64, 225, 238, 241, 253, 260, 261, 263, 265
Rubus idaeus, 9, 10, 11, 12, 36, 215, 222, 225, 226, 229, 234, 241, 250, 258, 259, 263, 265, 267, 271, 278, *pl.68*
Rubus spp., 31–32, 213
Rubus villosus, 10, 11, 157, 232, 233, 258, 263, 265, *pl.12*
Rumex crispus, 30, 45, 87–88, 213, 218, 233, 234, 235, 251, 257, 277, 278, *pl.96*
Ruta graveolons, 218, 220, 224

Salix alba, 227, 265, 276, 278, *pl.91*
Salix nigra, 265
Salix spp., 7, 132, 180
Salvia apiana, 152, 212, 215, 217, 219, 240, 241, 247, 249, 250, 251, 252, 260, 268
Salvia lyrata, 152
Salvia miltiorrhiza, 58

Salvia officinalis, 12, 74, 152, 201, 215, 217, 240, 241, 247, 251, 268
Salvia spp., 139
Sambucus canadensis, 53–54, 59, 72–73, 169–70, 215, 275, *pl.33*
Sambucus nigra, 7, 32, 39, 53–54, 59, 61, 72–73, 169–70, 199, 215, 275, *pl.33*
Sambucus spp., 10, 55, 58, 132, 212, 213, 246, 255, 256
Sanguinaria canadensis, 21, 214, 226, 239, 253, 254, 256, *pl.14*
Sanicula bipinnata, 95
Sanicula bipinnatifida, 95
Sanicula canadensis, 94
Sanicula crassicaulis, 95
Sanicula europaea, 214, 233, 240, 257, 259, 268, 272, 273
Sanicula marilandica, 95
Sassafras albidum, 7, 27, 178–79, 217, 224, 229, 237, 245, 247, 257, 273, *pl.71*
Sassafras officinale, 244
Sassafras variifolium, 7, 27, 178–79, 217, 224, 229, 237, 245, 247, 257, 273
Satureja hortensis, 12
Schisandra chinensis, 52
Scrophularia nodosa, 18
Scutellaria baicalensis, 58
Scutellaria lateriflora, 10, 17, 18, 58, 202, 215, 220, 240, 250, 253, 254, 259, 260, 261, 263, 270, 274, 278
Scutellaria spp., 10
Sempervivum tectorum, 135
Sequoia sempervirens, 187–88, *pl.74*
Serenoa serrulata, 219, 220, 229, 230, 248, 249, 250, 265, 270
Silybum marianum, 217, 235, 244, *pl.55*
Simaruba amara, 17
Smilacina racemosa, 42–43
Smilax ornata, 212, 214, 219, 228, 237, 244, 247, 250, 271
Smilax spp., 10
Solanum dulcamara, 10, 243, 245
Solidago odora, 43–44

Solidago spp., 33, 43–44
Solidago vigaurea, 43–44, *pl.39*
Sorbus americana, 158–59, *pl.57*
Sorbus aucuparia, 158–59, *pl.57*
Sorbus spp., 178
Spiraea tomentosa, 11
Stachys officinalis, 214, 237, 238, 242, 252, 253, 261
Stachys palustris, 240
Stellaria media, 21, 238
Stillingia sylvatica, 218
Styrax spp., 11
Symphytum officinale, 8, 9, 12, 13, 174, 201–2, 215, 226, 228, 230, 231, 232, 235, 238, 243, 250, 252, 255, 258, 260, 262, 267, 268, 269, 271, 272, *pl.28*
Symphytum spp., 170–71
Symplocarpus foetidus, 7, 44–45, 269, *pl.77*
Syzygium aromaticum, 135, 145, 201

Tabebuia avellanedae, 55
Tabebuia impetiginosa, 55
Tanacetum parthenium, 224, 251, 275, *pl.36*
Tanacetum vulgare, 12
Taraxacum officinale, 8, 12, 13, 18, 19, 22, 29, 39, 135, 212, 214, 216, 217, 226, 229, 231, 233, 235, 237, 243, 256, 268, 272, 273, *pl.30*
Thuja occidentalis, 194–95, 230, 231, 243, 248, 249, 254, 256, 265, 272, 274, *pl.23*
Thymus serpyllum, 8, 12, 19, 59, 135, 139
Thymus vulgaris, 8, 12, 19, 52, 59, 152–53, 240, 254, 270, 273
Tilia americana, 176
Tilia cordata, 228
Tragopogon spp., 9
Trifolium pratense, 8, 12, 13, 38, 39, 214, 216, 217, 242, 243, 244, 247, 257, 267, 270, 277, 278

Trigonella foenum-graecum, 216, 228, 231, 232, 238, 249, 258, 259, 262, 264, 269, 272
Trillium pendulum, 214, 223, 254
Tropaeolum majus, pl.60
Tropaeolum spp., 38
Tsuga canadensis, 23, 195
Tulipa spp., 28
Turnera aphrodisiaca, 212, 219, 222, 228, 249
Tussilago farfara, 12, 17, 241, 248, 250, 255, 264, 267, 269, 274
Typha spp., 21, 42

Ulmus campestris, 170
Ulmus fulva, 11, 36, 56, 58, 74, 170, 203, 232, 235, 239, 250, 252, 255, 258, 259, 260, 261, 262, 265, 266, 267, 270, *pl.78*
Ulmus procera, 170
Ulmus rubra, 74, *pl.78*
Ulmus spp., 170–71
Umbellularia californica, 143
Urtica dioica, 11, 55, 103, 212, 213, 215, 217, 218, 229, 230, 232, 235, 240, 242, 255, 267, 268, 273, *pl.61*
Urtica spp., 24–25
Urtica urens, 103, 217, 218, 229, 230, 232, 235, 240, 242, 255, 267, 268, 273
Usnea barbata, 269

Vaccinium spp., 31–32
Vagnera racemosa, 42–43
Valeriana officinalis, 8, 202, 252, 260, 267, 280
Veratrum album, 19
Veratrum viride, 45
Verbascum spp., 71–75
Verbascum thapsus, 10, 11, 226, 238, 241, 242, 252, 260, 270, 279, *pl.59*
Verbena hastata, 7, 13, 97, 214, 220, 221, 244, 247, 257, 258, 275, 278, *pl.15*

Verbena officinalis, 7, 13, 214, 220, 221, 244, 247, 257, 258
Veronica chamaedrys, 134
Veronicastrum virgincum, 233, 236
Viburnum opulus, 220, 222, 223, 224, 252, 260, *pl.29*
Viburnum prunifolium, 220, 222, 224
Vinca minor, 135
Viola canina, 134, *pl.85*
Viola cornuta, 29
Viola hybrida, 29
Viola odorata, 29, 39, 134, 214, 244, 247
Viola riviniana, pl.85
Viola spp., 19, 29
Viola tricolor, 17, 29, 39
Viola wittrockiana, 29
Viscum album, 227, 252, 260, *pl.56*
Vitex agnus-castus, 216, 224
Vitis vinifera, 10

Wasabia japonica, 148
Wisteria spp., 30
Withania somnifera, 52, 248
Wolfiporia extensa, 243

Xanthorhiza simplicissima, 270

Yucca aloifolia, 85
Yucca angustissima, 85
Yucca baccata, 85
Yucca filamentosa, 85, *pl.1*
Yucca glauca, 85–86, 86
Yucca spp., 227

Zanthoxylum americanum, 16, 218
Zanthoxylum clava-herculis, 16, 218, 270, 274
Zea mays, 231, 248, 249, 250, 272, 279
Zingiber officinale, 11, 16, 51–52, 54, 55, 58, 59, 132, 135, 137, 139, 147–48, 201, 202, 220, 224, 225, 228, 230, 234, 240, 245, 246, 255, 258, 259, 260, 262, 263, 266, 272, 279

INDEX OF
HEALTH CONCERNS

adrenal glands
  builders, 212
  cleansers, 212
  tonics, 212
ague, 103
alcohol cravings, 90
allergies, 24–25, 275
anemia, 35, 45
anti-inflammatories, 42–43
antioxidants, 56
aphrodisiacs, 110
arthritis, 16, 87, 107, 184
atherosclerosis, 53, 172–73

back and spine concerns, 74–75, 103
benign prostatic hypertrophy, 75
bites, 24, 26
bitters, 107
blood concerns and conditions
  anemia, 35
  blood builders, 87, 110, 212–13
  blood cleansers, 37, 41–42, 81, 92,
    213–14
  blood purifiers, 83, 176, 178
  blood sugar, 14
  blood tonic, 36
  blood tonics, 186, 214–15
  coagulation, 35
  internal bleeding, 36, 166–67, 175,
    185–86
  styptics, 37, 42–43, 175

bone issues, 13
  builders, 215
  cleansers, 215
brain issues, 10
  builders, 215–16
  cleansers, 216
  tonics, 216
breastfeeding, 89
  galactagogues, 36
breasts
  builders, 216–17
  cleansers, 217
bronchial problems. See pulmonary/
    respiratory concerns
bruises, 87, 95–96
bug repellants, 62–65

cancers, 14, 87, 168–69
candidiasis, 167
catarrh, 12, 99, 146
cellulitis, 97
children. See infants and children
chills, 102
cholera, 105, 108
cholesterol problems, 28
chronic obstructive pulmonary disease
    (COPD), 21
circulation
  builders, 217–18
  cleansers, 218
  tonics, 218

colds, 7, 16, 16–17, 23, 27, 51–52, 52–58, 83, 92–93, 98, 171
colic, 86, 91, 178
colitis, 44, 170
constipation, 19, 21, 96–97
contusions, 95–96
coronary heart disease, 53
cramps, 16, 27, 91, 106, 142, 149
croup, 178
cyanosis, 13

deodorants, 105
diabetes, 81, 104–5
digestive issues, 15, 22, 89–90, 142, 143–44, 168, 177, 179, 258–61
diphtheria, 178
distemper, 82–83
dysentary, 36, 94, 97, 103, 107, 108

ears, 73, 81, 105
elderly, 89–90
emmenagogues, 43–44
enteritis, 170
expectorants, 81, 86–87
exposure, 98
eyes, 44, 53, 94, 99, 106, 111, 218–19

fainting, 87, 102
fatigue, 81
fevers, 7, 19, 21, 27, 29, 34–35, 37, 43–44, 82, 102, 103, 167, 169, 171, 177, 179, 275–76
fractures, 171
frostbite, 98

galactagogues, 216–17
gallbladder, 172, 225
galls, 11
gallstones, 22
gastrointestinal system
    gas, 84, 142, 143, 145, 149
    large intestine, 232–35
    pain, 108
    small intestine, 258–261

stomach, 35, 82, 85–86, 141–42, 261–67
stomach cramps, 43–44
stomach disorders, 87–88
stomach ulcers, 44
ulcers, 12, 35, 37
upset stomach, 35, 87
see also digestive issues and stools
gingivitis, 26
glands, 34–35, 73–74, 91, 176–77
goiters, 176–77
gout, 18, 23, 35, 148–49, 184
gravel problems, 23
gums, 225–26

hair wash, 103
hangovers, 83
headaches, 10, 81, 82, 95–96, 98, 99, 102, 103, 110, 111, 142
heart conditions, 11, 26, 84, 87, 94
    angina, 172–73
    atherosclerosis, 172–73
    builders, 226
    cleansers, 226
    high blood pressure, 19, 104–5, 172–73
    myocarditis, 172–73
    tonics, 226–27
hemorrhoids, 75
hunger, 81

immune system, 51, 56, 61
infants and children
    bath, 94, 99, 105
    colic, 91, 94, 96–97, 178
    constipation, 96–97
    convulsions, 89, 99
    diarrhea, 97
    fevers, 89–90
    plants for common conditions, 278–79
    sore back, 89
    umbilical cord, 82, 107
infection, 37, 56, 89–91

inflammatory conditions, 18, 21–22, 26
influenza/flu/grippe, 16, 16–17, 90
    flu, 32, 43–44, 83
    remedies, 52–60
    stomach flu, 61
insect bites, 89–91, 90, 95–96, 185
insomnia, 10, 82, 145, 172–73
itching, 11–12, 21, 24

joints, 227

kidney issues, 37, 43–44, 81, 87, 92–93,
    100, 105, 176, 187
    builders, 228–31
    cleansers, 228–31
    infection, 231–32
    nervous system, 229–30
    solid waste, 230–31
    tonics, 229–32

laxatives, 28
lesions, 8, 11
liver conditions, 9, 12–13, 15, 19, 22,
    23, 81
    builders, 235, 237–38
    cleansers, 41–42, 236–37, 238
    tonics, 237
lungs
    builders, 241
    cleansers, 239–40, 242
    tonics, 241, 242
    See also pulmonary/respiratory
    concerns
Lyme disease, 23
lymph system, 242–47

measles, 27, 170
menstruation. *See* reproductive system-
    female
metabolism, 89–91, 145, 276–77
moist lesions, 11
mouth and throat concerns, 81–82
    builders, 268
    cleansers, 268–69

mouth sores, 102, 108–9
    pyorrhea, 171
    sore throat, 11, 23, 36, 44, 53, 53–54,
        56, 81, 91, 98, 102, 146, 171, 179
    thrush, 86–87
    tonics, 269–70
    tonsilitis, 91, 97
    tonsils, 179
    toothache, 81, 91, 180
mouthwash, 168, 179
mucous, 7, 12, 16, 19, 34–35
mucous membranes, 250–51, 258–60
mumps, 91, 102
muscles, 91, 180, 251

negativity, 68–69
nervous system, 251–53, 260–61,
    266–67
neuralgia, 92, 169
nose, 253–54
nosebleeds, 99, 103, 110
nutritional deficiencies, 277–78

pain, 9–10, 10–11, 11, 74–75, 83, 278
    chest, 100, 103–4
    neck, 91
    stomach, 82
pancreas, 254
parasites, 16
    lice, 166–67
    pinworms, 106
    ringworm, 101
    scabies, 166–67
    worms, 89, 99
piles, 104
pleurisy, 92–93
poisoning, 89–91, 105
pregnancy and labor, 82
    abortifacients, 81, 89–90, 93, 94, 95,
        98, 107
    cramps, 106
    induction, 88–89
    labor/delivery/birth, 36
    labor pains, 11

morning sickness, 36
obstetric, 221–222
placenta, 106, 107
postpartum hemorrhages, 36
postpartum pain, 107
recovery, 99
tonics, 105
water breaking, 97
weight gain, 14
womb weakness, 86
prostate issues, 173–74
psychological and emotional concerns, 19, 29
anger, 29
depression, 19, 29, 44–45
negativity, 68–69
nervous conditions, 10, 29, 44–45, 89–90, 98, 172–73
plants for common conditions, 280
pulmonary/respiratory concerns, 98
asthma/asthmatics, 21, 35–36, 44–45, 72–73, 81, 102
bronchitis, 21, 23, 29, 32, 34–35, 35–36, 44–45, 56, 169–70, 171, 177
builders, 238–39, 241
cleansers, 239–40, 242
coughs, 7, 27, 29, 42–43, 43–44, 53–54, 72, 81, 83, 91, 98, 102, 106–7, 176
lungs, 94, 168, 176
phlegm, 146, 177
pneumonia, 98, 105, 169–70
rheumatism, 35–36
sinusitis, 171, 254–55
tonics, 241, 242
tuberculosis, 35, 82, 102
whooping cough, 34–35, 35–36, 44–45, 82, 83
pus, 10, 11

reproductive system-female, 89–90
builders, 219, 220, 221, 221–22
cleansers, 219, 220, 221, 223–24

contraceptives, 100
douches, 36
fertility, 86, 93
gynelogical discharge, 110
hormonal system, 219–20
menstruation, 16, 27, 36, 42–43, 83, 89, 95, 111, 141–42
nervous system, 220–21
sore breasts, 89–90, 105
sterility, 35–36
tonics, 219–20, 220, 221, 224–25
uterine bleeding, 32
uterine prolapse, 81
uterine structure and cervix, 221–25
vaginal infections, 34–35, 35, 179
see also pregnancy and labor
reproductive system-male, 248–50
sterility, 35–36
rheumatic conditions
builders, 227
cleansers, 227
rheumatic parts, 37, 95–96, 103
rheumatism, 7, 19, 22, 27, 34–35, 42–43, 44–45, 83, 84, 87–88, 89, 92–93, 98, 148–49, 184
tonics, 227
ringworm, 179

saddle sores, 85–86
sexually transmitted diseases
gonorrhea, 35, 92, 176
herpes, 56
syphilus, 90
venereal disease, 82, 97, 108, 185–86
sinuses, 254–55. See also pulmonary/respiratory concerns
skin concerns and conditions, 9, 10
abscesses, 34–35
acne, 22, 41–42, 45, 53, 172
bites, 85
boils, 34–35, 35–36, 37, 42–43
builders, 255
burns, 24, 34–35, 37, 42, 44, 85, 92–93, 99

chancres, 83
cleansers, 255–57
cuts, 26, 34–35, 43–44, 45, 87
dandruff, 34–35, 82, 86, 185–86
demulcents, 44
eczema, 22, 166–67, 169, 172
inflammation, 75
insect bites, 43–44, 81–82, 185
itching, 42–43
poison ivy, 34, 41–42
poison oak, 41–42
psoriasis, 11, 169
rashes, 19, 24, 45
skin healers, 32
sores, 37, 41–42, 42, 83, 85–86
sunburn, 34–35
swelling, 35–36, 37, 81–82, 166–67
warts, 11, 84
wounds, 10, 30, 35, 36, 37, 42, 44,
    81–82
smallpox, 187
snakebite, 35–36, 84, 89–91, 90, 93,
    94, 95
sore muscles, 98, 176, 180
spleen, 242–45
splinters, 95–96, 187
sprains, 82, 85–86, 87, 171
stings, 26
stone problems, 23
stools
    constipation, 42–43, 45, 89, 142,
        185–86
    diarrhea, 18, 23, 36, 43–44, 81,
        87, 88–89, 97, 106–7, 107, 167,
        173–74, 176
    hemorrhoids, 75
    laxatives, 45, 101, 105, 168, 169, 178

stress, 61, 172–73
sunburn, 19

teeth, 267–68
thorns, 95–96
thyroid gland, 270–71
tissue regeneration, 271–72
tonics, 90
tonsilitis, 11
toothache, 88
tuberculosis, 81, 84, 97, 108
tumorous growths, 10
typhoid fever, 36
typhus, 90

urinary concerns
    bedwetting, 75
    bladder conditions, 21, 37
    bloody urine, 96
    builders, 272
    cleansers, 272–73
    cystitis, 75
    diuretics, 7, 28, 35, 42, 43–44, 100,
        145, 168, 173
    gravel, 83
    inflammation, 75
    milky urine, 107, 108
    tonics, 273–75
    urine retention, 103

varicose veins, 53, 176–77
vertigo, 86–87
vomiting, 102, 173

yellow fever, 88

GENERAL INDEX

Acorn Bread, 47
Acorn Cake, 47–48
Acorn Muffins, 48–49
acorns, 46–49
acute, 198
Adonis, 179
Air, 9, 17–19, 79
Algonquin Nation, 194
Ancient Beauty Aid, 140
animal spirits, 78–79
Anishnabe, 78
annuals, 9
antibiotics, 12
antihistamines, 24–25
anti-inflammatories, 15–16
Antibiotic Tea for Kids, 60
antiseptics, 12, 21
antispasmodics, 10, 202
antivirals, 15–16
Aphrodite, 167
apple cider vinegar, 32, 168
Aquarius, 114
Arapaho, 186
Aries, 114
Artemis, 164
astringents, 11
astrology, herbal
   nature of selected plants, 115–18
   properties by planetary body, 112–14
Atholl Brose, 136
avocados, 14

babies, herbs for, 200
bacteria, 131
bad spirits, 76
Balder, 164
bark, 16–17, 166
barley, 126–27
bath sachets, 194
bath scrub, 194
bat-they-naw, 186
bear fat, 174
bear medicine plants, 80–86
bedbugs, 63
beef tallow, 174
bee medicine. *See* honey
beer, 126–27
Beltaine, 154
berries, 16–17
Berry-Flavored Honey, 138
biennials, 9
bioflavonoids, 178
Birch Beer, 178–79
birdbaths, 62–63
bitter, 13, 15–16
Black Elk, Wallace, 4
blood purifiers, 10, 12
Bonewits, Isaac, 4
Book of Herbal Wisdom, The, 77
brandy, warming, 59
breastmilk, 200
bridge herb, 207–9, *208*

Brighid, 164
brooms, 168
bug repellants, 64–65
builders, 198, 204–10

calcium, 22
Cancer, 114
Capricorn, 114
capsules, 199
carbon dioxide, 165–66
carminatives, 203
carotene, 13
carrots, 13–14
Carson, David, 78
catastrophe, 101
caudles, 130
cautions, 20
Celts, 127
center of gravity, 204–10
charms, 72
cherries, 59
chi, 86
Chicken Soup, 57
Chinese plant classification, 15–17
chronic, 198
citric acid, 11
citrus fruits, 14
Clarified Pine Butter, 192–93
classification systems
    Chinese, 15–17
    doctrine of signatures, 6–15
    four humors, 17–19
cleansers, 198, 204–10
cockroaches, 63
cold and flu, 49–50
color, 12–13
colors, energetics of, 18
conifers, 181–95
constitutional prescribing,
    204–10
    common conditions, 275–80
    organs and systems of the body,
        212–74
contraindications, 281–96

cooling herbs, 204–5
Cough Syrup, 59

damp, 7
Dandelion Jelly, 29
Daylily Sides, 38
deciduous trees
    author and, 161–62
    as medicine, 166–80
    for our future, 165–66
    tree lore, 163–65
deer medicine plants, 100–101
deer tallow, 174
demulcents, 202–3
deodorizers, 12
devas, 119–23
Dioscorides, 128
disinfectants, 12
divining rods, 164–65
djasakee, 78
doctrine of signatures, 6–15
dolphins, 1
Dragon's Blood Ink, 69–70
drawing poultice, 201–2
Druid Clan of Dana, 4
Druid Fellowship, A (ADF), 4
Druid Isle, The, 3
Druids, 4, 163–64
*Druid's Herbal of Sacred Tree Medicine,
    A,* 163

Earth, 9, 17–19, 79
Earth Mother, 104
eggs, 14
Elderberry Elixir, Cooked, 54–55
Elderflower tea, 32
Elder Mother, 169
elementals, 119–23
elk medicine plants, 97–100
embalming fluids, 127
Erinyes, 164
Erraid, 3
essential oils, 64–65
Evans, Ron, 4, 195

fairies, 119–23
fasting, 80
fear, 101
Fennel Liqueur, 33
figs, 14
financial success, 173–74
Findhorn, Scotland, 3
Fine na Darach, 164
Fire, 9, 17–19, 69, 79
Fire Cider, 51
First Nations, 4
fish, 104
five flavors, 15–16
fleas, 62–65
Flower Cake, 38–39
flowers, 37–40
Flower Tea, 37–38
fomentation, 201
foods, signatures of, 13–14
formulas
    constitutional prescribing, 204–10
    delivery methods, 198–202
    Tierra's method, 202–3
    See also constitutional prescribing
fossil fuels, 166
four directions, 16–17
four temperatures, 15
Francis, Saint, 1–3
Frankincense, 128
free radicals, 131

Galen, 17
gallic acid, 11
Garlic and Honey Wound Dressing,
    132
Garlic Scapes and White Bean Dip, 147
Gemini, 114
germicides, 12
ghosts, 102
Gibbons, Euell, 4
Gifts from the Healing Earth, 163
Ginger Ale, 138
Gingerbread, 191–92
glycerites, 199–200

gnomes, 119–23
Golden Bough, The, 72
grapefruits, 14
gravel, 7
Grieve, Maude, 68–69
grounding, 9
Guanches, 68–71
gum, 185

habitat, 7–8
Hag's Tapers, 71–72
hara, 86
Harris I, 128
healing crisis, 203
heat, 7
Heather Ale, 136
Hebrides, 3
hedgerows, 154–61
Henge of Keltria, 4
herbal astrology
    nature of selected plants, 115–18
    properties by planetary body,
        112–14
herbal formulas. *See* formulas
herbal glycerites, 199–200
herbal tea, 200
Herb-Infused Honey, 138
herbs of spring, 20–30
herbs of summer, 31–40
Hickory Nut Oil/Milk, 49–50
hickory nuts, 49–50
Hindus, 127–28
Hoffman, Alice, 67
Hogmanay, 181
hollow stems, 8
honey, 126–40
    around the world, 126–27
    beauty aids, 140
    contraindications, 131
    cooking with, 137–40
    magical lore of, 128–29
    medicinal uses of, 131–35
    recipes, 128–29, 130, 132–34,
        135–40

as sacred, 127–29
Scottish remedies, 134–35
Honeyed Fruit, 138–39
hoodoo, 70–71
Hopman, Ellen Evert, 1–4, 76–79,
    162–63
Horse Chestnut Salve, 174–75
Hot Toddy, 135

incense, 69, 181, 193–94
Indra, 164
infants and children, 62–63
    cow's milk allergy, 170
intention, 121
intuition, 14–15
Iona, 3
iron, 13

Jelly, 29
John the Baptist, 128
Judaism, 128
jugleurs, 78
Juneberry Sauce, 161
Juniper Cookies, 182–83
Jupiter, 164
Jupiter-ruled plants, 113

kidney beans, 14
Kikonian, 164
kitchen medicines, 141–53
kupar, 128
Kybele, 164
Kyphi, 128–29
Kyphi Ebers Papyrus, 128

Lammas, 31
Land of Fairy, 165
leaves, 9–10
Lemon Flea Spray, 65
Leo, 114
LeSassier, William, 3–4, 74, 204–10
Libra, 114
lice, 63
lightning, 163–64, 168

liniments, 201
Little People, 77
Lughnasad, 31
lunar plants, 113
lymph cleansers, 14

Madhu Purnima, 127–28
Maenads, 164
magic, 72, 120–21
Maha Mrityunjaya mantra, 121–22
Make Your Own Vicks VapoRub Salve,
    60
malic acid, 11
Manetho, 128
Mars, 69
Mars-ruled plants, 113
Maya, 129
Maypoles, 165
medicated oils, 202
Medicine Cards, 78
Menes, King, 126–27
Mercury-ruled plants, 113
Midewiwin, 78
Min, 127–28
Modern Herbal, A, 68–69
Moerman, Daniel E., 77–78
Mohawk, 189, 220
Mojo Bag, 70–71
molds, 11
Monongye, David, 119
mosquitoes, 62–65
mouthwash, 151
Mullein Poultice, 74–75
mushrooms, 16
Myrrh, 128

Nasturtium Flower Sandwiches,
    38
Native American Medicinal Plants,
    77–78
Neptune-ruled plants, 114
nervines, 10
nervous system, 8
Nettle Bread, 25

neutral, 15
nuts, 46–50

Odin, 164
oils, medicated, 202
olives, 14
omega-3 fatty acids, 26
On-Niona, 164–65
oranges, 14
Order of the White Oak, 164
Ord Na Darach Gile, 164
overdose, 203
oxalic acid, 30, 45

paal, 186
Pagan Spirit Gathering, 4
Paiute, 186
pancreas, 13, 14
parasites, 131
perennials, 9
Perkunas, 164
Perun, 164
pets, 62–65
Pine Butter, 192–93
Pine Elixir, 192
Pine Gingerbread, 191–92
Pine Oxymel, 193
Pine Syrup, 192
Pine Vinegar, 193
Pisces, 114
Pitawanakwat, Lillian, 78, 80
plant singing, 121–23
plants in groups, 8
plant spirits, 119–23
plaster, 201
Pluto-ruled plants, 114
poisonous plants, 13
pomegranates, 14
Poor One, the, 1–2
potted plants, 62–63
poultices, 79, 201–2
powdered herbs, 200
prethrum, 63
purification, 154, 181, 194

Pyramid Texts, 128
Pythagoras, 204

Qur'an, 128

Ra, 127–28
rabbit medicine plants, 101–4
Ragnarok, 164
recipes
    Ancient Beauty Aid, 140
    Ancient Method of Making Kyphi,
        128–29
    Antibiotic Tea for Kids, 60
    Atholl Brose, 136
    Berry-Flavored Honey, 138
    Birch Beer, 178–79
    bug repellants, 64–65
    Caudle, 130
    Chicken Soup, 57
    Cooked Elderberry Elixer, 54–55
    Cooked Honeyed Fruit, 139–40
    conifers, 182–83, 190–94
    Daylily Sides, 38
    Dragon's Blood Ink, 69–70
    Elderberry Elixir, 54–55
    Fennel Liqueur, 33
    flowers, 37–40
    Flower Cake, 38–39
    Flower Salad, 39
    Flower Tea, 37–38
    Garlic and Honey Wound Dressing,
        132
    Garlic Scapes and White Bean Dip,
        147
    Ginger Ale, 139
    Golden Honey Immune Booster, 133
    Hag's Tapers, 71–72
    Heather Ale, 136–37
    Herb-Infused Honey, 138–39
    honey, 128–29, 130, 132–34, 135–40
    Honey Flu and Bronchitis Remedy,
        132
    Honey Throat Syrup, 133
    Horse Chestnut Salve, 174–75

Hot Toddy, 135
Jelly (Violet, Rose, or Dandelion), 29
Juneberry Sauce, 161
Juniper Cookies, 182–83
Make Your Own Rosewater, 40
Make Your Own Vicks VapoRub
    Salve, 60
Medicinal Onion Honey Syrup for
    Coughs, 133
Mojo Bag, 70–71
Mullein Poultice, 74–75
Nasturtium Flower Sandwiches, 38
Nettle Bread, 25
No-Cook Honey Syrups, 137–38
nuts, 47–50
Old-Fashioned Remedy for
    Bronchitis and Whooping Cough,
    133
Queen of Hungary Rosemary
    Cologne, 39–40
Red Clover Blossom Tea Sandwiches,
    38
Scottish Highland Remedies Using
    Honey, 134–35
Shagbark Hickory Syrup, 27
Violet Flower Syrup, 134
Warming Winter Brandy, 59
White Pine Cookies, 190–91
Wild Berry Syrup, 31–32
Red Clover Blossom Tea Sandwiches,
    38
resin, 11
Rig Veda, 122
Robertson, Olivia, 4
rocks, 7
roots, 8–9, 16–17
Rosebud reservation, 76–79
Rose Jelly, 29
rosewater, 40
Rosh Hashanah, 128
Rowan Berry Jam, 159

safety, 20
Sagittarius, 114

sained, 181
salicylic acid, 180
salt and vinegar, 200–201
salty, 15–16
Samhaim, 154
sammapo, 186
Sams, Jamie, 78
San Masseo, 2–3
Saturn-ruled plants, 113–14
Saxons, 127
Scabwort, 17
Schaef, Anne Wilson, 196
Scorpio, 114
Scottish remedies, 134–35
seaweeds, 16
seed germination, 121
seeds, 16–17
Sequoyah, 187–88
shade plants, 7
Shagbark Hickory Syrup, 27
Shiva Purana, 122
Shoshone, 186
side effects, 203
signatures, doctrine of, 6–15
silica, 35
silverfish, 63
singing, 121–23
smells, 12
snake medicine plants, 89–91
solar plants, 112–13
solitary plants, 8
sorcery, 110
sour, 15–16
spicy, 15–16
spinach, 13
spleen, 13
stems, 8–9
stimulants, 202
stomach, 13
Subasio, Mount, 2–3
sulfur, 13
summer herbs, 31–40
sun, 7
sweet, 15–16

sweet potatoes, 14
sweet taste, 13

tannins, 11
Taranis, 164
taste, 13
Taurus, 114
teas, 79
thiamine metabolism, 35
thin soil, 8
Thor, 164
thorns, 10–11
ticks, 62–65
Tierra, Michael, 198, 202–3
tinctures, 199
tobacco ties, 76
tomatoes, 13–14
tonics, 198, 204–10
Tree Medicine, Tree Magic, 4, 163
triangle system, 204
Tribe of the White Oak, 4, 164
Turtle Island, 78, 104
turtle medicine plants, 104–9

Ukho, 164
Uranus-ruled plants, 114

Venice turpentine, 175
Venus-ruled plants, 113
vinegar, 193, 200–201
Violet Flower Syrup, 134
Violet Jelly, 29
Virgo, 114
viruses, 131
vitamin A, 178

vitamin C, 13, 21, 57, 178, 189, 194
vitamin D, 61
voodoo, 70–71

Wabeno Society, 78
walnuts, 14
wapi, 186
warming herbs, 204–5
Warming Winter Brandy, 59
Washoe, 186
Water, 17–19, 79
water, 121
wheat, 126–27
Whiteoak Druid Order, 4
White Pine Cookies, 190–91
Whitman, Walt, 125
wild, 109
Wild Berry Syrup, 31–32
Winston, David, 75
wishes, 177
witches, 102
wolf medicine plants, 109–11
Wood, Matthew, 77, 204
woodland herbs, 34–37
World Tree, 194

Yahweh, 164
yang, 15
Yavapai, 183
Yggdrasil, 164
yin, 15

Zeus, 164
zinc, 57
zodiac, plant properties, 114

BOOKS OF RELATED INTEREST

The Sacred Herbs of Spring
Magical, Healing, and Edible Plants to Celebrate Beltaine
by Ellen Evert Hopman

The Sacred Herbs of Samhain
Plants to Contact the Spirits of the Dead
by Ellen Evert Hopman
Foreword by Andrew Theitic

The Real Witches of New England
History, Lore, and Modern Practice
by Ellen Evert Hopman
Foreword by Judika Illes

A Druid's Herbal for the Sacred Earth Year
by Ellen Evert Hopman

A Druid's Herbal of Sacred Tree Medicine
by Ellen Evert Hopman

Sacred Plant Initiations
Communicating with Plants for Healing and Higher Consciousness
by Carole Guyett
Foreword by Pam Montgomery

Plant Spirit Healing
A Guide to Working with Plant Consciousness
by Pam Montgomery
Foreword by Stephen Harrod Buhner

Witchcraft Medicine
Healing Arts, Shamanic Practices, and Forbidden Plants
*by Claudia Müller-Ebeling, by Christian Rätsch,
and Wolf-Dieter Storl, Ph.D.*

Inner Traditions • Bear & Company
P.O. Box 388
Rochester, VT 05767
1-800-246-8648
www.InnerTraditions.com

Or contact your local bookseller